AIDS, Poverty, and Hunger:
Challenges and Responses

AIDS, Poverty, and Hunger: Challenges and Responses

Edited by Stuart Gillespie

Highlights of the International Conference on HIV/AIDS and
Food and Nutrition Security, Durban, South Africa, April 14–16, 2005

International Food Policy Research Institute
2033 K Street, N.W.
Washington, D.C.

International Food Policy Research Institute
2033 K Street, N.W.
Washington, D.C. 20006–1002
U.S.A.
Telephone +1–202–862–5600
www.ifpri.org

How to cite this book:
Gillespie, Stuart, ed. 2006. *AIDS, poverty, and hunger: Challenges and responses.* Highlights of the International Conference on HIV/AIDS and Food and Nutrition Security, Durban, South Africa, April 14–16, 2005. Washington, D.C.: International Food Policy Research Institute.

Library of Congress Cataloging-in-Publication Data

AIDS, poverty, and hunger : challenges and responses / edited by Stuart Gillespie.
    p.   cm.
    "Highlights of the International Conference on HIV/AIDS and Food and Nutrition Security, Durban, South Africa, April 14–16, 2005."
    Includes bibliographical references and index.
    ISBN 0-89629-758-6 (alk. paper)
    1. AIDS (Disease)—Social aspects—Congresses.   2. AIDS (Disease)—Economic aspects—Congresses.   3. Nutrition policy—Congresses.
I. Gillespie, Stuart (Stuart R.)   II. International Conference on HIV/AIDS and Food and Nutrition Security (2005 : Durban, South Africa)
RA643.76.A35   2006
362.196′9792—dc22   2006020877

Contents

Tables

Figures

Boxes

Foreword

More than a quarter-century after HIV was identified, the long-wave, intergenerational nature of AIDS epidemics is becoming starkly evident. We may have passed the peak of the infection wave in many countries, but the multiple impact waves continue to gather momentum. Advances are indeed being made in prevention, treatment, care, and support. Yet, in 2006 in many of the hardest-hit countries, fewer than one in eight people living with HIV have sustained access to lifesaving drugs. At the same time, we are learning more about the intertwining of HIV and AIDS with poverty, nutrition, and agriculture. It is now clear that, if the Millennium Development Goals on hunger and AIDS are to be met, especially in eastern and southern Africa, we need to continue to research these dynamics and proactively address them through better, AIDS-responsive food policy and programming.

Against this backdrop, the International Food Policy Research Institute convened the "International Conference on HIV/AIDS and Food and Nutrition Security: From Evidence to Action" in Durban, South Africa, April 14–16, 2005. The conference provided a forum for stakeholders to collectively review emerging knowledge of the interactions between AIDS and hunger and to better understand what it implies for poverty, food, and nutrition-relevant policy and programs. As highlights from the conference, the chapters in this book amply illustrate the diversity of activity and the imperative for interdisciplinary work in this new field. Economists, nutritionists, anthropologists, health specialists, and other development professionals have approached the issue from different angles, often using innovative methods, to generate important new findings.

It is hoped that this book will serve as a benchmark and a resource for researchers, policymakers, and practitioners who continue to grapple with the combined threats of AIDS, poverty, and hunger.

Joachim von Braun
Director General, IFPRI

Chapter 1

AIDS, Poverty, and Hunger: An Overview

Stuart Gillespie

The AIDS epidemic is a global crisis with impacts that will be felt for decades to come. More than 28 million people have died since the first case was reported in 1981. In 2005, AIDS killed 2.8 million people, and an estimated 4.1 million became infected, bringing to 38.6 million the number of people living with the virus around the world; 24.5 million of these people live in Sub-Saharan Africa (where in some countries one in three adults are infected) and 8.3 million live in Asia (UNAIDS 2006).

AIDS epidemics are multidimensional, long-term, and phased phenomena. First comes the wave of HIV infection itself, followed by a wave of opportunistic infections, the most common one being tuberculosis. This is followed several years later by AIDS illness and death. And finally, depending on the prevalence of the disease and availability of treatment, there is an accumulation of macroeconomic and social impacts at household, community, and national levels. A few countries have brought down infection rates. However, no country has yet seen a downturn in AIDS mortality, and the fourth phase is only just beginning for the majority of affected countries. These multidimensional, long-wave characteristics, linked to the fact that AIDS disproportionately strikes the most productive members of society, are what sets HIV and AIDS apart from many other health shocks.

We do not know how severe the impacts of the third and fourth phases will be because little about this epidemic is linear over time, and little is generalizable across contexts. But we do know that, for many countries, impacts will continue to be felt for years to come. Because of the vast numbers of people currently infected with the virus and the slow rollout of antiretroviral therapy (currently only 1 in 10 Africans who need the drugs actually have access to them), this would still be the case even if HIV transmission magically ceased overnight.

Attempts to attenuate these various waves are conventionally grounded in the three core pillars of AIDS policy: prevention, treatment and care, and mitigation. As direct interventions are scaled out patchily and slowly, there is an urgent need for a deeper understanding of the integral role that food and nutrition can and should play. And there is a corresponding urgency to use this understanding to improve responses at all levels.

Against this backdrop, the International Food Policy Research Institute (IFPRI) decided to bring researchers and practitioners together to review the existing evidence and its implications for future food- and nutrition-relevant policy and to highlight remaining knowledge gaps. In so doing, it also aimed to forge links between countries, sectors, and perspectives in both research and action.

Conference and Book

The "International Conference on HIV/AIDS and Food and Nutrition Security: From Evidence to Action" was held April 14–16, 2005, in Durban, South Africa, following broad consultation with a range of partners within national governments, the Consultative Group for International Agricultural Research (CGIAR), the United Nations, civil society, academia, along with bilateral and international donors. Around 200 international researchers and practitioners participated over three days, during which over 50 papers were presented in a series of parallel and plenary sessions. Most papers were selected by an external review panel on the basis of a competitive call for abstracts in October 2004 that yielded nearly 300 abstracts. The ensuing papers were revised and resubmitted following the Durban discussions, rigorously peer reviewed, with the final selection being brought together in this book in early 2006.

The IFPRI conference was deliberately planned to follow directly from the WHO Consultation on Nutrition and HIV/AIDS in Africa (April 10–13). Extensive discussions were held between organizers of the two conferences to maximize their complementarity, with the hope that this would help bring researchers and practitioners working on clinical nutrition in the context of HIV and AIDS together with others focusing at the broader level of household- and community-level food and nutrition security in the context of people's livelihoods. In this way the food and nutrition causes and consequences of HIV epidemics, and their policy and program implications, were systematically and comprehensively addressed over the full week.

The conference adopted a thematic approach, with structure, format, and conference participation being driven by the key issues and questions to be addressed, namely:

- *Interactions.* What is known about the interactions between agriculture and other rural livelihood systems, the spread of HIV, and the impacts of AIDS at different levels?

- *Local responses.* What is known about the capacities and strategies of households and communities to reduce infection risk (resistance) and to respond effectively to the impacts of HIV/AIDS (resilience)? What do these strategies imply for the types of support needed from governments, civil society, the private sector, and international agencies?

- *Policies, programs, interventions.* What is known about the processes and impacts of food- and nutrition-relevant policies, programs, or interventions that have sought to prevent the spread of HIV and/or mitigate the impacts of HIV/AIDS?

In short: what is happening, how are people responding, and how can external support be best applied?

This book applies a similar structure using some of the key chapters under each of these themes to highlight what is known and not known about interactions, local responses, interventions, and policy responses, identifying along the way the key challenges for research and action. Theme 2 on local responses is the critical interface between the dynamic impacts of HIV and AIDS at household and community level (Theme 1), and the necessary responses on the part of governments and other development actors (Theme 3). Many impacts are revealed through the responses that households make, with the response itself often classified as an impact. The treatments of Themes 1 and 2 thus tend to merge in many studies, and this has been reflected here in the division between two main sections of this book—first, understanding interactions (primarily Themes 1 and 2), and second, responding to interactions (primarily Theme 3).

Concepts

In order to begin to answer these questions, to know what to look for and where, the conference took as its starting point the conceptual framework in Figure 1.1. The framework depicts the universe of factors and processes conditioning the

Figure 1.1 The universe of HIV/AIDS determinants, impacts, and responses

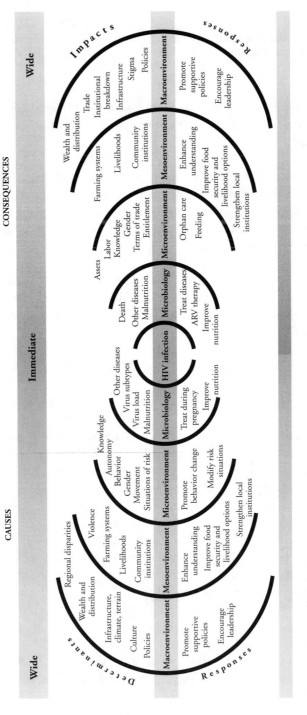

causes and consequences of AIDS epidemics. With time broadly flowing left to right, it shows the waves of determinants of HIV infection, from macro to micro levels, and the subsequent waves of impacts, from micro to macro (Loevinsohn and Gillespie 2003).[1]

In the top left quadrant, we can see the various levels and sources of susceptibility, that is, risk of exposure to HIV and risk of infection by the virus. Infection is at the epicenter of Figure 1.1 and is followed, in the top right quadrant, by the various sources and levels of vulnerability to AIDS-related impacts. In the bottom half of the diagram, we can see various responses: those that are broadly preventive (or aimed at strengthening resistance) in the bottom left, and those aimed at mitigating impacts (or strengthening resilience) in the bottom right.

It is also useful, as many authors did, to sharpen the focus on household, community, and institutional interactions. This can be done by folding these concepts into an adaptation of the livelihoods framework (Carney 1998; Gillespie, Haddad, and Jackson 2001) that is complementary to the universe map (see Figure 1.2). Such

Figure 1.2   Adapting the livelihoods framework to HIV and AIDS

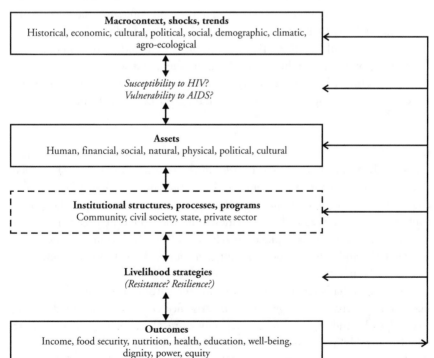

a framework is a useful organizational tool, a synthetic framework that shows how HIV and AIDS affect, and are affected by, people's livelihoods in an iterative cycle. It captures the diversity of interactions at different scales while providing a simple, common frame of reference to enable researchers and practitioners (often from quite different disciplines) to communicate effectively.

Starting from the top of Figure 1.2, the macro context and its conditions, shocks, and trends will to a certain extent determine both the susceptibility and vulnerability of different livelihood systems to HIV and AIDS. (Such a context will, of course, determine other vulnerabilities, some of which may overlap and interact with HIV/AIDS.) The risks that people face of contracting HIV will be partly governed by the susceptibility of the livelihood system on which they depend (e.g., agriculture), and the downstream effects of HIV and AIDS on assets and institutions will be conditioned by the vulnerability of the system. After HIV has entered a household or community, the type and severity of its impacts on assets, mediated by various institutional structures, processes, and programs, will determine the type of strategies that the household adopts. These strategies will differ, among other ways, in terms of the resistance to HIV or resilience to AIDS that they confer on the household. Such strategies and responses in turn lead to various outcomes, nutrition and food security among them, and these outcomes will themselves condition future susceptibility and vulnerability (the upward feedback loop).

This is the pathway that HIV takes through households and communities. But it is important, as will be repeatedly emphasized, that we do not lose sight of the many factors driving vulnerability, including such macro-level conditions and trends as climate change, debt, international trade policy, and governance.

Context

Overall, AIDS epidemics are most severe in the region of the world where food insecurity is most severe, Sub-Saharan Africa, although there are significant differences between countries. The majority of participants were from Africa, though the conference was designed to be international in order to ensure opportunities for cross-regional learning. Examples of such learning from the past include the Junior Farmer Field and Life Schools, an approach pioneered in Cambodia and now being scaled out across eastern and southern Africa.

In Asia, India is fertile terrain both for the spread of the virus and for its impacts on poverty and hunger, given the existence of many known predisposing factors (gender and socioeconomic inequality, caste, class, religious divisions, high population mobility, urban–rural linkages, food insecurity, and malnutrition). It should also be remembered that in just 10 years from 1990 to 2000, the HIV preva-

Table 1.1   Prevalence and numbers of people infected with HIV in selected countries (end 2003)

Country	Estimated total numbers of adults and children	Estimated prevalence among adults 15–49 years (%)
India	5,700,000	0.9
Malawi	940,000	14.1
Mozambique	1,800,000	16.1
Rwanda	190,000	3.1
South Africa	5,500,000	18.8
Zambia	1,100,000	17.0
Zimbabwe	1,700,000	20.1

Source: UNAIDS (2006).

lence in South Africa rocketed to 25 percent from 1 percent (the present prevalence in India). Using the case of India, one chapter in this book looks at how biostructural livelihood interventions may reduce risk of people's exposure to HIV.

The latest available national-level HIV data for the countries highlighted in this book are provided in Table 1.1. Most chapters focus on single countries, but others are more regional and/or synthetic in nature. Though the conference was not geographically restricted in any way, it was inevitable that most paper submissions, and ultimately most studies featured in this book, originated from the region where most research and programmatic experience are under way: southern Africa. There are thus geographic as well as thematic gaps in the evidence base. Not enough is known about the situation in western Africa, for example. Though the spread and the impacts of HIV and AIDS are less pronounced in this region, there are some hot spots (e.g., Cote d'Ivoire, parts of Nigeria) where more research is needed.

Nothing is static in the pandemic. In representing the proportions of a given population living with HIV, the prevalence data in Figure 1.1 are delayed snapshots of incidence. Prevalence could decline because of high mortality rates and/or reduced incidence of new cases of infection. Barnett and Topouzis (2003) delineate three principal stages that a community may pass through: *AIDS-initiating,* with very low HIV prevalence rates and no AIDS impacts; *AIDS-impending,* where HIV prevalence rates are rising but the majority of infected people are still in the asymptomatic phase before becoming ill; and *AIDS-impacted,* when households and communities feel the impact of AIDS as infected people succumb to AIDS-related illnesses and eventual death. Clearly, response strategy needs to be tailored to stage of epidemic, with preventive approaches, aimed at strengthening resistance, taking precedence in the early stages (e.g., India, Ethiopia), whereas impact mitigation or the strengthening of household and community resilience needs to be at the fore in the latter stages of epidemics (e.g., Uganda, which long ago reached its peak HIV prevalence, is now in the midst of the death wave). Another limitation of such national data is they mask often huge subnational variations, as some of the following chapters will demonstrate.

Content

The conference was subtitled "From Evidence to Action" for two reasons. The first was to signal its scope, with several detailed academic studies of interactions being balanced with descriptions of approaches and interventions aimed at responding to these interactions. The second was to signal that we are now, in a sense, at a watershed. The evidence base, though still incomplete and in some places a little murky, has grown enormously in the past 5 years. In the time between the conference in mid-2005 and this book being published, numerous new studies have emerged, and more are in the pipeline. Because of this, and because of the context specificity of interactions and necessary responses, it is not the intention here to generate definitive policy conclusions. Rather, this overview attempts to build on earlier work (for example, that summarized in Gillespie and Kadiyala 2005) to map the evolving breadth and depth of this field, capture new knowledge, and generate ideas to be built on and operationalized in future work. In this way the dual agenda of research and action may be better advanced. Key emerging research priorities are highlighted in boxes as they apply to various parts of this overview.

The first nine chapters that follow this overview are mainly concerned with examining impacts and interactions (as described in the section on "Understanding Interactions" below), and subsequent chapters focus primarily on policy and program responses to these interactions. The book concludes with the big challenges for the future, as set down by Tony Barnett in his riveting keynote address. Several chapters, however, derive from work that examines both impacts and responses.

The chapter ordering is thus based on the original thematic structure: from interactions to responses, from evidence to action. Chapters range from studies focusing on risks of HIV infection (Chapoto and Jayne), on the impacts of HIV and AIDS on rural livelihoods, including agriculture (Dorward and Mwale, Donovan and Bailey, Masanjala, Jayne et al.), to chapters seeking to unravel interactions between HIV, AIDS, and nutritional status (Stillwaggon). Most chapters rely primarily on quantitative data, but some are largely informed by qualitative data (e.g., Bryceson and Fonseca, Bond, Bishop-Sambrook et al., Senefeld and Polsky). Of the latter, Binswanger, Gillespie, and Kadiyala and Gavian, Galaty, and Kombe present broad-brush analyses of the policy and programming environment, highlighting the various limitations of the status quo, and Drimie and Mullins offer an NGO perspective and approach to mainstreaming. Two chapters focus on innovations in response: Loevinsohn's on biostructural interventions, and Djeddah, Mavanga, and Hendrickx on Junior Farmer Field and Life Schools, while Egge and Strasser consider approaches to monitoring the impact of food aid on HIV-affected groups.

Contributions also reflect the diversity of disciplinary involvement in this field and the varied methodological approaches being applied to it. Many professional backgrounds are represented, including agricultural economics, epidemiology, sociology, anthropology, public health, nutrition, program management, and policy, and in some cases, studies themselves are interdisciplinary. Not surprisingly, given such professional diversity, a variety of methods are employed. Econometric analyses of longitudinal quantitative panel data are balanced by qualitative techniques that aim to elicit the interpretation and understanding of those who are directly and indirectly affected. Although neither econometric models nor local people's responses are themselves fully satisfactory for establishing causality, the triangulation and cross-checking of these methods can greatly increase the trustworthiness of interpretations. Differences in approach, "language," and method can bring challenges (some of which are discussed later), but they can also foster insights and innovations that help unravel the pathways of HIV through people's livelihoods and through their lives and deaths.

Understanding Interactions

Poverty, Food, and Nutrition Security and the Risk of Being Infected with HIV

Looking at the top left quadrant of Figure 1.1, in investigating the risk of an individual being infected with HIV, we[2] need to ask *what* social, economic, political, cultural factors and processes are responsible for the spread of HIV (and specifically how are food and nutrition implicated, if at all), *who* is most susceptible, and *why* are they susceptible. A few important papers shed light on these questions (though this aspect remains relatively underresearched; see Box 1.1).

Who Is at Risk, and Why?

In line with earlier evidence of the disproportionate risks faced by women, especially younger women, more than 60 percent of the prime-age deaths observed in a nationally representative rural Zambian sample between 2001 and 2004 were women (Chapoto and Jayne, this volume). The marginal probability of dying from disease and AIDS-related causes rises steeply from age 15, peaking between ages 30 and 34 for women and 50 and 54 for males. Young, single women were at most risk.

Box 1.1 Research Priority: HIV Spread and Food Insecurity

What is the role of poverty and food insecurity in driving risky behaviors? How prevalent is transactional sex, and how linked is it to food poverty? Is food insecurity a major determinant of migration, and are migrants at heightened risk of being exposed to HIV? Can efforts aimed at enhancing food security and livelihood options of susceptible groups make a cost-effective and timely contribution to preventing the spread of HIV? Can options be identified that are economically and environmentally sustainable, that make use of local opportunities?

Addressing the question of whether poverty puts people at greater risk of being exposed to the virus, Chapoto and Jayne (this volume) find, in line with with findings in the early stages of the epidemic, that men in the upper half of the assets distribution are more likely to die of disease-related causes than poorer men. In contrast, poor women are equally likely to die as better-off women. Digging deeper, they find that within the group of relatively poor women, those having some form of formal or informal business income are 15 percent less likely to die of disease-related causes than those without any such income, suggesting that efforts to provide greater income-earning opportunities for poor women may make at least a modest contribution to reducing female prime-age mortality.

The link between poverty and HIV risk may be mediated through the need to move in search of work. In Malawi, the search for work and food is conflated in the term *kusokola,* or "looking for food" (Bryceson and Fonseca, this volume). Mobility here is not inherently risky, but it is a marker of increased risk. In Zambia, low-income men living away from home 1 month or more per year are more than twice as likely to die as men living at home (Chapoto and Jayne, this volume). Among richer women, who are also more mobile, it is possible that the protection conferred by their greater financial independence may to some extent be negated by the heightening of mobility-induced risk. In Ethiopia, though there are significantly lower levels of HIV infection in rural communities than in urban areas, the disease is concentrated in higher-risk "bridging populations" that have substantial links with other, more risk-averse subpopulations (Bishop-Sambrook et al., this volume).

At the macro level there is no obvious relationship between national wealth and HIV prevalence. Southern Africa is richer than other regions in Sub-Saharan

Africa but has countries with particularly high prevalences, such as Botswana and South Africa. Physical dislocation of families, driven by the need to find work, coupled with the ability to move around via relatively good transport routes, probably plays a large part in this. Men tend to live away from home for long periods, increasing the chances of both partners engaging in commercial sex. Strong urban–rural economic linkages in southern Africa may thus translate into both higher incomes and higher infection rates.

The links between livelihoods and risk suggest that HIV is an "occupational hazard" for particular economic categories of people (Bryceson and Fonseca, this volume). But again, preconceptions may be challenged: for example, Campbell's (2003) South African study found commercial sex workers to be less vulnerable to HIV infection than miners or youth because of their insistence on condom use.

In Malawi, poverty and HIV risk do seem to be increasingly linked against a backdrop of major livelihood shifts. Bryceson and Fonseca (this volume) highlight the ongoing collapse of the peasant household's coherence as a unit of production as livelihood portfolios have veered: (1) from self-sufficient unpaid labor performed within the household (especially by women and children) toward cash-earning piecemeal work (or *ganyu*); (2) from agriculture toward nonagriculture, with income-earning turning increasingly to trade and services, including sexual services; and (3) from household toward individualized work, whereby every able-bodied person works, including women and youth, to earn cash to cover their subsistence needs. Women and girls are now undertaking *ganyu* labor beyond the confines of the village, with poor women at particular risk as transactional sex is increasingly incorporated into *ganyu* contracts (Bryceson and Fonseca, this volume).

A religious leader in a patrilineal village in Khongoni captured this well: "HIV/AIDS is not very threatening compared to the hunger which most households face. In fact it is hunger, which is contributing to the rise in HIV infections in the area" (Bryceson and Fonseca, this volume).

Another major source of risk, and one that sets HIV apart from most other diseases, is the prior death of at least one adult in the same household. In Zambia, this was found to be the single most important factor influencing the probability that a prime-aged individual would die (Chapoto and Jayne, this volume). Irrespective of gender and income status, individuals experiencing a prior death in their household are six to seven times more likely to die of disease-related causes than individuals in households with no prime-age deaths in the past 8 years.

Malnutrition and Ill Health as Risk Factors

Nutrition is the pivotal interface between food security and health security. An individual's susceptibility to any disease depends on the strength of the immune system, which among other factors is affected by nutrition, stress, and the presence of other infections and parasites. The risk of infection with HIV is heightened by high prevalences of such cofactor conditions, which decrease immune response in HIV-negative persons and increase viral load in HIV-infected persons (Stillwaggon, this volume). Worms cause malnutrition through malabsorption and intestinal bleeding, and they weaken the immune response by forcing its chronic reaction to the nonself invaders. Infectious and parasitic diseases and malnutrition thus create an environment of enhanced risk.

Occupational hazards extend to domestic environments. Stillwaggon (this volume) paints a picture of risk in Africa as a child gathering water for the family in a slow moving stream, or helping with the family laundry at the riverside. Any resulting schistosome colonization of the genitourinary tract may render him or her, as an adult, at much higher risk of sexual transmission of HIV than a healthy person with similar sexual behavior.

HIV/AIDS Impacts on Food and Nutrition Security

We now move from a focus on the risk of being infected to the downstream or postinfection impacts (i.e., the top right quadrant of Fig. 1.1). How did the conference enhance our understanding of these impacts and the ways in which households and communities are responding?

The literature on the impacts of HIV and AIDS has grown very rapidly in recent years (with numerous studies recently reviewed in Gillespie and Kadiyala 2005). Impacts are multiple, often interrelated, and often highly determined by context. In Rwanda, Donovan and Bailey (this volume) find death-affected households to show few significant differences in crop production from matched nonaffected households without a death or illness. All crops show lower production amounts for households with a death, but with variability between households, significant differences were found only for beans, beer bananas, and fruit bananas. The difference in bean production (18 percent lower in death-affected households), however, might be important because beans are a key food security crop for Rwandan households. Also, beer bananas are traditionally a major source of income for women, so this difference implies a relative decline in women's income-earning potential in affected households.

Donovan and Bailey also highlight an important point that many earlier studies failed to take into account. Relatively small "death effects" may be a reflection that predeath measurements occurred during the illness period, when the household was already adjusting to AIDS. The measured "death effect" in such cases would thus be an underestimate of the extent to which the household was initially affected and had to change. Measuring the effects of adult illness and death separately provides insight into the possible need for interventions before death to mitigate the most severe effects (e.g., irreversible asset disposal), which may cause permanent livelihood declines. In a study in Zimbabwe, Senefeld and Polsky (this volume) found that households with chronically ill adults were more likely to have their children drop out of school and more likely to resort to migration strategies to "cope."

Because many impacts are revealed in actual responses that households and communities make in the face of HIV/AIDS, we need to examine these responses for their effectiveness and sustainability. Where households are not subject to additional stresses such as drought, and when they are viewed over a relatively short reference period (e.g., a couple of years), there are some indications from the literature that traditional responses can mitigate the worst effects of AIDS. However, complex factors determine the success of these strategies. These include the sex, age, and position in the household of the ill/deceased person, the household's socioeconomic status, the type and degree of labor demand in the production system, the availability of labor support to affected households, other livelihood opportunities, available natural resources, the availability of formal and informal sources of support including credit and interhousehold transfers, the length of time that the epidemic has been impacting the rural economy, and the existence of concurrent shocks such as drought or commodity price collapses (Gillespie and Kadiyala 2005).

This all shows the complexity and the context-specificity of impacts. But what happens when the household is subjected to multiple stresses over the longer term, including those relating to macro, meso, and micro processes depicted in Figures 1.1. and 1.2? And what happens to communities when the proportion of such struggling households increases significantly? Though HIV/AIDS is different in several important ways from other shocks and stresses, where it is most prevalent in Sub-Saharan Africa, it is one among many concurrent stresses. We need to learn more about how increasing numbers of households and communities are struggling to respond to multiple overlapping vulnerabilities and interacting processes of change (see Box 1.2).

One distinct aspect of AIDS as a stress is its long-acting, slow-burning nature. AIDS can exert its effects over a relatively long period of time while rendering other stresses/shocks both more likely and more severe in their effects. Following a shock to household income, households in Malawi affected by HIV/AIDS were found to take up to 18 months to stabilize, with a new equilibium income that was about half the preshock income levels (Masanjala, this volume). Similar findings had been reported earlier in Kenya (Yamano and Jayne 2004). Such limited resilience is likely to increase vulnerability to other shocks.

Households are often perceived as "coping," but it is often not clear that households themselves would classify their responses in this way, nor that such "coping"

Box 1.2 Research Priority: HIV/AIDS, Multiple Stresses, and Overlapping Vulnerabilities

How does HIV/AIDS, as a source of vulnerability to food and nutrition insecurity, intersect and interact with other sources of vulnerability? How should one go beyond identifying who is "vulnerable" to better understand why households are, or why they become, vulnerable? Conversely, why are certain households more resilient than others in similar situations? What are the implications of this for vulnerability-monitoring systems? How should one develop approaches to identify options for households to reduce their vulnerability? What are the implications of overlapping vulnerabilities for approaches to addressing HIV/AIDS and food and nutrition insecurity?

---

is sustainable. "Coping" may be an illusion, a dangerous misnomer, according to several prominent commentators: "Coping is a way of escaping from the challenge of confronting how people's capabilities are stunted, how their entitlements are blocked, and how their abilities to function as full human beings with choices and self-definitions are frustrated" (Barnett and Whiteside 2002). More recently, Marais (2005) refers to the "coping fetish that exalts the presumed pluck and grit of the poor. . . . the discourse of 'coping' is an acceptance, an endorsement even, of the way things are, a patronizing gloss on a reality of privation and marginality." The fact is that "coping" is an externally applied value judgment that may or may not correspond to what is actually happening. Many responses are those of distressed households without much conscious strategy, "struggling not coping," as Rugalema (2000) pointed out. Responses may have a veneer of coping, but the costs may need to be paid further down the line (e.g., a child denied schooling).

Broader Impacts on the Agricultural Sector

The prevailing narrative of major declines in agricultural output for the region as a direct result of the impacts of HIV and AIDS has gained much momentum. Though many studies do show that significant negative impacts are being experienced at the individual and household levels as a direct result of AIDS-related labor losses (morbidity and mortality), there is as yet no conclusive support for the net decreases in agricultural output that might be expected as the impacts of HIV and AIDS increase (Larson et al. 2005). Second, it is not clear whether the major constraints being faced by agriculture-dependent households in the contexts of AIDS relate to labor, cash, or a combination of other resource deficits.

Using demographic projections and household survey evidence, Jayne et al. (this volume) consider the likely consequences of the AIDS pandemic for the agricultural sector of the hardest-hit countries of Eastern and Southern Africa. They suggest that although AIDS is projected to erode population growth to roughly zero in the seven hardest-hit countries, the net result is a roughly stable number of working-age adults over time. AIDS-related agricultural labor shortages are likely to induce labor migration out of the urban informal sector into agriculture. For poorer smallholder households, they argue that land will remain a primary constraint on income growth. AIDS-induced decapitalization of highly afflicted rural communities, meaning a loss of savings, cattle assets, draft equipment, and other assets, may come to pose the greatest limits on rural productivity and livelihoods for these communities.

In Malawi, Dorward and Mwale (this volume) highlight the challenges in determining the nature and magnitude of broader impacts of HIV/AIDS on labor markets and wages. Although affected households may face increased labor shortages, widespread reductions in household incomes and increased cash constraints will also depress labor and nontradable demand in rural communities with high HIV incidence. Reductions in family labor may also lead to a shift out of more labor-demanding cash crops. Depressed labor demand could cause wages to fall, posing serious problems even for poor households not directly affected by HIV/AIDS. They find some evidence for such a shift, driven primarily by reductions in labor hiring by better-off households with HIV-induced cash constraints. The introduction of labor-saving technologies in such a context could be damaging, as discussed later. Cash transfers to help bolster labor hire may be more appropriate here.

Moreover, where HIV/AIDS does depress unskilled wages, this is likely to increase inequality within rural communities and impose further pressures on poor people and their livelihoods. Jayne et al. (this volume) also point to the inequality-driving aspect of capital asset loss. Unlike the loss of labor and knowledge, which represent a loss to entire communities, capital assets lost by afflicted households are generally redistributed within the rural economy rather than lost entirely.

Macroeconomic Impacts, Poverty, and Inequality

At a macro level, the impacts of HIV and AIDS are not clear, at least not within current models and/or not yet. Several researchers have criticized the use of per capita GDP growth rate as a metric of AIDS impacts, along with the assumptions underlying common macroeconomic models (e.g., McPherson 2002). Earlier models tended to assume an early peak in the epidemic, and they omitted households that dissolved because of AIDS. Many important aspects of development are econometrically invisible, including women's work, the loss of information in social systems including intergenerational knowledge fracture, the loss of social capital as networks and information channels erode, relational goods, misery/ happiness, and others. What, for example, is the long-term cost to communities and nations of millions of psychologically damaged, poorly socialized children growing up as orphans? Put another way, looking at Figure 1.1, the indicators conventionally used at the macro level often fail to pick up the aggregated effects of changes at the meso- and micro-level environmental levels.

Because of the long incubation period between HIV and AIDS, no country has yet reached the peak of AIDS impacts. A full timeline of impacts is thus not even available to use as a basis for projections in other countries (notwithstanding the possible problems in extrapolating from one country to another). Possible social unraveling as the AIDS impact waves hit suggests that the development of macroeconomic effects may be nonlinear, and may be some way off.

Because our concern is primarily with deprivation, manifested by food insecurity and malnutrition, we should not be overly focused on aggregates or means that effectively mask subnational differentials. There is strong evidence, first, that inequalities (socioeconomic, gender) drive the spread of HIV infection, and, second, that AIDS itself increases these inequalities, a potentially vicious cycle that is not captured by measuring income means.

Two drivers of inequality have been discussed above: declining unskilled wage rates and decapitalization of affected households. Land acquisition by better-off households is likely to increase as widows and orphans fail to keep access and/or ownership rights to land after the death of the husband/father. The fear of such a loss may also foreclose the option of renting out land as a response, another example of the enmeshing of vulnerabilities and inequities (in this case, relating to gender and HIV). The AIDS epidemic is thus intertwined with the way in which power, authority, value, and opportunity are distributed within societies. Such land acquisition trends could even lead to aggregate production increases at the "community" level while simultaneously increasing inequality, poverty, and malnutrition.

The majority of impact studies are at the household level. As well as suffering from an inability to track the dynamics of interactions over time (see "Research Gaps and Challenges" below), household-level effects do not relate well to more aggregated sector-level or national-level impacts. Nor do they shine a clear light on what is happening within households, such as intrahousehold division of labor, caregiving, and other resources, especially impacts on women and children. Yet another problem with the notion of "household coping" is its implication of intrahousehold homogeneity of those affected. A conference participant highlighted this well in pointing out how the "extended family" in most cases meant "extended women."

AIDS, Poverty, and Stigma

Stigma itself is an impact of HIV/AIDS that may adversely affect the ability of individuals or households to respond: both a consequence of HIV and AIDS as well as a cause of future vulnerability. Depending on the social environment, disclosure of HIV status may lead to stigma, or it may open up other response options. Where there is openness, disclosure may be a gateway to community support (Norman and Chopra 2005).

Stigma and poverty are mutually reinforcing (Bond, this volume). Stigma may not be primarily associated with promiscuity and reckless behavior, but it may be increasingly linked to the sense of being overwhelmed by the work, expense, and emotional strain of having to care for sick people in the context of declining household resources. Bond (this volume) quotes a 15-year-old boy who describes how in a "biting economy," people living with HIV and AIDS are considered a "burden" because they are not able to contribute to household income when they are sick, and they soak up money, energy, and time. Both they and relatives who come to visit them take up space. The fact that illness takes a long time drags households down.

The AIDS impact literature has spawned a variety of labels including "afflicted households" (containing an individual infected with HIV), "affected households" (possibly caring for an orphaned child), along with the label PLWHA ("persons living with HIV and AIDS"). But given the diversity of risk factors and processes, and the fact that HIV/AIDS is one among many interacting sources of vulnerability, these terms are increasingly questioned. They may in themselves stigmatize.

Research Gaps and Challenges

Geographic gaps in the evidence base were mentioned earlier, with data tending to be somewhat overconcentrated on smallholder farming households in southern and eastern Africa. But there are also thematic gaps and challenges. First, although the two-way nature of AIDS–food insecurity interactions is increasingly recognized, far more attention remains focused on the impacts of AIDS on food security than on the other direction, how food and nutrition-security outcomes, policy, and practice may contribute to the spread of HIV. Methodological challenges include how to measure the actual presence of HIV without testing (is "chronic illness" or adult death an appropriate indicator?), how to disentangle HIV/AIDS effects from other stresses and shocks, how to go beyond cross-sectional studies to effectively track the dynamic interactions between HIV and food security and their micro–macro links, and how to monitor and evaluate the various remedial responses and interventions? Though progress is being made, as reflected in the authorship of chapters here, more interdisciplinary studies are needed involving collaborations between researchers from different disciplines and perspectives in order to truly understand why the interactions between HIV/AIDS and food and nutrition security play themselves out differently in different contexts.

Old methods and tools may in some cases not suffice. As with the example of macroeconomic impact assessment, Stillwaggon (this volume) asserts that global health policy is trammeled by reliance on tools of epidemiology and health economics that are too rudimentary for understanding a complex epidemic. Public health problems of populations in poverty are interrelated, synergistic, and they are virtually ubiquitous in poor populations. Attempts to isolate the effects of vitamin A or malaria or worms on HIV transmission may be confounded by other endemic conditions, and treatment of any one condition may be constrained by the persistent impact of others. Global AIDS policy is paralyzed because epidemiologic methods demand a "smoking gun" as evidence of relationships between HIV and the endemic conditions of malnutrition, parasites, and infectious disease. Such a burden of proof is inappropriate because interventions to reduce malnutrition, parasite load, and infectious diseases are beneficial in themselves (Stillwaggon, this volume).

Propensity score matching (PSM) may be useful in the measurement of the impacts of adult illness and death on crop production. In Rwanda, Donovan and Bailey (this volume) used a combination of cross-sectional and panel data to construct the counterfactual situation required to estimate HIV/AIDS impacts. This application demonstrates that, given appropriate variables and sample size, PSM enables analysts to estimate the impacts of adult illness and death using cross-sectional data with recall complemented with a small amount of panel information. Although panel data are preferred for the econometric estimation of impacts, governments and development practitioners cannot always wait for the ideal data to inform local policy decisions.

An overriding challenge lies in capturing the diversity and context specificity of impacts and interactions without thwarting action. How can one achieve a policy-amenable synthesis of multiple findings that reflect the context specificity of interactions? And how, against a backdrop of thousands of AIDS deaths every day, can one do this in real time? Though research on impacts has grown enormously over the last few years and much has been learned, more case study research is needed to respond to the diversity of interactions in different settings at different points on the epidemic curve. Tools such as the HIV/AIDS lens accommodate the ground realities and facilitate the use of local knowledge to generate appropriate responses in a timely way. Parallel to this, a well-publicized and accessible library of documented experience needs to be built up.

Responding to Interactions

Work aimed at elucidating the interactions between HIV/AIDS and food and nutrition security has been highlighted above. In this section, the focus switches to the responses being made by households and communities and, through policies and programs, by governments and international agencies.

To ensure food and nutrition security in the context of HIV/AIDS, there is a growing consensus, reinforced in Durban, on what is essentially a three-pronged strategic approach: to strengthen household and community resistance and resilience, preserve and augment livelihood opportunities for affected communities, and ensure that there are safety nets in place for those who need them. The emphasis in mitigation strategy needs to be on strengthening resilience, the ability of households and communities to adapt livelihood strategies so as to bounce back from the shock of AIDS. Policy needs to draw on what is working already in communities where proactive responses are under way. This is quite distinct from any notion of leaving it to the communities to "cope." Rather, it is to maximize learning from community innovations (for reasons described in "Community-Driven Responses" below) as to what works where and why. Where households' and communities' capacity to respond effectively has been exceeded, a broad-based social security system offering minimal benefits or specifically targeted support programs will in the short and medium term be important for mitigation. These three strategies should be pursued simultaneously, based on the different comparative advantages of all stakeholders from households to national governments and international agencies.

Given the evidence of interactions described in the first section, what type of options exist for responding to the AIDS–food insecurity nexus? After a discussion of community responses and the potential of renewed attention to community-driven development, the key issues of scaling up, multisectoralism, and mainstreaming are discussed below. This is then followed by discussion of specific intervention options highlighted in Durban. Again, the intention is to capture and synthesize the key conference presentations and discussions, not to provide a comprehensive review. It is also worth remembering the two mutually reinforcing rationales for responding to interactions: first, to improve the chances that food and nutrition security policies and programs can achieve their original objectives in a heavy AIDS context, and second, to contribute to the multisectoral response to HIV/AIDS.

Community-Driven Responses

The Durban conference highlighted the differentiated impacts of HIV and AIDS on communities and the variety of attempts they make to improve their resistance to HIV spread and their resilience to AIDS impacts. Communities have responded in innovative ways, including labor sharing, orphan support, community-based childcare, community food banks, credit schemes for funeral benefits, and new ways of reducing the time and energy of domestic tasks such as fuel and water collection and food preparation, to name but a few (see Gillespie and Kadiyala 2005).

In the context of high HIV prevalences and associated stigma, community-driven approaches, with their advantages of local knowledge, may represent an untapped resource for addressing the HIV/AIDS–food insecurity nexus. Like the problem itself, community-led approaches are naturally more "multisectoral" and cross-cutting. Unlike vertical sectoral programs that tend to focus narrowly on infected individuals, they focus on affected communities.

The issue of capacity to respond is critical, particularly as AIDS itself is eroding local capacity. Tony Barnett warns against defaulting to "installed capacity"— the fact that certain vertical program infrastructures are in place does not mean these are the most appropriate ones to employ. Binswanger, Gillespie, and Kadiyala (this volume) point to evidence from the field on the existence of latent community-level capacity including unemployed or underemployed youth. Resources could be applied to developing appropriate community responses to AIDS, thus obviating constraints on personnel experienced in scaling up vertical programs. Investing in local institutions through support to decentralization could go a long way in addressing remaining evidence gaps too, as communities have local knowledge, but they often lack power and resources. To support such new approaches, donors need to alter their time horizons, and they need to be more flexible.

In the context of AIDS, this is new ground. Important remaining questions include: What scope is there for new approaches to pooling labor and resources in affected communities? Can win-win approaches be found? Can communities find ways to protect the entitlements of affected households, enabling them to equitably exchange what they have (e.g., land they can no longer cultivate) for what they need (e.g., food)?

Scaling Up

Responses need to recognize the diversity of impacts, but they also need to be large-scale. In a study of a community-led program in Malawi cited by Binswanger, Gillespie, and Kadiyala (this volume), contextual factors for scaling up, including an enabling policy environment and a strong governmental commitment, were important. The adoption of a community mobilization model through capacity strengthening of district, community, and village AIDS committees, a commitment to documenting and disseminating lessons learned, and the drive to reach more affected populations through establishing partnerships were key organizational factors. Community-specific factors include leadership within the community, whether the communities are urban or rural (rural communities being easier to mobilize), the nature of livelihoods, and the history and culture of the communities with respect to collective action. Joint planning with communities for a phasing down of NGO presence and scaling up of the role and responsibilities of the local AIDS committees and funding mechanisms were also identified as critical in enabling and sustaining the scaling up of collective action (Kadiyala 2004).

Scaling up may be pursued along various dimensions. Quantitatively, it may be viewed as the rolling out of various programs to reach more people who can benefit from them. The development of networks for research and action (e.g., RENEWAL) is another approach to simultaneously increase capacity, communications, and the coherence and scale of response. Community radio and Internet portals are useful for communicating, strengthening capacity, and scaling up ideas and innovations. Another approach to increasing the scale of the organizational response is through mainstreaming.

Multisectoral Approaches and Mainstreaming

AIDS is a multisectoral issue requiring a multisectoral response. Several rationales have been invoked. Multisectoral programming is needed to increase the organizational scale of the response to HIV/AIDS for the following reasons:

- Because the difference between behaviors of people in high- and low-prevalence areas is smaller than that between their environments, which in turn are shaped by many sectors. Many sectors both affect, and are affected by, AIDS. The fact that HIV epidemics are endogenous to livelihood systems, not exogenous, implies a responsibility for different sectors to be part of the solution.

- Because there are positive synergies among prevention, care and treatment, and mitigation that may be better exploited in a multisectoral approach.

- Because original international and sectoral goals (e.g., the Millennium Development Goals in many countries) may not be achieved unless HIV/AIDS implications are taken on board.

- Because it is simply not enough to mainstream HIV/AIDS within only one or two sectors (e.g., just health and agriculture).

UNAIDS has recognized this in its promotion of the "Three Ones" principle: one agreed national framework of action against AIDS, one national AIDS coordinating authority with a broad multisectoral mandate, and one agreed country-level monitoring and evaluation system.

Multisectoral approaches to HIV/AIDS control will involve (but not be limited to) mainstreaming of HIV implications into the policy and practice of many sectors. But, as Gavian, Galaty, and Kombe (this volume) stress, multisectoralism is more than simply "many sectors," and it goes well beyond policy mainstreaming. Communities are not sectors, but they are, or they should be, part of multisectoral responses. Binswanger, Gillespie, and Kadiyala (this volume) highlight lessons learned from "Integrated Rural Development," a failed centralized and state-driven approach to rural development, and show why highly decentralized and community-driven approaches (as discussed above) with strong private sector involvement, hold great potential for avoiding difficulties in the coordination and execution of multisectoral programs.

Mainstreaming is not a one-time event but a continual process of learning, synthesizing, and acting. It has two dimensions. The first is the personal: adjusting the mindsets of the organization and its individual staff in order to internalize the HIV/AIDS issue into the core of their perceptions and programming. The second (professional) is specifically technical or operational: identifying the most beneficial ways of giving practical expression to these concerns through the design and delivery of appropriate project activities. In addition to workplace policies, mainstreaming HIV/AIDS encompasses strategic planning and all stages of the program cycle from situation analysis and project design to implementation, monitoring, and evaluation.

Mainstreaming does not imply that an organization should suddenly start undertaking new tasks for which it is not equipped. Rather, it should continue to focus on its core business but view it through the lens of its interactions with HIV/AIDS. Drimie and Mullins (this volume) employ a livelihoods approach to focus on risk and vulnerability (and their positive flipsides, resistance and resilience) using an HIV/AIDS lens but move on to use a more generic "health and development" lens.

Reviewing progress on the ground, Gavian, Galaty, and Kombe (this volume) found an upswing in the number of countries with comprehensive, multisectoral national AIDS strategies, but that implementation lags. The World Bank's (2004) "Turning Bureaucrats into Warriors" publication and Multicountry AIDS Program (MAP) Interim Review 2004 speak of a "somewhat half-hearted" introduction into many ministries, with "cookie cutter" sectoral plans tending to ignore the local context; line ministries adopting workplace action plans yet failing to consider programs for their constituencies and failing to submit fundable proposals and workplans. A 2003 UNAIDS survey in 63 countries found that only 13 percent had actually made progress in implementing sectoral plans.

Tracking the progress or the bottlenecks in multisectoral implementation requires appropriate HIV-relevant indicators to be built into routine monitoring and evaluation systems of many sectors, including gender-sensitive indicators of livelihoods, food and nutrition security, and stigma.

Enhancing Learning and Innovation

The large-scale, long-wave, and cross-cutting nature of AIDS epidemics has challenged both learning and implementation processes, creating tensions between research and action, between researchers and activists, as well as between proponents of different strategies such as prevention versus treatment. In the face of complex interactions, researchers are hesitant to generate policy recommendations. And yet, the epidemic (or "endemic," as Barnett terms it) continues regardless.

There are lags between HIV and AIDS and there are lags between policy change and results. Because many policies and programs take years to implement and provide tangible results, there is urgency to put in place an appropriate set of public investments and programs that can cushion the blow by the time the long-wave impacts of AIDS are in full force (Jayne et al., this volume). Proactivity not reactivity is the emphasis to ensure that policy gets ahead of the epidemic curve. To facilitate this, there is thus an urgent need for research to be linked with action, both ways: with research informing action while implementation generates challenges and questions for operational research. This is the essence of action research.

Part of the shift "from evidence to action" will come through a wider adoption of learning-by-doing approaches. Policy needs to support and encourage timely and locally relevant community responses that naturally respond to diversity. But for the "doing" to actually be accompanied by real-time "learning," good systems of process and outcome monitoring and communications are required.

In his keynote address, Tony Barnett spoke of a 5- to 10-year window of opportunity presented by the ongoing (albeit slow-moving) antiretroviral drug rollout. Because of likely difficulties for large numbers of people meeting and sustaining drug adherence thresholds of greater than 95 percent, there is a significant likelihood that viral resistance will develop and spread, undermining the efficacy of existing drug regimens. During this window of time, Barnett asks, how do we literally get ahead of the epidemic curve and promote/enable the development of innovations that will be useful for current and future AIDS control? Such innovations, moreover, will need to be for collective, not simply personal, gain.

The Farmer Life Schools approach is one example of an innovative modification of an earlier approach to agricultural extension (Djeddah, Mavanga, and Hendrickx, this volume). Farmer Life Schools originated from Farmer Field School discovery-based learning approaches to help groups of farmers gain a deep understanding of ecological concepts as well as their practical implications. In the Farmer Life Schools adaptation, this was extended to human ecology, and the same processes have been translated to HIV/AIDS and other livelihood issues. Its latest incarnation, the Junior Farmer Field and Life Schools (JFFLS), has made the link to youth, often orphaned children, who have not been able to learn new agricultural skills and practices from their parents who died too young.

Biostructural intervention is another example of innovation. In this case, simultaneously maximizing the benefits people derive from living natural resources (e.g., through agriculture) while ensuring they are protected from HIV (Loevinsohn, this volume). In India, rural "distress migrants" are at heightened HIV risk and may spread the virus when they return home. Such risky migration has been reduced by some watershed development (WSD) programs through efforts to restore degraded soils and vegetation, capture rainfall, and extend irrigated cultivation. Drawing on recent data from South India, Loevinsohn uses an epidemiologic model to simulate various scenarios. Results suggest that WSD, through reducing migration, may already be preventing significant numbers of HIV infections, in some contexts at a cost per infection averted comparable to single-purpose interventions such as condom promotion. But such programs may also harm the landless, so securing these benefits and avoiding any adverse effects require attention to precisely those issues that have challenged large WSD: interinstitutional cooperation, sustained and flexible local management, equitable sharing of benefits, and effective participation by women, the landless, and other marginalized groups. Loevinsohn concludes that AIDS effectively sharpens the incentives to get WSD "right."

Interventions

When it comes to interventions aimed at combating the HIV/AIDS–food insecurity nexus, the evidence base remains weak. Little is known about designing cost-effective solutions, scaling them up, situating them in the larger strategies for obtaining complex development objectives, or monitoring the full multidimensional nature of such interventions. "Best practices" are often announced that have never been properly evaluated or compared. Where organizations have launched interventions, they are usually isolated, small scale, with minimal monitoring, and they are rarely well evaluated.

The conference made a plea for more rigorous evidence of what works, where, and why. Better links are needed between programmers and researchers to achieve informed action. Interventions with well-functioning management information systems that are amenable to operational research become more effective over time, as well as promoting wider learning. Many NGO participants in particular recognized the need for learning, documentation, and dissemination to become higher priorities in their work.

Interventions aimed at responding to the interactions described earlier may be categorized in various ways. A multiplicity of impacts translates into a potential role for many interventions. Again, without any claims to being comprehensive, here are three of the main intervention options.

Agriculture
Conventional wisdom prioritizes technologies and crops that save labor in the context of HIV/AIDS. Jayne et al. (this volume), however, believe this to have been overgeneralized, although such technologies may be appropriate for certain types of households and regions. Dorward and Mwale (this volume) concur, arguing that laborsaving technologies may even be harmful if they further drive down wage rates that are already falling as a result of HIV-induced cash constraints on ability to hire. Emphasis may need to be placed on other ways of assisting these households, such as cash transfers to help them with labor hire.

With high population density and very small average agricultural holdings, Donovan and Bailey (this volume) found that Rwandan households appear to use labor replacement strategies rather than laborsaving technologies to deal with labor shortages. They found a disturbing trend of households shifting away from crops that provide erosion control, thus endangering future soil fertility. Because affected households consequently tend to be in the lower income groups, agricultural policy that can generate rural income growth from diverse sources will assist these and other poor households.

Raising living standards of households and communities over the long-run through productivity-enhancing investments in agricultural technology generation and diffusion, improved crop marketing systems, basic education, infrastructure, and governance will improve their ability to withstand the social and economic stresses caused by HIV/AIDS (Jayne et al., this volume).

But what types of modifications are needed to ensure that agriculture is "HIV-responsive" and that it plays its part in strengthening resistance and resilience to HIV/AIDS? Bishop-Sambrook et al. (this volume) address this through applying an HIV/AIDS lens to the commercialization of agriculture in Ethiopia. Initiatives to strengthen the market orientation of agricultural production present both an opportunity and a threat in the context of a rural AIDS epidemic. Although any contributions toward reducing poverty and the need to migrate to find work may reduce susceptibility to HIV, the authors state that there are very real risks that the additional cash and the stimulus to travel further afield to market produce could have the opposite effect. Hence, activities associated with promoting the marketing of agricultural products need to be designed with care to ensure that they play a role in arresting, rather than hastening, the spread of the disease in rural communities. They go on to outline several opportunities for addressing HIV/AIDS through market-led growth strategies. Examples include the following:

- Raising awareness and understanding about HIV and AIDS among groups associated with agricultural production and marketing initiatives who are traditionally overlooked because they do not usually belong to formal associations (such as petty traders and retailers, itinerant traders, transporters, owners of hotels and drinking houses).

- Reducing risk of exposure to HIV infection. For example, reducing the need and desire to migrate by improving livelihood options in and around the community, extending the growing season through developing small-scale irrigation, product diversification, agroprocessing, strengthening existing, and creating new, market linkages, and developing the farm input supply chain.

- Reducing vulnerability to AIDS impacts. For example, overcoming barriers to participating in agricultural production and marketing by affected households, such as their depleted resource base, their need to be close to home to tend to the sick, loss of key skills, and their inability to take on risk; using cooperatives and farmer organizations as entry points for mitigation, care, and support activities in communities by, for example, developing income-generating activities, savings, health insurance, or establishing a social fund to provide care for orphans.

Jayne et al. (this volume) conclude their extensive work by discussing four types of potential agricultural policies and programs: factor use and input markets, agricultural research and extension systems, commodity markets, and gender-differentiated resource allocation. In each category they describe clear options for strengthening the HIV-responsiveness of these policy instruments.

Another element of earlier conventional wisdom in this field suggested that AIDS was driving a shift to less labor-intensive and less nutritious crops among smallholders, such as cassava. But how much of this is actually driven by AIDS? Jayne et al. (this volume) point to major changes in agricultural policy that have shifted some farming systems from maize toward tuber crops. Many countries in eastern and southern Africa had formerly implemented state-led maize promotion policies and subsidies on fertilizer distributed on credit to small farmers along with hybrid maize seed. These policies were either eliminated or scaled back significantly in the 1990s as part of economy-wide structural adjustment programs, reducing the financial profitability of growing maize. Cropping incentives prioritize other food crops, especially those relatively unresponsive to fertilizer application, such as cassava.

Social Protection

AIDS can be viewed as a "long-wave crisis" (Barnett, this volume) where, unlike classic, fast-onset emergencies, people do not recover well between crises, or it can be viewed as a "slow-onset disaster" (Wisner et al. 2004) or an urgent development challenge that requires a large-scale long-term response. Until now, AIDS has tended to be addressed either as a humanitarian issue (notably during the 2001–02 food crisis in southern Africa) or as an ongoing threat to development. In recent years, however, discussion has turned to whether these two perspectives need to be better linked. The notions of "developmental relief," "relief in development," and a contiguum approach (as opposed to an emergency to development continuum) have gained currency. Barnett (this volume) also argues for the need to review current paradigms of development and relief and strengthen the ability to switch rapidly between activities as people's needs and priorities change. Oxfam, too, is firmly behind such a contiguum approach, viewing the concept of a development path periodically interrupted by short emergencies as a fiction in the context of AIDS. Oxfam's support to social protection is predicated on the likelihood that at all times in all places people require access to support and interventions in relief, rehabilitation, and development to ensure that their basic needs are covered in the short term while longer term development opportunities are made available.

"Social protection" means different things to different people. Definitions differ with regard to the degree to which the envisioned protection extends to enhancing livelihoods, includes social insurance as well as assistance, and the degree to which it is advocated as a right rather than a reactive form of relief (Adato, Ahmed, and Lund 2004). Increasingly recognized as an essential part of social policy, social protection systems have been used to enable individuals, families, and communities to reduce risk and/or mitigate the impacts of stresses and shocks to their livelihoods. They may also be used to support people who suffer from chronic incapacities to even secure livelihoods, including people living with HIV. Interventions may include conditional and unconditional cash transfers, direct distribution of food or nutritional supplements, school-based food programs, price subsidies, agricultural inputs, public works programs, social health insurance, asset insurance, life insurance, and microfinance. In the context of AIDS, however, there is still little experience to build on, though there are signs that this is now changing. Several issues, including nutrition security, are important operational research priorities (Box 1.3).

Box 1.3 Operational Research Priority: Nutrition Security and HIV/AIDS

In addition to food security, nutrition security[a] has emerged as an important dimension in the prevention, care, treatment, and mitigation of HIV/AIDS. A focus on nutrition security can help reveal opportunities for effectively linking health services with food and nutrition policy in the context of HIV/AIDS. Current research indicates that good nutrition is important to the efficacy of medical interventions as it is to peoples' ability to resist and mitigate infection. There is currently a strong focus on clinical nutrition and HIV/AIDS in the context of issues such as infant feeding and the efficacy of antiretroviral therapy among malnourished populations (see Annex). This relates primarily to interactions within the individual body and their implications for health policy. Yet there have been few attempts to link nutritionists with agricultural economists and/or program managers to investigate the broader issue of community-level nutrition security and food policy and programming in the context of HIV/AIDS. Many of the food responses to date have revolved around delivery of food aid. What other longer-term options exist for ensuring nutrition security within affected communities? What does nutrition "through an HIV lens" look like, and what are the operational implications of rethinking nutrition from this perspective? Does nutrition offer an entry point for forging better links between public health and agricultural responses to AIDS?

[a] Food security here is concerned with physical and economic access to food of sufficient quality and quantity. Food security is necessary, but by itself insufficient, for ensuring nutrition security. Nutrition security is achieved for a household when secure access to food is coupled with a sanitary environment, adequate health services, and adequate care to ensure a healthy life for all household members.

In contrast, food assistance is a widely employed safety net in the context of HIV and AIDS, despite a paucity of evaluations of impacts on HIV-related target groups (Egge and Strasser, this volume). Key areas of expected effect include increases in daily food consumption by all household members and in money available for other needs and an overall increase in household food security. These key effects should in turn generate a cascade of secondary effects measurable by indicators such as anthropometrics, treatment adherence, school attendance, productivity, and the degree of reliance on risky response strategies and on caregivers. Food aid–targeting design, however, tends to be oriented by certain types of people rather than the determinants of vulnerability, and this may lead to significant inefficiencies. Not all female-headed or orphan-fostering households, for example, are vulnerable. Where food assistance is required, there is an emerging consensus on the need for multiple criteria to target beneficiaries. Analyzing community health surveillance data, Egge and Strasser (this volume) suggest targeting efficiency could be improved by first differentiating households according to wealth category (using, for example, assets as a proxy) and then applying other criteria such as chronic illness. Drimie and Mullins (this volume) discuss ways in which a livelihoods approach can guide analysis to go further, to a better understanding of who is actually at risk or vulnerable, why, and how to improve their resilience.

Nutrition and Public Health
"AIDS is a development issue" may be an oft-repeated mantra, yet even in the health sector itself, accumulated knowledge and experience in the field of public health has hardly influenced AIDS policy and programming. Stillwaggon (this volume) argues that it is the same conditions that promote high prevalence of other infectious diseases and parasites that are responsible for the spread of the AIDS epidemic in poor populations. She calls for AIDS policy to address the mundane risks of growing up in environments that burden people with sickness and make them more susceptible to HIV. Programs to prevent HIV transmission are unlikely to succeed unless they address the underlying causes of its spread. HIV prevention must be based on scientific evidence regarding cofactor conditions, not, as they currently are, on unproven assumptions about the primacy of behavioral factors. In addition to food security, deworming, schistosomiasis prevention and treatment, and malaria control programs should thus be integrated as critical components of a broad-based approach to HIV prevention (Stillwaggon, this volume).

The WHO Consultation on Nutrition and HIV/AIDS in Africa (April 10–13, 2005) that preceded the IFPRI conference concluded with several key nutrition-relevant recommendations detailed in the Annex. In sum, these were aimed at strengthening political commitment and improving the positioning of nutrition in national policies and programs; developing practical tools and guidelines for nutritional assessment for home, community, health facility–based, and emergency programs; expanding existing interventions for improving nutrition in the context of HIV; conducting systematic operational and clinical research to support evidence-based programming; strengthening, developing, and protecting human capacity and skills; and incorporating nutrition indicators into HIV/AIDS monitoring and evaluation plans.

Conclusions

In many ways, HIV/AIDS is exposing the fragility of people's livelihoods, a fragility that derives from multiple sources of vulnerability, many of which interact and are worsened by AIDS. Poverty, malnutrition, and hunger have been around a lot longer than the virus. We should thus not be blind to AIDS, but nor should we be blinded by it. An HIV lens, not a filter, needs to be employed. Any move toward "AIDS exceptionalism" will not improve understanding of these important interactions and may even close off some important opportunities for effectively responding.

Three overlapping sets of problems therefore need to be kept in focus: HIV/AIDS, food insecurity, and malnutrition. Not only do these problems overlap significantly, they interact too. We need to keep track of the nature, magnitude, and outcomes of these interactions so that responses are appropriate and effective in the context of high or rising HIV prevalences.

Geographically and disciplinarily, there is a need for breadth as well as depth. Much past work on the HIV/AIDS–hunger nexus has been undertaken in Sub-Saharan Africa where the risks and impacts are most common and most serious and where there is more experience to build on. But it is imperative that future work extends beyond Africa, especially to Asia, in order to be better prepared in other areas where such impacts may soon be experienced. In terms of disciplinarity, diversity of impacts needs to be matched by diversity of researchers, working collaboratively. In order to come to grips with this dynamic new universe, and effectively fill these knowledge gaps, bridges need to be built between social scientists, epidemiologists, public health specialists, nutritionists, and agricultural economists.

Large-scale responses to the diversity of impacts and that are relevant to the local context are now needed. These responses must go well beyond the addition of components to existing vertical programs and structures.

Greater emphasis needs to be placed on learning from, supporting, and enabling community-driven responses and innovations. Communities have better, more relevant information (that responds to the diversity and context-specificity), and they often have latent, untapped capacity. Transparency and accountability may also be enhanced through local peer oversight. Communities have incentives to act, and they are responding, albeit not always optimally. But in general there is a need to start with an understanding of which community-driven responses are working before looking at ways to provide relevant support where local capacity is exceeded. This in turn requires a clear articulation of roles of other stakeholders, including the state, in a broad-based system of social protection.

In the face of the challenges posed by the interactions among HIV/AIDS, food, and nutrition security, there is no convenient magic bullet intervention and no blueprint. The fact that "business as usual" is not working well, however, does not mean that everything needs to change. Rather, a truly multisectoral involvement is required, not the perfunctory addition of more (usually vertical) HIV activities on to sectoral plans. Mainstreaming starts with decisionmakers internalizing AIDS as a development issue, leading in turn to a critical review of existing policies and programs through the lens of their growing knowledge of AIDS interactions. It is a process involving continual reflection, and the progressive application of principles and processes for responding rather than pulling predesigned interventions off the shelf.

Mounting awareness of the links between HIV/AIDS and food and nutrition security creates an opportunity for food and nutrition professionals to develop the conceptual links that, as Gavian, Galaty, and Kombe (this volume) point out, are lacking in current multisectoral frameworks, to provide an empirical basis to assess impacts and costs, propose indicator and monitoring systems, and design appropriate food- and nutrition-relevant interventions.

In all this we must collectively balance the need to know more with the urgent need for large-scale action. As Binswanger, Gillespie, and Kadiyala (this volume) caution, we must not fall into the "evidence trap"; a lack of knowledge is rarely an impediment to action. Although gaps remain in the literature that will require dedicated research to address, there is need for a shift in emphasis toward "learning-by-doing," or action research. For the "doing" to be accompanied by learning, as mainstreamed programs come on stream, the development and maintenance of strong systems of HIV-relevant monitoring, evaluation, and communications will be crucial. The heterogeneity of much recent evidence may preclude generic policy recommendations, but the fact that knowledge gaps remain is no excuse for inaction.

Notes

1. The scope of the IFPRI conference essentially spanned the micro- to macroenvironmental levels, whereas the WHO consultation primarily focused on the two inner circles: the individual-level microbiological and microenvironmental levels.

2. The word "we" is used throughout this overview to denote the primary audience of this document, namely policymakers; national, regional, and international planners; program managers; representatives of civil society; community-based organizations; and researchers whose work (actually or potentially) contributes to combating food and nutrition insecurity, HIV/AIDS, or both.

References

Adato, M., A. Ahmed, and F. Lund. 2004. *2020 Africa Conference Brief 12.* Washington, D.C.: IFPRI.

Barnett, T., and D. Topouzis. 2003. *FAO and HIV/AIDS: Towards a food and livelihoods security based strategic response.* Rome: FAO.

Barnett, T., and A. Whiteside. 2002. *AIDS in the 21st century: Disease and globalization.* New York: Palgrave Press.

Campbell, C. 2003. *"Letting them die": Why HIV/AIDS prevention programmes fail.* Oxford: James Currey.

Carney, D., ed. 1998. *Sustainable rural livelihoods: What contribution can we make?* London: Department for International Development.

Gillespie, S. R., and S. Kadiyala. 2005. *HIV/AIDS and food and nutrition security: From evidence to action.* Food Policy Review 7. Washington, D.C.: IFPRI.

Gillespie, S., L. Haddad, and R. Jackson. 2001. HIV/AIDS, food and nutrition security: Impacts and actions. In *Nutrition and HIV/AIDS.* Nutrition Policy Discussion Paper 20, United Nations SCN, Geneva.

Kadiyala, S. 2004. *Scaling up HIV/AIDS interventions through expanded partnerships (STEPs) in Malawi.* Food Consumption and Nutrition Division Discussion Paper 179. Washington, D.C.: IFPRI.

Larson, B., S. Rosen, P. Hamazakaza, C. Kapunda, and C. Hamusimbi. 2005. Adult health, labour availability and smallholder productivity in Zambia. Draft, available from Dr. Bruce Larson, BLarson@wtnairobi.mimcom.net.

Loevinsohn, M. E., and S. Gillespie. 2003. *HIV/AIDS, food security and rural livelihoods: Understanding and responding.* RENEWAL Working Paper no. 2/IFPRI Discussion Paper no. 157. Washington, D.C.: IFPRI.

Marais, H. 2005. *Buckling: The impact of AIDS in South Africa,* University of Pretoria.

McPherson, M. F. 2005. Asset preservation in African agriculture in the face of HIV/AIDS. *American Journal of Agricultural Economics* 87 (5): 1298–1305.

Norman, A., and M. Chopra. 2005. *HIV disclosure in South Africa: Enabling the gateway to effective response.* Washington, D.C.: IFPRI/RENEWAL (draft).

Rugalema, G. 2000. Coping or struggling? A journey into the impact of HIV/AIDS in southern Africa. *Review of African Political Economy* 28 (86) (December).

UNAIDS. 2006. *Report on the global AIDS epidemic.* Geneva: UNAIDS.

Wisner, B., P. Blaikie, T. Cannon, and I. Davis. 2004. *At risk: natural hazards, people's vulnerability and disasters.* 2nd edition. London: Routledge.

World Bank. 2004. *Turning bureaucrats into warriors.* Washington, D.C.: World Bank.

Yamano, T., and T. S. Jayne. 2004. Measuring the impacts of working-age adult mortality on small-scale farm households in Kenya. *World Development* 32 (1): 91–119.

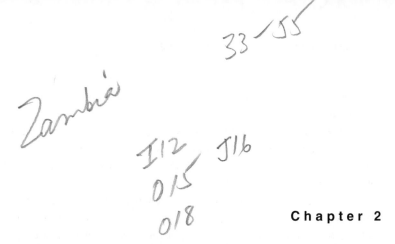

Chapter 2

Socioeconomic Characteristics of Individuals Afflicted by AIDS-Related Prime-Age Mortality in Zambia

Antony Chapoto and Thomas S. Jayne

Introduction

Campaigns to prevent the spread of HIV/AIDS require accurate knowledge of the characteristics of those most likely to contract the disease. Studies conducted in Sub-Saharan Africa during the 1980s generally found a positive correlation between socioeconomic characteristics such as education, income, and wealth and subsequent contraction of HIV (see Ainsworth and Semali 1998; Gregson, Waddell, and Chandiwana 2001). However, as the disease has progressed, the relationship between socioeconomic status and HIV contraction may have changed in many areas of Sub-Saharan Africa, although there is little hard evidence to support this. For example, it is increasingly believed that poverty forces some household members to adopt more risky behaviors that contribute to HIV infection, which could mean that AIDS-related mortality is disproportionately affecting relatively poor households. This chapter seeks to determine the ex ante socioeconomic characteristics of individuals who die between the ages of 15 and 59 years of age (hereafter called "prime-age" mortality), using nationally representative panel data on 18,821 individuals in 5,420 households surveyed in 2001 and 2004 in rural Zambia.

We estimate several probit models of disease-related mortality of prime-age (PA) individuals in rural Zambia between May 2001 and May 2004. The results of these models are used to report the probabilities of mortality over a three-year period for a range of individual profiles that differ according to their gender, level of income, education, months residing away from home, distance to district town, and other individual and household characteristics.

Generally, we find that single women are two to five times more likely to die of disease-related causes as women who are the heads or spouses of their households. Somewhat consistent with findings in the 1980s and early 1990s, relatively wealthy men are more likely to die of disease-related causes than men from poor households. When ranked by asset levels, relatively nonpoor men are 43 percent more likely to die of disease-related causes than men in poor households. In contrast, women in the lower and upper halves of the asset distribution are equally likely to die of disease-related causes, with the probability of mortality over the 3-year period being roughly 1.0 percent regardless of their households' income or asset levels. However, among relatively poor women, those having some form of formal or informal business income are 15 percent less likely to die of disease-related causes than those without any form of business income, but this effect is statistically weak. Although among relatively nonpoor women, those with business income were 7 percent more likely to die than those without any business income. This finding, coupled with the finding that poor and nonpoor women are equally likely to die of disease-related causes, calls into question the view that poverty leading to risky behavior is the major pathway through which the disease is spread, although this may certainly be one of many pathways. There is no clear relationship between educational attainment and probability of dying; both well-educated and poorly educated men and women should continue to be targeted for HIV/AIDS behavior change campaigns. Prime-aged men and women experiencing a prior death in their household are more likely to die of disease-related causes than men and women in households with no prime-age deaths in the past 8 years. These findings will help policymakers and development agencies better understand the transmission pathways of HIV/AIDS, which should help in the formulation of AIDS prevention and mitigation strategies.

Data and Methodology

Data and Attrition

The study uses nationally representative longitudinal data on 18,821 prime-age individuals (15–59 years of age) in 6,922 households in 393 standard enumeration areas (SEAs)[1] in Zambia surveyed in May 2001 and May 2004. The survey was carried out by the Central Statistical Office (CSO) in conjunction with the Ministry of Agriculture and Cooperatives (MACO) and Michigan State University's Food Security Research Project. For sampling procedures see Megill (2004). Of the

6,922 households interviewed in 2001, 5,420 (78.3 percent) were reinterviewed in May 2004. If attrition caused by enumerators not revisiting several SEAs in 2004 that were included in the 2001 survey is excluded, the reinterview rate rises to 88.7 percent. And if attrition caused by adult household members being away from home during the enumeration period and those refusing to be interviewed is excluded, the reinterview rate rises to 94.5 percent.

An examination of the relationship between household attrition, dissolution, and household size in 2001 shows that the percentage of households lost to attrition is inversely related to household size. Whereas 8.4 percent of the households sampled in 2001 contained either one or two members, these households accounted for over 12 percent of the cases of attrition and 18 percent of the cases of household dissolution. In contrast, 65.5 percent of the sample contained households with five or more members, and among these households, only 47 percent of attrition as a result of dissolution is observed. In addition, the results show that dissolution was a more important cause of household attrition among smaller households than among larger households. By contrast, larger households were more likely to incur a prime-age adult death. This is because the probability that a household will incur a prime-age adult death is positively correlated with the number of adult members in the household.

Basic information on the households surveyed, reinterview rates, and prevalence of disease-related mortality over the 2001–04 period is presented in Table 2.1. Of the 5,420 households successfully reinterviewed, 362 of these households (6.3 percent) had at least one disease-related prime-age (PA) death over the 3-year period.[2] Of these 362 households incurring a prime-age disease-related death, 53 of them suffered multiple prime-age deaths, with 45 households experiencing two deaths, 6 households experiencing three deaths, and 2 households experiencing four prime-age deaths. Survey design problems made it difficult to determine the relationships between the deceased in households suffering multiple deaths. Using the World Health Organization (WHO) standard algorithm for diagnosis of HIV infection in the absence of blood tests, 24 percent of the deaths from diseases are estimated to be AIDS related.[3] However, because information was not collected on all of the WHO minor symptoms, it is likely that our classification of AIDS and non-AIDS deaths underestimates the percentage of deaths related to AIDS. Therefore, our analysis is confined to correlates of prime-age mortality from disease in general.

There were 419 prime-age deaths recorded in the sample, 21 of which resulted from accidents or homicide, and 398 cases of illness-related PA mortality. Of the 398 cases of illness-related PA mortality, 165 (41 percent) were men, and 233 (59 percent) were women.[4] Of the 18,821 prime-age adults recorded in 2001, 36 percent

Table 2.1 Prevalence of prime-age (PA) mortality[a] by province, rural Zambia, between 2001 and 2004

Province	Households interviewed in 2001 (a) Number	Households reinterviewed in 2004[b] (b) Number (%)	Households from column (b) with at least one prime-age adult death in 2001–04 (c) Number (%)	Prime-age deaths from illness				Predicted AIDS-related deaths[d]		Median age of adults dying from diseases from 15–59 years of age (h) Years
				Male (d) Number	AMR[c]	Female (e) Number	AMR[c]	By WHO classification[e] (f) Number (%)	One major sign and at least one minor sign (g) Number (%)	
Central	714	573 (80.3)	50 (8.7)	27	12.1 (14.4)	26	13.7 (16.1)	10 (18.9)	13 (24.5)	34
Copperbelt	393	312 (79.4)	16 (5.1)	6	11.1 (14.8)	10	11.2 (14.6)	4 (25.0)	6 (37.5)	36
Eastern	1331	1126 (84.6)	71 (6.3)	31	12.4 (14.6)	45	15.4 (18.5)	15 (19.7)	27 (35.5)	35
Luapula	777	619 (79.7)	41 (6.6)	19	9.7 (12.1)	27	12.1 (15.1)	11 (23.9)	22 (47.8)	36
Lusaka	214	161 (75.2)	15 (9.3)	5	15.7 (19.2)	10	13.3 (16.6)	3 (20.0)	6 (40.0)	36
Northern	1363	1027 (7503)	55 (5.4)	27	8.0 (10.3)	29	10.3 (13.1)	14 (25.0)	18 (32.1)	38
Northwestern	472	324 (68.6)	15 (4.6)	9	6.1 (9.3)	8	6.8 (10.0)	2 (11.8)	3 (17.6)	36
Southern	872	690 (79.1)	55 (8.0)	25	12.0 (15.1)	36	14.0 (17.3)	15 (24.6)	25 (41.0)	32
Western	786	588 (74.8)	51 (8.7)	16	12.5 (16.4)	42	12.6 (17.7)	22 (37.9)	31 (53.4)	33
Total	6922	5420 (78.3)	362 (6.7)	165	11.1 (14.0)	233	12.2 (15.4)	96 (24.4)	151 (38.3)	35

Source: CSO/MACO/FSRP Post Harvest Survey, 1999/2000, and Supplemental Survey, 2001 and 2004.

Notes: [a]Prime-age is defined as ages 15–59 for both men and women. [b]Of the 21.7 percent not reinterviewed, 0.2 percent were refusals, 10.2 percent moved out of standard enumeration area (SEA), 5.7 percent were recorded as dissolved, and 5.2 percent noncontact. [c]AMR (adult mortality rate) = (Prime-age deaths/1000 prime-age person years). Figures in parentheses are AMR including individuals who joined the household and died between 2001 and 2004 but were not in the first survey. [d]Cause of death is defined as HIV/AIDS using lay diagnosis data of the deceased. [e]WHO classification: two major signs (weight loss greater than 10 percent of body weight in a short period of time, chronic diarrhea for more than a month) and at least one minor sign (persistent cough for more than 1 month, itching skin rash, fungal infection of mouth and/or throat, history of herpes zoster, generalized herpes simplex infection, and enlarged lymph nodes).

had left the sample between 2001 and 2004 for causes other than death, such as moving to another location, getting married, and starting another household elsewhere. Excluded from this analysis are 211 prime-age individuals who joined the household after the 2001 survey and died between 2001 and 2004. Strictly speaking, the relevant sample is composed of prime-aged adults who were residents of sampled households in 2001. Including individuals joining sampled households later might overestimate the prevalence of prime-aged mortality, as indicated in Table 2.1, columns d and e (figures in parentheses). Other studies have found that a high proportion of HIV-positive individuals returned to their rural families to receive terminal care after becoming ill (e.g., Kitange, Machibya, and Black 1996).

To test for possible bias in results caused by household attrition, the mean levels of control variables measured in May 2001 were compared for households that were reinterviewed versus those that were lost to attrition. The means of many variables differ statistically between reinterviewed and lost households. For example, households not reinterviewed had slightly younger household heads (43 years vs. 45 years), smaller household sizes with fewer children age 5 and below, fewer boys and girls age 6 to 14, fewer prime-age men and women, and fewer elderly men, slightly smaller landholdings, less farm equipment and animals, and slightly higher rates of chronically ill adults in 2001. This is not surprising given the fact that the households lost to follow-up were smaller to start with in 2001. Systematic differences between those reinterviewed and those not, coupled with a high attrition rate, may cause concern about inference with these data. Also, if the lost households suffered a higher incidence of PA mortality between 2001 and 2004, there would be attrition bias in estimating the ex ante socioeconomic characteristics of individuals who died of AIDS-related causes.[5] So one should be worried about the possibility of systematic attrition leading to selection bias.

In order to deal with potential attrition bias, the inverse probability weighting (IPW) method is adopted, which assumes that the probability of being reinterviewed as a function of observables information is the same as the probability of being reinterviewed as a function of observables, plus unobservables that are observable only for nonlost observations (see Wooldridge 2002).[6] In general, the IPW method works well if the observations on observed variables are strong predictors of nonattrition and if the observations on unobserved variables are not strong predictors of nonattrition. Interview-quality variables are used to predict interview; in particular, 59 enumeration teams are used to predict reinterview. Each enumeration team was headed by a supervisor who was authorized to decide how much effort enumerators make to contact designated households after not finding a valid respondent at home after the first visit. The reinterview model is specified as follows:

$$\text{Prob}(R_{kht} = 1) = f(HIV_{t-j}, I_{hk,2000}, X_{h,2000}, E_{ht}, P) \qquad (2.1)$$

where R_{kht} is 1 if individual (k) is in a household (h) that is reinterviewed at time t, conditional on being interviewed in the previous survey and 0 otherwise; HIV_{t-j} is the district HIV prevalence rate at the nearest surveillance site in 1999; $I_{hk,2000}$ is a vector of individual characteristics in 2000; $X_{h,2000}$ is a set of household characteristics in the 2001 survey including landholding, productive assets, demographic characteristics (number of children ages 5 and under, number of prime-age men and women), and ownership of various assets; E_{ht} is a set of 59 enumeration team dummies; and P is a set of nine provincial dummies. Note that all of the variables in equation 2.1 are observable even for individuals in households that were not reinterviewed in 2004.

Equation 2.1 is estimated with probit for attrition between the 2001 and 2004 surveys, obtaining predicted probabilities (Pr_{2001}). Then, the inverse probability ($1/\text{Pr}_{2001}$) is computed and applied to the probit models, estimating the determinants of prime-age (PA) mortality. Because of space restriction we do not discuss the results from the reinterview models.

Estimation Strategies and Variables

In order to examine the relationship between socioeconomic characteristics and the probability of PA death, all individuals in households interviewed in 2001 were used, and it was determined whether they died between 2001 and 2004. Probit regressions were run for a dichotomous (0/1) dependent variable that equals 1 if the person died of disease-related causes and 0 otherwise. The base model for the analysis is as follows:

$$\text{Prob}(A_{it} = 1) = g(I_{i2000}, X_{h2000}, HIV_{t-j}, C) \qquad (2.2)$$

where A is a binary variable that equals 1 if individual i died between 2001 and 2004, 0 otherwise; I_{i2000} is a set of individual characteristics in 2000; X_{h2000} is a set of household characteristics in 2000; HIV_{t-j} is the lagged district HIV prevalence rate in 1999; and C is a set of community variables including 393 village dummies. Because initial 2000 conditions associated with subsequent mortality are being measured, all of the variables are observable even for individuals in households that were not reinterviewed in 2004 but were contained in the 2001 survey. The vector of individual characteristics includes relationship of the deceased to the person who was household head in 2000, marital status, age, years of education, and months residing away from home. Ages are entered as 5-year age groups up to the age of 59, with ages 15 to 19 as the reference group. Years of schooling are also included in dummy variable form for lower primary (1 to 3 years), upper primary (3 to 6 years), completed primary (7 years), and secondary and higher schooling (8 years and above), with the reference group being those with no formal schooling. Months away from home are divided into three binary variables: 0, 1, and 2 or more months away during the 2000/01 survey season. Individuals who died in 2001 are excluded in computing months away from home variables because 86 (22 percent of total prime-age deaths) of those who died in 2001 were at home all the time in 2000, suggesting that these individuals were already chronically ill and were more likely to be at home throughout the year.

Household characteristics include landholding size, a dummy variable for prior prime-age death between 1996 and 2000, value of productive assets (farm equipment and farm animals), and ownership of durable assets (housing quality, radio, motor vehicles, and water source).

Community variables include distance of the village from the nearest tarmac road and district town and whether the district is located on a railroad line (proxies for degree of interaction between local residents and extent of contact with outsiders passing through the area). The inclusion of quadratic terms of landholding size, productive assets, and distance of village from the nearest tarmac road and district town are tested for because their marginal effect on the probability of being afflicted may be nonlinear. However, specification tests rejected the nonlinearity hypotheses in all cases, so no quadratic terms are included in the reported model results.[7]

Potential regional differences in factors associated with prime-age adult mortality in terms of wealth and income were also tested for, but there was very limited evidence of this through specification tests, so the pooled national sample is used, which is further stratified by gender and assets and/or income status.[8]

Equation 2.2 is estimated with probit using the inverse probabilities from the reinterview model as weights. We run province and village effect models on the full sample as well as estimate separate models for prime-aged men and women and for individuals in the top versus bottom half of the 2001 assets distribution in order to understand whether the socioeconomic correlates of adult mortality vary by gender and wealth status. Provincial fixed-effects models allow us to examine the effects of variables measured at the district level, such as lagged HIV prevalence rates and indicators of market access (distance to the nearest town, distance to the nearest tarmac road, and district on a railroad line). These models also provide more accurate estimates of probability of death over the 3-year survey interval because the full sample is utilized.[9] All findings pertaining to probability of mortality are derived from these models. By contrast, the advantage of village–fixed-effects models is that they control for intervillage differences in the attributes of mortality and thus may provide a more accurate indication of the importance of household-level and individual-level correlates of mortality within communities. Because of space restrictions we report results only from provincial fixed effects.

It is likely that individual participation in nonfarm income activities, having formal or informal business income, months away from home, and prior prime-age death, are likely to be endogenous because they may be related to household's wealth status and individual's educational attainment, which may increase or decrease the likelihood of contracting and dying from AIDS-related cause. Therefore, to check the robustness of our results we run two sets of models, with and without these variables. However, the results on the impact of wealth and education on the likelihood of death from illness were not statistically significant even when we exclude the likely endogenous variables. Therefore, we report the results from the two models side by side but discuss in detail only the findings from the longer models.

Results

Adult Mortality and HIV Prevalence in Zambia

We begin by investigating the correlation between prime-age mortality rates from the Zambia panel household survey data and district HIV prevalence rates from antenatal clinics as reported in Zambia's Demographic Health Survey (CSO, MoH, and Macro International 2003).[10] A strong relationship between prime-age mortality and HIV prevalence rates would suggest that a large proportion of prime-age mortality observed in our household data is indeed from AIDS-related causes.

Figure 2.1 presents a scatter plot of provincial HIV prevalence and rural adult mortality rates from our provincially representative household data. The strength of these correlations is notable, especially considering that the provincial HIV prevalence rate is not disaggregated by urban/rural classification. The Pearson correlation coefficient of 0.84 suggests that the adult mortality rates observed in our survey data is closely associated with HIV prevalence.

Descriptive Analysis

Table 2.2 presents characteristics of the prime-aged individuals who died in sampled households. The following features are discernible. First, more women die from prime-aged disease (and, most likely, from AIDS) than men. The first row of Table 2.2 reports absolute numbers of prime-aged men and women having died compared to individuals remaining in the sample. After weighting of the results to the national level, results indicate that 61 percent of the illness-related prime-age deaths in Zambia's small- and medium-scale farm sector between 2001 and 2004 were

Figure 2.1   Correlation between provincial adult mortality rates from CSO 2001 and 2004 household survey data and 2001 HIV Prevalence Rates, Zambia

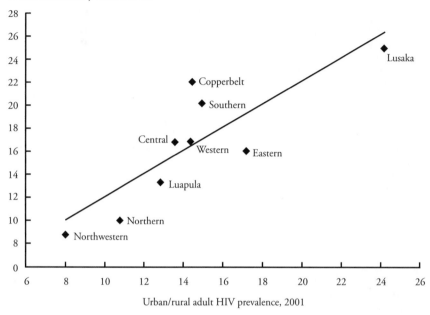

Note: Pearson correlation coefficient is 0.84.

Sources: Adult mortality rates are derived from the 2001 and 2004 household surveys. HIV prevalence rates are from 2001 Sentinel Surveillance Site information published by the Ministry of Health and Zambia Demographic and Health Survey, respectively.

women. These results are also consistent with emerging evidence that a higher proportion of women are dying of AIDS than men in Southern Africa (UNAIDS 2003). Women's mortality rates are expected to be somewhat higher than men's in low-income countries even in the absence of HIV because of maternal-related mortality, but these figures count only illness-related deaths. An important question is whether this 61 percent finding is explained by the physiological differences between men's and women's susceptibility to contracting the disease,[11] or whether it also reflects gender differences in the use of ARV therapy. Because the use of ARV therapy was known to be extremely low during the survey period (fewer than 1 percent of all HIV-positive individuals), it is likely that physiological difference is the primary explanation for this finding. In addition, prime-age female mortality is occurring predominantly among single women in the younger age groups. These

Table 2.2 Descriptive statistics among PA[a] adults who died from illness in 2001–04 and remaining PA adults in the sample

Attributes	PA adult deaths from illness in 2001–2004		PA adults remaining in the sample	
	Male	Female	Male	Female
Number prime-age adults (unweighted)	165	233	5,735	5,851
Number prime-age adults (weighted)	17,801	27,730	659,478	677,593
Individual characteristics in 2000				
Relationship of deceased to the household head in 2000 (%)				
Head/spouse	55.5	54.6	61.5	76.4
Others (sons and daughters, uncles, etc.)	44.5	45.4	38.5	23.6
Marital status 2000 (%)				
Single	43.5	55.4	38.3	32.5
Married	56.5	44.6	61.7	67.5
Age (years)	35.6	33.5	31.2	32.7
Completed school (%)				
No formal education	7.5	21.9	9.8	22.9
1–3 years	11.6	16.7	10.6	16.1
4–6 years	20.9	22.7	25.4	25.2
7 years and above	60.1	38.7	54.2	35.7
Salaried/wage employment (%)	11.3	3	14.2	4.1
Informal/formal business activities (%)	21.2	13.2	18.5	13.3
Months spent away from home (median)	0.4	0.5	0.4	0.3
Household characteristics				
Female-headed households in 2000 (%)	17.7	32.6	12.3	22.8
Prior death of adults 1996–2003 (% of households)[b]	68.4	65.5	6.0	5.9
Landholding size in 2000 (hectares)	3.4	2.7	3.0	2.9
Draft animals and equipment (000 Zkw)	641.9	588.1	729.2	664.4
Per capita household income quartiles in 2000 (%)				
Poor (bottom 50%)	47.6	56.1	49.0	50.7
Nonpoor (top 50%)	52.4	43.9	51.0	49.3
Community characteristics in 2000				
Distance to the nearest town (km)	31.4	33.1	33.4	34.4
Distance to the nearest tarmac road (km)	23.7	22.9	24.1	24

Source: CSO/MACO/FSRP Post Harvest Survey, 1999/2000, and Supplemental Survey, 2001 and 2004.
Notes: [a]Prime age is defined as ages 15–59 for both men and women. [b]Refers to other adults aged 15 to 59 in household who died up to 8 years before the individual under analysis.

results are consistent with the findings of a five-country study by Mather et al. (2004). Moreover, men and women who died between 2001 and 2004 were somewhat more likely to be better educated.

Attributes of Deceased Prime-Age Individuals
The probabilities of PA death for men and women were roughly 0.6 percent and 1.1 percent, respectively (see Chapoto 2006). However, the probability of death for

relatively nonpoor men was 0.9 percent and 0.6 percent (depending on whether the sample is stratified in terms of 2001 income or asset levels), whereas for relatively poor men, the death probabilities were 0.5 percent and 0.8 percent. There was little variation in probability of death between poor and nonpoor women (Table 2.3).

For both relatively poor and nonpoor women, being married and/or the head or spouse of the household significantly reduces the likelihood of death. Among men, the effects of being married in 2001 on the probability of mortality between 2001 and 2004 are weak but still negative. In the village fixed-effects models, relatively poor men who are heads of households are significantly less likely to die than other poor men.

Other variables that affect the probability of death are whether the individual resided at home throughout the year, whether the household experienced prior prime-age mortality, and education (for nonpoor women mainly). Variables that had little effect or ambiguous effects on the probability of dying included whether the individual was engaged in formal or informal business activities, landholding size of the household, and community indicators of proximity to towns and markets.

To aid in understanding the magnitude of the impact of these variables on death probabilities, the provincial–fixed effects model results reported in Table 2.3 were used to compute estimated probabilities of dying over the 3-year period for 20 different individual "profiles." These simulations are reported in Table 2.4 and discussed in the remainder of this chapter.

Relationship of Deceased to Head of Household
Single and relatively young women are much more likely to die than married women. Individual profiles 1 and 2 in Table 2.4 are identical in every respect except for their marital status. According to the probit model results, women fitting the "profile 2" category have a 1.09 percent likelihood of dying over a 3-year period, compared to 0.45 percent for women fitting the "profile 1" category. With other attributes constant, single women are about 2.4 times more likely to die of disease-related causes than married women. Married men are also less likely to die from disease-related causes than single men. As seen in profiles 12 and 13 in Table 2.4, single men with the specified characteristics are 59 percent more likely to die than married men with otherwise similar characteristics.

Age Groups
Age is one of the more important determinants of death from illness as shown by the marginal probabilities in Table 2.3 (where the 15- to 19-year-old age group dummy is omitted). The marginal probability of dying from disease rises steeply

Table 2.3 Probit models[a] of PA mortality in 2001–04 by gender and wealth status (provincial–fixed effects models) corrected for attrition

	Deceased prime-age adult (= 1, 0 otherwise)							
	Asset poor (bottom 50%)				Asset nonpoor (top 50%)			
	Male		Female		Male		Female	
	(a)	(b)	(c)	(d)	(e)	(f)	(g)	(h)
Individual characteristics in 2000								
Head/spouse (= 1)	-0.004	-0.004	-0.007	-0.005	0.003	0.003	-0.007*	-0.006*
	(1.00)	(1.10)	(1.16)	(0.94)	(0.46)	(0.50)	(0.98)	(1.05)
Currently married (= 1)	-0.009	-0.005	-0.007	-0.005	0.004	0.005	-0.003	0.001
	(1.80)	(1.35)	(2.37)	(2.41)	(1.03)	(0.94)	(1.86)	(1.92)
Never married (= 1)	-0.009	-0.005	-0.007	-0.005	0.004	0.005	-0.003	0.001
	(1.70)	(1.18)	(1.38)	(1.11)	(0.43)	(0.55)	(0.34)	(0.12)
Age groups in 2000 (= 1)								
Age 20–24	0.017*	0.011*	0.009	0.008	0.003	0.002	0.008	0.007
	(2.09)	(2.01)	(1.09)	(1.08)	(0.52)	(0.36)	(1.07)	(1.01)
Age 25–29	0.030**	0.022**	0.015	0.016	0.043**	0.042**	0.038**	0.041**
	(2.74)	(2.50)	(1.51)	(1.80)	(3.68)	(3.64)	(3.23)	(3.75)
Age 30–34	0.027*	0.015*	0.041**	0.042**	0.037**	0.032*	0.029*	0.032*
	(2.28)	(1.94)	(2.95)	(3.22)	(2.75)	(2.47)	(2.02)	(2.29)
Age 35–39	0.036**	0.028*	0.025*	0.024*	0.042*	0.040**	0.060**	0.063**
	(2.60)	(2.44)	(2.10)	(2.21)	(2.84)	(2.76)	(2.98)	(3.35)
Age 40–44	0.090**	0.080*	0.023	0.027*	0.044**	0.044**	0.038*	0.041**
	(3.59)	(3.59)	(1.84)	(2.20)	(2.97)	(2.91)	(2.35)	(2.74)
Age 45–49	0.087**	0.077**	0.031*	0.031*	0.073**	0.068**	0.001	0.004
	(3.14)	(3.18)	(1.98)	(2.08)	(3.81)	(3.65)	(0.10)	(0.36)
Age 50–54	0.097**	0.087**	0.003	0.004	0.101**	0.096**	0.029	0.033*
	(3.78)	(3.74)	(0.28)	(0.38)	(3.54)	(3.47)	(1.75)	(2.06)
Age 55–59	0.108**	0.100**	0.021	0.023	0.079**	0.078**	0.031	0.031
	(3.81)	(3.90)	(1.50)	(1.70)	(3.76)	(3.70)	(1.65)	(1.78)
Years of education in 2000 (= 1)								
1–3 years	0.005	0.003	0.009	0.008	0.034*	0.032*	-0.009	-0.009*
	(0.83)	(0.57)	(1.45)	(1.33)	(2.14)	(2.12)	(1.76)	(2.08)

	(1)	(2)	(3)	(4)	(5)	(6)	(7)	(8)
4–6 years	0.003	0.001	0.003	0.002	0.022*	0.021*	-0.010*	-0.009*
	(0.55)	(0.26)	(0.52)	(0.33)	(2.03)	(2.05)	(2.03)	(2.23)
7 years	0.017**	0.012**	-0.003	-0.003	0.012	0.011	-0.007	-0.007
	(2.60)	(2.21)	(0.49)	(0.54)	(1.32)	(1.29)	(1.21)	(1.40)
8 years and above	0.006	0.003	0.014	0.013	0.010	0.008	-0.009	-0.010**
	(1.07)	(0.77)	(1.65)	(1.58)	(1.27)	(1.06)	(1.91)	(2.58)
Salary wage income in 2000 (= 1)	–	0.008*	–	-0.008	–	0.002	–	-0.009
	–	(2.27)	–	(1.44)	–	(0.56)	–	(1.41)
Business activity in 2000 (= 1)[b]	–	0.002	–	-0.002	–	-0.002	–	0.002
	–	(1.13)	–	(0.47)	–	(0.64)	–	(0.42)
Resided in home throughout the year in 2000 (= 1)[b]	–	0.002	–	-0.002	–	-0.002	–	0.002
	–	(3.85)	–	(4.44)	–	(2.65)	–	(6.02)
One month spent away from home in 2000 (= 1)	–	-0.002	–	-0.012*	–	-0.007	–	-0.012**
	–	(0.90)	–	(2.37)	–	(1.12)	–	(2.99)
Household characteristics in 2000								
Polygamous household (= 1)	-0.006	-0.005*	-0.001	-0.001	0.002	0.001	0.002	0.003
	(1.91)	(2.25)	(0.11)	(0.17)	(0.35)	(0.26)	(0.39)	(0.59)
Prior PA death in 1996–2003[c] (= 1)	–	0.140**	–	0.169**	–	0.079**	–	0.111**
	–	(11.77)	–	(14.37)	–	(10.43)	–	(9.96)
ln[Landholding size (hectares)]	-0.000	-0.000	-0.001	-0.001	-0.003	-0.003	-0.005*	-0.005**
	(0.19)	(0.17)	(0.34)	(0.48)	(1.48)	(1.49)	(2.42)	(2.70)
Community characteristics								
District HIV prevalence rate in 1999	-0.000	-0.000	0.000	0.000	0.001	0.001	0.002*	0.002*
	(0.48)	(0.37)	(0.45)	(0.51)	(0.66)	(0.72)	(2.29)	(2.57)
District on the line of rail (= 1)	-0.000	-0.001	-0.005	-0.004	0.001	0.000	-0.006	-0.008
	(0.07)	(0.36)	(0.83)	(0.79)	(0.17)	(0.05)	(1.21)	(1.72)
Distance to the nearest tarmac road (km)	-0.000	-0.000	-0.000	0.000	0.000	0.000	0.000	0.000
	(0.39)	(0.13)	(0.00)	(0.03)	(0.50)	(0.53)	(0.41)	(0.47)
Distance to the district town/boma (km)	0.000	0.000	0.000	0.000	0.000	0.000	0.000	0.000*
	(0.55)	(0.44)	(0.24)	(0.21)	(0.79)	(0.66)	(1.63)	(1.97)
Provincial dummies included	Yes	Yes	Yes	Yes	Yes	Yes	Yes	Yes
Predicted probability of dying from disease-related causes[d]	0.006	0.005	0.013	0.012	0.009	0.009	0.012	0.011
Number of observations	3,596	3,596	3,977	3,977	3,812	3,812	3,711	3,711

Source: CSO/MACO/FSRP Post Harvest Survey, 1999/2000, and Supplemental Survey, 2001 and 2004.

Notes: [a]Absolute z-scores, calculated using heteroskedasticity robust standard errors clustered for households. ** indicates 1 percent significance level; * indicates 5 percent significance level. [b]Formal or informal business activities. [c]Refers to other adults ages 15 to 59 in household who died up to 8 years before the individual under analysis. [d]The probability of dying from disease related causes, setting all explanatory variables at their mean values.

Table 2.4 Simulations[a] of the probability of mortality based on specific individual and household attributes

Individual profile	Gender	Marital status	Income group	Age group	Education	Months away from home per year	Salary wage income	Formal/ informal business income	Prior death of adult in household, 1996–2004	Predicted P of mortality in 3-year period	
										Assets (%)	Income (%)
1	Female	Married	Low	25–29	4–6 years	0	No	No	No	0.45	0.59
2	Female	Single	Low	25–29	4–6 years	0	No	No	No	1.09	2.17
3	Male	Married	Low	25–29	4–6 years	0	No	No	No	0.01	0.66
4	Male	Single	Low	25–29	4–6 years	0	No	No	No	0.34	1.50
5	Female	Married	High	20–24	4–6 years	0	Yes	No	No	0.03	0.05
6	Female	Single	High	20–24	4–6 years	0	Yes	No	No	0.28	0.20
7	Female	Single	High	20–24	1–3 years	0	No	No	No	0.66	0.95
8	Female	Single	High	20–24	1–3 years	0	No	Yes	No	0.73	1.41
9	Female	Single	Low	20–24	1–3 years	0	No	No	No	1.25	1.33
10	Female	Single	Low	20–24	1–3 years	0	No	Yes	No	1.11	0.82
11	Female	Single	Low	20–24	1–3 years	≥ 2	No	Yes	No	4.69	3.45
12	Male	Married	High	45–49	≥ 8 years	0	No	No	No	0.90	0.44
13	Male	Single	High	45–49	≥ 8 years	0	No	No	No	2.09	1.93
14	Male	Single	High	45–49	≥ 8 years	≥ 2	Yes	No	No	7.76	8.67
15	Male	Single	High	45–49	≥ 8 years	0	Yes	No	No	3.61	2.69
16	Male	Single	Low	45–49	≥ 8 years	0	No	No	No	1.58	1.14
17	Male	Married	High	45–49	≥ 8 years	0	No	No	No	0.90	0.44
18	Male	Married	High	45–49	≥ 8 years	0	No	No	Yes	12.8	14.9
19	Female	Married	High	35–39	≥ 8 years	0	No	No	No	0.72	1.29
20	Female	Married	High	35–39	≥ 8 years	0	No	No	Yes	12.2	18.8

Source: CSO/MACO/FSRP Post Harvest Survey, 1999/2000, and Supplemental Survey, 2001 and 2004.

[a]Simulation outcomes based on regression models in Table 2.3. For purposes of the simulation, married men and women are simulated as being heads and spouses of their households.

from age 15, peaking between ages 30 and 39 for poor females and 45 to 59 years of age for men, regardless of their poverty status. This finding confirms previous findings showing that women are more likely to die at an earlier age than their male counterparts. The predicted probability of dying from diseases for women residing in relatively high-asset households rises from age 15, peaks between ages 50 and 54, and then declines. However, among women in relatively poor families, the probability of mortality peaks in the 30- to 34-year age range. The predicted probability of disease-related mortality for a relatively poor woman in the 30- to 34-year age range is roughly twice as high as for a poor woman in the 20- to 24-year age range. The probability of mortality for a relatively nonpoor woman in the 30- to 34-year age range is only 1.3 times higher than a nonpoor woman in the 20- to 24-year age range.

Education, Mobility, Income, and Household Wealth Indicators
Unlike earlier studies in Sub-Saharan Africa that generally found a positive correlation between education and HIV-related deaths (e.g., Ainsworth and Semali 1998; Gregson, Waddell, and Chandiwana 2001; Hargreaves and Glynn 2002), the results in Table 2.4 show a much weaker relationship between educational attainment and the probability of mortality from disease. There is no statistically significant relationship for men in households with either low or high income and/or assets even after exclusion of all potentially endogenous variables as discussed earlier. This appears to be in contrast to earlier findings showing that highly educated men were the most likely to die of disease-related death (Ainsworth and Semali 1998). Among women, the findings generally indicate a negative relationship between educational attainment and the probability of disease-related death, especially for relatively nonpoor women. These findings are consistent with de Walque (2004), who found that over time, susceptibility to HIV/AIDS in Uganda declined for relatively well-educated people more than for poorly educated people, as information regarding precautionary measures spread. One apparent implication of this finding is that well-educated and (especially) poorly educated men and women should continue to be targeted for HIV/AIDS education campaigns.

The results are somewhat consistent with findings in the 1980s and early 1990s indicating that prime-age mortality is more likely to affect men in the upper income brackets. This can be seen in Table 2.4 by comparing profiles 13 and 16, which are identical in all respects except for assets and/or income. Nonpoor men with the attributes shown in profile 13 are 1.3 times more likely to die of disease-related deaths compared to men in the bottom half of the assets distribution (nonpoor men have a probability of mortality over a 3-year period of 2.09 percent compared to 1.58 percent for men in the bottom half of the assets distribution). Although poverty might be expected to raise the probability of infection of sexually transmitted diseases and HIV because men with low incomes may be less able to afford condoms or STD treatment, our findings indicate that the influence of high economic and social status tends to predominate for men. As shown in Table 2.3, women in the lower and upper half of the asset distribution are equally likely to die of disease-related causes, with the probability of mortality over the 3-year period being roughly 1.0 percent regardless of their households' income or asset levels. This may vary somewhat according to age group. For example, comparison of profiles 7 and 9 shows that women in the bottom half of the asset distribution (with the particular characteristics specified for these profiles) have a probability of mortality over a 3-year period of 1.25 percent compared to 0.66 percent for women in the top half of the assets distribution. If the age group of profiles 7 and 9 is changed from 20–25 to 35–39 and all other characteristics are kept the same, the opposite result is obtained: women in the bottom half of the asset distribution have a probability of mortality over a 3-year period of 2.2 percent compared to 3.2 percent for women in the top half of the assets distribution. This finding highlights the sensitivity to age group of the relationship between poverty and probability of death.

Women from relatively poor households who have some form of formal or informal business income are less likely to die of disease-related causes than poor women who did not have any formal or informal business activity (profiles 9 vs. 10). This finding seems to support Epstein (2002, 2003), who contends that female members in poorer households with few employment opportunities are more likely to engage in riskier sexual activities for economic reasons, exposing themselves to HIV infection.

So efforts to provide greater income-earning opportunities for poor women may make at least a modest contribution to reducing female PA mortality. However, Epstein's argument is contradicted by our finding that women from relatively nonpoor households having some formal or informal business income are 10 percent more likely to die of disease-related causes than women with similar characteristics not having business income. Nonpoor women with businesses are more likely to spend more time away from home and have more social interactions than poor women with and without businesses. Other things equal, working women with their own income sources may be less vulnerable (along the lines of Epstein's argument), but working may also involve being outside the village or working away from home more, which may in turn increase certain risk factors. Recent research demonstrates that relative economic disadvantage is found to significantly increase the likelihood of a variety of unsafe sexual behaviors and experiences in KwaZulu-Natal Province, South Africa (Hallman and Grant 2004). However, the findings from rural Zambia provide mixed evidence, which calls into question the view that poverty leading to risky behavior is the major pathway through which the disease is spread, although this may certainly be one of many pathways. Among rural prime-aged Zambian women, there appears to be no clear relationship between income and asset levels, access to business income, and probability of dying.

The results show that irrespective of poverty status, men and women living 2 months or more away from home per year in the 2000/01 period are more likely to die of disease-related causes between 2002 and 2004 than men and women of the same characteristics who spent all the time at home. For example, comparison of profiles 14 and 15 shows that nonpoor men who spend 2 months or more away from home in 2000/01 have a probability of mortality over a 3-year period of 7.8 percent, whereas men of the same characteristics who spend all their time at home and did not die in 2001 had a probability of mortality over the same period of 3.6 percent. In contrast, comparison of profiles 10 and 11 showed that poor women living 2 months or more away from home are four times more likely to die of disease-related deaths than women of the same characteristics who resided at home throughout the year.

Finally, the probit results show that the prior death of at least one adult in the household over the past 8 years is the single most important factor influencing the probability that a prime-aged individual will die as a result of illness.[12] Irrespective of income or assets status, men and women experiencing a prior death of a prime-age person in their household are 14 to 16 times more likely to die of disease-related causes than the average prime-age individual. This is shown by comparing Table 2.4 profiles 17 and 18 for men and profiles 19 and 20 for women. The probability that men and women with the profiles shown in rows 18 and 20 would die over a 3-year period is 12.8 percent and 12.2 percent, respectively. In this way, AIDS differs from other kinds of diseases (e.g., malaria) that do not appreciably raise the likelihood of subsequent death in the family after one member contracts the disease. To the extent that the death of two prime-age members from the same household within a few years of each other causes extreme hardships on remaining members, especially for children, the implication of this finding is that special programs to target and support AIDS-afflicted households are likely to become an important component of poverty reduction strategies, especially in areas hard hit by AIDS, such as most of eastern and southern Africa.

Household variables that appeared to be largely unrelated to the probability of an individual dying from disease include several indicators of rural wealth such as landholding size and livestock assets. As reported in Table 2.3, indicators of market access, such as the village's distance to the nearest tarmac road or district town, were largely unrelated to the probability of an individual dying from disease. This indicates that the disease has moved far into the interior of rural Zambia, such that proximity to towns and highways that initially were the main locations where the disease was transmitted no longer has a significant bearing on the probability of death. District-level HIV prevalence rates are correlated strongly only with the probability of death among women in the nonpoor groups. This is perhaps not surprising because HIV prevalence rates are derived from blood tests of women (not men) who visit antenatal clinics in periurban and urban areas, who are more likely to be nonpoor than most women contained in this sample.

Conclusion

This study has identified important ex ante socioeconomic conditions of individuals and households in rural Zambia who die between the ages of 15 and 59 years of disease-related causes, using nationally representative panel data on 18,821 individuals surveyed in 2001 and 2004 in rural Zambia. The findings of the study can help policymakers and development agencies better understand current transmission pathways of HIV/AIDS, which should help in the formulation of up-to-date AIDS prevention and mitigation strategies.

Overall, the probability that a prime-aged (i.e., 15- to 59-year-old) woman would die of disease-related causes was roughly 1.0 percent over the 3-year period, whereas the comparable probability for men was 0.6 percent. Just over 60 percent of the prime-age deaths observed in this nationally representative rural sample were women, supporting other findings that women are being disproportionately afflicted by the disease.

Consistent with findings in the 1980s and early 1990s, we find that men in the upper half of the assets distribution are more likely to die of disease-related causes than men residing in poor households. In contrast, women in the lower half of income/assets distribution are equally likely to die of disease-related causes as women residing in the upper half of assets/income distribution. An emerging strand of the social science literature on HIV/AIDS in Africa stresses the relationships among poverty, risky sexual behavior, and subsequent contraction of the disease. It has been argued that single women unable to sustain themselves through wage labor or agriculture are more likely to resort to transactional sex for survival. If this is an important social pathway contributing to the spread of the disease in Africa, then we expected to find a relationship over time between household- and individual-level indicators of poverty, especially for single women, and subsequent chronic illness and death. We find that, regardless of the initial poverty status of their households, women who have some form of formal or informal business income are about as likely to die of disease-related death as women with no formal or informal business activity, after controlling for other socioeconomic characteristics. This finding suggests that efforts to provide greater income-earning opportunities for poor women may make a modest contribution at best to reducing female prime-age mortality. These findings also suggest that the social factors driving the spread of AIDS are considerably more complex than simply poverty-based explanations, although poverty may certainly contribute to risky behavior and poor health, which are important pathways by which the disease is spread.

By contrast, there are several other socioeconomic variables that do have a major influence on probability of mortality. Single women and men in poor households are twice as likely to die of disease-related causes as poor women and men who are the heads or spouses of their households. Single women and men in relatively nonpoor households are 3.7 and 4.5 times more likely to suffer a disease-related death compared to married nonpoor women and men who are the heads or spouses of their households. Individuals who spend 2 months or more away from home are 2 to 10 times more likely to die of disease-related causes in succeeding years than individuals with similar socioeconomic attributes who reside at home all year. Mobility is thus a significant risk factor. It is possible that the creation of business opportunities that involve men and women spending more time away from home for extended periods may exacerbate the AIDS problem in rural Zambia and negate the positive effects of greater financial independence for women, unless progress is made in public health and educational campaigns to promote the use of condoms, other forms of safe sex, and prevention interventions.

Years of formal education was found to be largely unrelated to vulnerability to death for men. For women, the evidence is not robust, but the data tend to show that educational attainment reduces somewhat women's vulnerability to disease-related death, especially for nonpoor women. This result may indicate that public health information is indeed working for the more educated strata of rural Zambian society because earlier studies in the region found that HIV rates were much higher for relatively well-educated men and women (Ainsworth and Semali 1998). This finding suggests that education coupled with public health campaigns may be an important empowerment tool for women and may help to reduce the risk of HIV contraction among women. Also, HIV/AIDS education campaigns should still target both the literate and illiterate because men of any education level have roughly the same risk of contracting HIV.

Most importantly, the prior death of a prime-aged person in the household substantially increases the probability of another prime-aged member dying. Irrespective of poverty status, prime-aged men and women experiencing a prior death in their household are 23.0 and 18.1 times more likely to die of disease-related causes than men and women in households with no prime-age deaths in the past 8 years. The predicted probability of death was 12.4 percent and 16.3 percent for men and women experiencing a prior disease-related death in their household in the past 8 years versus 0.54 percent and 0.90 percent for men and women not experiencing a prior prime-aged death. Of the 362 households experiencing prime-age mortality between 2001 and 2004, 15 percent of them suffered multiple prime-age deaths. In this way, AIDS differs from other kinds of diseases (e.g., malaria), which does not appreciably raise the likelihood of subsequent death in the family after one member contracts the disease. To the extent that the death of two prime-age members from the same household within a few years of each other causes extreme hardships on remaining members, especially for children, the implication of this finding is that programs and strategies to support the care and education of orphans and children in AIDS-afflicted households may need to become a critical component of poverty reduction strategies in areas hard hit by AIDS, such as most of eastern and southern Africa. More research is necessary to understand the longer-term impacts of the disease on household behavior and welfare and to develop programs that can mitigate the adverse consequences. At this time, the research community still knows very little about the cost-effectiveness of alternative ways of mitigating the impacts of AIDS, but a solid understanding of the socioeconomic factors associated with the disease is likely to help considerably in designing appropriate risk messages and prevention strategies.

Notes

This research has been funded through the USAID/Zambia Mission and USAID/Global Bureau, Office of Agriculture and Food Security, and the Africa Bureau Office of Sustainable Development. This chapter draws from Chapoto's Ph.D. dissertation (see Chapoto 2006).

1. "Standard enumeration areas" (SEAs) are the lowest geographic sampling unit in the Central Statistical Office's sampling framework for its annual Post Harvest Surveys. Each SEA contains roughly 150 to 200 rural households.

2. This includes only households with individuals in both the first and second surveys. A small number of recorded deaths were the result of violence or accidents; these were excluded from the analysis.

3. A review of literature on verbal autopsies and lay diagnoses shows that there is no "ideal" method of measuring AIDS-specific mortality in a Zambian population-based sample. Therefore, we cannot get a "gold standard" diagnosis on a true population basis because the validation of verbal autopsy studies in literature are flawed (the validation samples come from a clinical sample and therefore are not likely to be representative of the population) (G. Birbeck, Michigan State University, personal communication, November 2004).

4. After weighting, women accounted for 61 percent of PA mortality.

5. Available evidence on attrition rates in longitudinal surveys in developing countries range from 5 to 30 percent for two rounds (see Alderman et al. 2001; Duncan, Frankenberg, and Smith 2001; Yamano and Jayne 2004). For a discussion of IPW, see Wooldridge (2002).

6. The literature addressing the detection and correction of selection bias is extensive, and a complete review of this literature is beyond the scope of this chapter. Overviews of sample selection models can be found in Fitzgerald, Gottschalk, and Moffit (1998) and Alderman et al. (2001).

7. In addition to the linear terms, the quadratic terms of landholding size, productive assets, and distance of village from the nearest tarmac road and district town are added to the models, and a test of joint significance is done in order to determine whether to include the quadratic term in addition to the linear term.

8. In order to test for regional wealth and/or income differences, we rank household wealth distribution (value of productive assets such as farm equipment and livestock) into terciles and then run two sets of models having two wealth dummies (top and bottom wealth distribution with the middle group as the reference), eight provincial dummies, and interaction terms of wealth distribution dummies and provincial dummies and other household and community variables in the second model. The joint test of significance of wealth and provincial dummies was rejected even at a 20 percent level of significance. A similar approach is done with household income (sum of value of productive assets, gross value of crop output, formal/informal business income, and nonfarm income), but the test for joint significance showed no regional difference by income status as well.

9. By contrast, when estimating models with village dummies, the estimation program automatically drops those households where no within-village variation in the dependent variable exists, which restricts the sample somewhat. Of the 393 villages in the sample, 118 villages experienced no prime-age disease-related mortality among their households. Estimating probability of mortality from such models will generate upwardly biased probabilities because of the many cases dropped of individuals residing in villages where there were no recorded disease-related deaths over the survey interval.

10. National estimates of HIV prevalence in Sub-Saharan Africa are almost exclusively based on surveys of antenatal clinics, the majority of which are located in urban areas. The Zambia Demographic Health Survey figures are derived from blood sample testing of a randomly selected national sample of PA adults.

11. Because of women's greater surface area where infected blood can be exchanged during sexual activity, the risk of HIV transmission from an infected male to a susceptible female is 2-4 times higher than the risk of HIV transmission from an infected female to a susceptible male (Chin 2003, drawing from Gray et al. 2001 based on findings from Rakai, Uganda).

12. Respondents in the 2001 survey were asked about prior deaths in the household back to 1996, whereas respondents in the 2004 survey were asked about deaths experienced in the household since the 2001 survey. A binary variable equaling 1 if the household experienced a death between 1996 and 2004 is then computed.

References

Ainsworth, M., and I. Semali. 1998. Who is most likely to die of AIDS? Socioeconomic correlates of adult deaths in Kagera Region, Tanzania. In *Confronting AIDS: Evidence for developing world*, eds. M. Ainsworth, L. Fransen, and M. Over. Brussels: European Commission.

Alderman, H., J. Behrman, H.-P. Kohler, J. Maluccio, and S. Watkins. 2001. Attrition in longitudinal household survey data: Some tests for three developing country samples. *Demographic Research* 5: 78–124.

Central Statistical Office, Ministry of Health, and Macro International. 2003. *Zambia Demographic Health Survey (ZDHS), 2001/2002*. Lusaka, Zambia.

Chapoto, A. 2006. *The impact of AIDS-related prime-age mortality on rural farm households: Panel survey evidence from Zambia*. Ph.D. dissertation, Michigan State University, East Lansing, Michigan.

Chin, J. 2003. *Understanding the epidemiology and transmission dynamics of the HIV/AIDS pandemic*. School of Public Health, University of California/Berkeley. Paper presented at USAID, Washington, D.C., October 2003.

De Walque, D. 2004. *How does the impact of an HIV/AIDS information campaign vary with educational attainment? Evidence from rural Uganda*. Policy Research Working Paper Series 3289. Washington, D.C.: World Bank.

Duncan, T., E. Frankenberg, and J. P. Smith. 2001. Lost but not forgotten: Attrition and follow-up in the Indonesia Family Life Survey. *Journal of Human Resources* 36: 556–592.

Epstein, H. 2002. The hidden cause of AIDS. *New York Times Review of Books* 49 (8), May 9, 2002.

———. 2003. AIDS in South Africa: The invisible cure. *New York Times Review of Books* 50 (12), July 17, 2003.

Fitzgerld, J., P. Gottschalk, and R. Moffitt. 1998. An analysis of sample attrition in panel data. The Michigan Panel Study on Income Dynamics. *Journal of Human Resources* 33: 251–299.

Gray, R. H., M. J. Wawer, R. Brookmeyer, N. K. Sewankambo, D. Serwadda, F. Wabwire-Mangen, T. Lutalo, X. Li, T. VanCott, T. C. Quinn, and the Rakai Project Team. 2001. Probability of HIV-1 transmission per coital act in monogamous, heterosexual, HIV-1 discordant couples in Rakai, Uganda. *Lancet* 357: 1149–1153.

Gregson, S., H. Waddell, and S. Chandiwana. 2001. School education and HIV control in Sub-Saharan Africa: From discord to harmony? *Journal of International Development* 13: 467–485.

Hallman, K., and M. Grant. 2004. *Poverty, educational attainment, and livelihoods: How well do young people fare in KwaZulu Natal, South Africa?* Horizons Research Summary. Washington, D.C.: Population Council.

Hargreaves, J. R., and J. Glynn. 2002. Educational attainments and HIV-1 infection in developing countries: A systematic review. *Tropical Medicine and International Health* 7 (6): 489–498.

Kitange, H. M., H. Machibya, and J. Black. 1996. Outlook for survivors in Sub-Saharan Africa: Adult mortality in Tanzania (abstract). *British Medical Journal* 312: 216–220.

Mather, D., C. Donovan, T. S. Jayne, M. Weber, E. Mazhangara, L. Bailey, K. Yoo, T. Yamano, and E. Mghenyi. 2004. *A cross-country analysis of household responses to adult mortality in rural sub Saharan Africa: Implications for HIV/AIDS mitigation and rural development policies*. Michigan State University International Development Working Paper, IDWP 82. East Lansing, Michigan.

Megill, D. J. 2004. *Recommendations on sample design for post harvest surveys in Zambia based on the 2000 census.* Working Paper 10. Lusaka, Zambia: Food Security Research Project/Zambia.

UNAIDS. 2003. *AIDS epidemic update.* Geneva, Switzerland: WHO.

Wooldridge, J. M. 2002. Inverse probability weighted M-estimators for sample selection, attrition and stratification. *Portuguese Economic Journal* 1: 117–139.

Yamano, T., and T. S. Jayne. 2004. Measuring the impacts of working-age adult mortality on small-scale farm households in Kenya, *World Development* 32 (1): 91–119.

Chapter 3

HIV/AIDS, Household Income, and Consumption Dynamics in Malawi

Winford H. Masanjala

Introduction

A survey of recent writings on the interactions between the AIDS epidemic and livelihoods in Africa leaves one with the impression that development practitioners, academics, and even casual observers of developments in Africa are hell-bent on pinning most of Africa's economic stagnation on the AIDS epidemic. This is all the more troubling because, although in the past 15 years economists have attempted to systematically link AIDS and poverty and to test the strength of those linkages, the relationships among livelihoods, poverty, and the AIDS epidemic remains so complex that we still know little about the actual contribution of AIDS in explaining observed cases of persistent poverty and divergent economic fortunes in Africa. For instance, a number of macro-level forecasts, from the pioneering studies (Ainsworth and Over 1992; Cuddington 1993; Cuddington and Hancock 1994) to more recent ones (e.g., Bloom and Mahal 1997; Greener, Jefferis, and Siphambe 2000; Arndt and Lewis 2001; Haacker 2002; Crafts and Haacker 2003) have generated an almost universal consensus that the AIDS epidemic will have an immense impact on the macroeconomies of hard-hit countries, significantly slowing economic growth and worsening poverty and income distribution (also see summaries in UNFPA 2002; UNAIDS 2002). Yet recent experience seems to suggest that because the HIV population is still a relatively small proportion of the total population, even in hard-hit countries, macro-level economic impacts of AIDS are likely to be barely visible in national statistics (Desbarats 2002).

In contrast, relatively more worthwhile efforts have been made at the micro level, where a number of studies have systematically investigated the link among the AIDS epidemic, rural livelihoods, and the socioeconomic systems through which those livelihoods are embedded and mediated (see summaries in Haddad and Gillespie 2001; Loevinsohn and Gillespie 2003; Gillespie and Kadiyala 2005). However, although these studies have managed to impose some structure on our understanding of the linkages between AIDS and livelihoods, to date the underlying causal processes are still poorly understood and, with few exceptions, not formulated in precise ways. More importantly, the divergence of findings, positions, and policy implications from these studies seems to highlight the difficulty attendant to any attempt to disentangle the economic stagnation that may be caused by the AIDS epidemic from that produced by a host of other debilitating features of the African landscape such as missing or imperfect factor, product, and financial markets or reliance on rain-fed subsistence agriculture. Yet the design of appropriate public policies depends critically on this knowledge.

This chapter seeks to examine the pathways through which the AIDS epidemic can cause poverty traps in rural agrarian households. A poverty trap is defined as any self-reinforcing mechanism that causes poverty to persist (see Azariadis 1996). Poverty traps do not refer to situations in which it is simply difficult to escape low incomes but to a situation where the evolution of household wealth or well-being is governed by a path-dependent process such that, depending on initial conditions, otherwise identical individuals or households may remain for long periods of time (if not indefinitely) "locked into" poverty or affluence. A key characteristic of a poverty trap is that "good" and "bad" outcomes are self-enforcing, so that small interventions or chance events will not alter the long-term outcome. Using data from the Malawi Integrated Household Survey (GOM 2000) and the Complementary Panel Survey (CPS) of 2000–02, this chapter seeks to capture how the AIDS epidemic can create conditions such that negative economic shocks can cause previously nonpoor households to become poor and to stay poor indefinitely or cause moderately poor households to fall into persistent destitution.

HIV/AIDS as a Possible Source of Poverty Traps

There are a number of pathways through which HIV and AIDS can cause a farm household to fall into perpetual poverty. First is the AIDS-expectations pathway. Because the probability of death from AIDS is unity, knowledge that a household member is infected with HIV inevitably changes the affected household's sense of time–preference, which in turn impacts its intertemporal resource allocation and utility maximization. Knowledge that a household member is infected with HIV will reduce the expected return from various social and economic investments and force affected households either to trade off lower risk for lower return or to heavily discount investments with long-term returns for current consumption. The second pathway works through labor productivity. HIV-linked illnesses or AIDS affect the health and productivity of those infected with the virus because a person suffering from debilitating HIV or AIDS is unable to do a full workload, resulting in reduced income and reduced capacity for future production. Moreover, HIV-linked illness and AIDS have a depressing effect on the productivity of healthy people because of the absenteeism caused by caregiving or attending funerals. These effects can also conspire to trap a household in perpetual poverty through either diversion of productive resources toward caring for the sick, reductions in household income as a result of illness, or the death of a breadwinner (see Serpell 1999; Bollinger et al. 1999).

Another pathway is through physical capital. The accumulation of voluntary savings and access to reasonable credit has never been easy for the poorest sections of African communities, and seldom has it been easy for women. Yet HIV/AIDS has made it harder. When faced with the costs associated with increase in morbidity and mortality from AIDS, households cope by using up savings, taking additional debt at penal rates of interest, or searching for additional sources of income. However, when households deplete their savings and exhaust debt sources, the next step in the course of impoverishment is to dispose of unproductive assets before ultimately disposing of productive assets such as land, draft animals, and equipment, that is, disinvestment and a nonreversible strategy. The fourth pathway is through vulnerability. Even when HIV-linked illness or AIDS does not immediately throw a farm household into poverty, it nonetheless increases the likelihood of livelihood collapse from other shocks. A characteristic of rural livelihoods across Africa is covariance of risk. Because households rely on rain-fed subsistence agriculture to derive their livelihoods, alternative income-earning opportunities open to farm households in particular locations exhibit high correlation between risks in returns attached to them. Reliance on rain-fed subsistence agriculture renders most farm households vulnerable to the risk of livelihood collapse in the face of weather-related shocks such as droughts or floods because these shocks simultaneously affect all income streams available to the household, be it own-farm or income from casual employment on other people's farms. As a shock, HIV/AIDS might be expected to increase the risk of income failure overall by diluting the diversity of household portfolio and to increase intrayear income variability by amplifying covariate risks and sensitivity of livelihood outcomes.

Poverty and HIV/AIDS in Malawi

Malawi presents a classic example of how untimely action and policy contradictions can provide a catalytic environment for faster spread of HIV and entrenchment of poverty. Although agriculture is the backbone of Malawi's economy, accounting for

40 percent of GDP and 85 percent of exports and formal employment, recent studies suggest that half of all farm households are food insecure, and 60 percent of farm households earn incomes below the official poverty line (GOM 2000). This is because until 1990 the agricultural sector was characterized by the coexistence of estate and smallholder sectors, which were differentiated by land tenure and regulations concerning the production and marketing of different crops. The estate sector was characterized by relatively capital-intensive production of export crops, such as tobacco, tea, and sugar while the smallholder sector was oriented toward subsistence production, accounting for 80 percent of food production. Under the Tobacco and Special Crops Act of 1972, smallholder farmers were prohibited from growing burley tobacco, a labor-intensive cash crop whose expansion underpinned Malawi's high growth rates of the 1960s and 1970s (World Bank 1994). Whereas estate output was marketed at the auction floors at farm-gate export parity prices, smallholder output was marketed through the Agricultural Development and Marketing Corporation (ADMARC) (Kydd and Christiansen 1982). Land cultivated by estates is privately owned (freehold land) or leased from the state on long-term leases (leasehold land), whereas land cultivated by smallholder farmers is governed by customary law (Diagne and Zeller 2001).

In the grand scheme of things, it was assumed that the relationship between the estate and smallholder sectors would be mutually beneficial or benign at worst, as smallholder farmers would benefit from technological spillovers and income diversification from estate employment while at the same time alleviating pressure on their own land (T. Mkandawire 1999). In reality, Malawi's agricultural policy resulted in an agriculture sector with a dual structure, involving a few thousand commercially oriented estates with privileged access to credit and extension and producing for export markets, on the one hand, and a smallholder sector with nearly 2 million farm households producing mainly for subsistence, on the other (GOM 1995). The lack of access to grow cash crops coupled with a lack of appropriate high-yielding food technologies and inadequate supplies and use of inorganic fertilizer reduced the real rate of return to smallholder agriculture, thereby increasing distributional inequity between the estate and smallholder sectors (Kydd and Christiansen 1982; Pryor 1990).

A national economic soul-searching subsequently concluded that "a lack of viable cash crop was keeping rural people poor . . . and that burley tobacco, a crop that is labor intensive and well suited within the smallholder farmers' technical ability, could enable smallholders to participate in the cash-crop economy" (M. Mkandawire 1999). However, implicit in the explanation of agriculture's redefined role in achieving the dual objective of promoting economic growth and rural poverty reduction was an understanding that smallholder agriculture needed to undergo a process of liberalization and commercialization. Under this framework, two scenarios have come to characterize Malawi's poverty alleviation strategies in the 1990s: the Green Revolution and burley tobacco liberalization (Orr and Orr 2002). Under the Green Revolution scenario, poverty alleviation is premised on growth in small-holder income, which, in turn, is predicated on increasing the production of maize, by far the most important crop in terms of area cultivated, number of growers, and food security. To this end, a program of large-scale distribution of free fertilizer and hybrid maize was implemented under the umbrella of the Starter Pack, a targeted input program that supplies farm households with free improved seed and fertilizers (Orr and Orr 2002). Poverty alleviation through burley tobacco liberalization is based on removal of the long-standing legal and institutional constraints that pre-cluded smallholder farmers cultivating on customary land from growing burley tobacco. According to the World Bank, "the objective of this element was to allow smallholders access to a broader means of increasing their incomes, in order to reduce poverty and, simultaneously, provide farmers with a means of financing the intensification of their maize production" (World Bank 1994, p. 14). To this end, under the World Bank–funded Agricultural Sector Adjustment Credit (ASAC) of 1990, the production of burley tobacco by smallholder farmers on customary land was first permitted on a pilot basis during the 1990/91 growing season.

It was during this time of structural transformation and policy uncertainty that HIV/AIDS waylaid the Malawi population with disastrous consequences for household structure (Floyd et al. 2003), agricultural production and rural liveli-hoods (Bryceson, Fonseca, and Kadzandira 2004; Harvey 2004), and provision of public services, especially in the ministries of health and education. Since the first case of AIDS was diagnosed in 1985, epidemiologic evidence portends an escalat-ing epidemic. In samples of pregnant women attending antenatal clinics in urban Blantyre, HIV seroprevalence rose from 2.6 percent in 1986 to over 30 percent in 1998, decreasing only slightly to 28.5 percent in 2001. According to the latest national data from UNAIDS/WHO (2004), adult HIV prevalence (15–49 years) in Malawi is estimated at 14.2 percent, with a total of 900,000 adults and children living with HIV. Annual deaths caused by HIV/AIDS are estimated at over 83,000, amounting cumulatively to 555,000 deaths since 1985 (National AIDS Commis-sion of Malawi 2001). In addition, HIV has also increased crude death rates from tuberculosis and other opportunistic diseases.

The extent to which HIV/AIDS and livelihoods are intricately intertwined is exemplified in two recent studies. In explaining the 2001/02 famine in Southern Africa, de Waal and Whiteside (2004) cite the case of Malawi as typifying the new variant famine thesis. They argue that unlike past famines, which could be ex-plained in terms of drought or breakdown of entitlement systems, the HIV/AIDS epidemic was the major factor explaining why many households faced food short-ages and few were able to recover in the most recent famine. In contrast, Bryceson and Fonseca (2005) argue that actually it is poverty and famine that may be the major drivers of the spread of the HIV/AIDS epidemic in Malawi. They observe that during the famine period, because of inadequacy of traditional coping mecha-nisms, farm households on the margin of destitution were forced to adapt and broaden the scope of long-established traditional coping strategies to include risky coping strategies such as transactional sex.

Data and Methodology

In order to explore the differential impact of negative economic shocks on HIV/AIDS-affected and nonaffected households, we use a panel survey of Malawian households. We use data from the Malawi Integrated Household Survey (GOM 2000) and the Complementary Panel Survey of 2002. The IHS was a nationally representative survey implemented between September 1997 and October 1998 by the Malawi government's National Statistical Office in collaboration with the National Economic Council and the Center for Social Research with technical assistance from the International Food Policy Research Institute. The IHS was administered in two parts. The first involved a large questionnaire administered to respondent households on a single visit, consisting of a dozen modules including those on household composition, educational attainment, health and nutritional status, agriculture, and home-produced and purchased consumption items. The second part was an expenditure diary, maintained over a period of 14 days by liter-ate household heads or through twice-weekly visits by enumerators to the survey households to record any expenditure since their previous visit. Although the sur-vey was administered to 12,960 households, only 6,586 households were adjudged to have reliable consumption and expenditure data. For the CPS, four rounds of additional survey were administered between January 2000 and September 2002 on a subsample of 758 households selected from the 6,586 households enumerated in the IHS. Unfortunately, rather than derive a panel of data, the four rounds collected different modules of data that complemented the IHS but were not repeated. Only CPS round 4 attempted to collect consumption and expenditure data that were comparable to those in IHS.

Measurement of Household Welfare

In the analysis that follows, we use an expenditure-cum-consumption-based mea-sure of household welfare. The use of an expenditure- and consumption-based measure rather than an income-based measure was motivated by two factors. First was the recognition that expenditure and consumption are smoother measures of welfare than income. Because farm households are wholly dependent on rain-fed agriculture, income is lumpy and seasonal as farm households receive a large lump-sum amount after harvest and little else during the year. Second, given the subsistence nature of rural livelihoods and that a lot of exchange of goods and services takes place outside markets, income understates the value of goods and services consumed by the household. To adjust for the effect of inflation and also fully account for market-based and non-market-based dimensions of household welfare, our measure of welfare is expressed in real terms with the value of consumption normalized to the April 1998 base and is made up of four components:

- Total food consumption: imputed value of all food consumption reported by the household, normalized to a daily consumption of individual food items.

- Total nonfood, non-durable-goods expenses: a daily value in Malawi Kwacha was determined for all nonfood, nondurable goods consumed by the household including the value of outgoing income transfers.

- Estimated use-value of durable goods such as vehicles, furniture, appliances: the value was derived using an imputed value of daily rental rate for each good. The rental rate was computed by taking into account the rate of depreciation for an item, the opportunity cost locked up in the durable good, and the replacement cost of the durable good. The formula is given as: UseValue = current replacement value*((interest rate + depreciation rate) /(1 − depreciation)).

- Actual or imputed value of housing for the household

Table 3.1 summarizes household characteristics and welfare measures for our sample. The top section of the table shows that about 22 percent of all households reported an AIDS-related death. The mean household size among HIV/AIDS-affected households is larger than the nonaffected one, suggesting that household members may have been relocated within the extended family system. Both in 1998 and 2000, the HIV/AIDS-affected households in the sample appear relatively better-off than the average household in the sample, from the viewpoint either of per capita daily expenditure or per capita monthly income. Although, two-thirds of all households in the sample experienced some negative economic shock between 1998 and 2000, the data seem to indicate that HIV-affected households were better able to cope with shocks than nonaffected households. For instance, whereas

Table 3.1   Household characteristics and welfare dynamics in Malawi

Household characteristic	Affected households	Nonaffected households	All households
Demographics			
Mean household size	5.38	5.12	5.18
Female-headed households (%)	14.00	22.00	20.00
Mean age of household head (years)	42.62	43.81	43.55
Dependency ratio	0.44	0.48	0.47
Mother's mean years of education	4.43	3.35	3.59
Maximum years of education in h/hold	5.45	4.50	4.71
H/holds where relative died of AIDS (%)	100	0.00	22.34
Welfare dynamics			
Per capita daily expenditure, 1998 (MKwacha)	14.66	13.20	13.52
Per capita daily expenditure 2002 (MKwacha)	21.32	18.02	18.75
Per capita monthly income 2002 (MKwacha)	184.01	115.33	130.67
H/holds that experienced economic shocks (%)	60.00	59.73	59.79
H/holds dropped 2+ welfare quintiles (%)	12.31	17.70	16.49
H/holds rose 2+ welfare quintiles (%)	24.62	16.37	18.21
Productive activity			
Per capita acreage cultivated (hectares)	0.55	0.46	0.47
Household grows hybrid maize (%)	35.00	38.00	37.00
Household grows tobacco (%)	15.00	14.00	14.00
Household uses fertilizer (%)	30.77	33.19	32.65
Value of inputs used (MKwacha)	1,355.67	937.53	817.27
Per capita livestock value (MKwacha)	314.94	254.64	268.10
Employment			
H/hold head is employer (%)	0.00	0.00	0.00
H/head is self-employed (%)	43.00	41.00	41.00
H/hold head is employee (%)	51.00	48.00	48.00
H/hold member employed by government (%)	17.00	8.00	10.00
H/hold members with agric occupations (%)	40.00	36.00	37.00

about 18 percent of nonaffected households dropped by two or more welfare quintiles between 1998 and 2000, only 12 percent of households affected by HIV/AIDS experienced a welfare decline of two quintiles or more. Similarly, whereas 24 percent of households affected by AIDS improved in welfare by over two welfare quintiles, only 16.37 made any welfare gains in the rest of the population. We hypothesize that these counterintuitive statistics arise from the fact that although both groups have roughly the same proportions in employment, for some reason, HIV/AIDS-affected households in the sample had twice as many household members with government jobs as the rest of the sample. Alternatively, because most people dying of HIV/AIDS are from the city, on death, the recipient households in the rural areas inherit both members and some property, which raises both household size and, for people living on the margin of destitution, household welfare.

Retrospective Measurement of Shocks

In the module on shocks, household heads were asked whether they had experienced any of a set of events during the previous 2 years (i.e., 1999 and 2000). These shocks included events affecting individuals within or connected to the household (e.g., death, serious illness, injury, or loss of a job), property losses suffered by the household (e.g., through theft, crop failure, loss of livestock, or business failure), and declines in resource flows to the household (e.g., decline or cutoff in private or government remittances). In addition, the module also attempted to assign a value to the economic loss each event caused. For each event that occurred, the household provided information regarding (1) the year it occurred, (2) duration in months, (3) the monthly decline in household income, (4) the total once-off expenditure, and (5) the value of items lost.

Table 3.2 provides the frequency distribution of the various shocks reported for the 758 households. The evidence shows that the most commonly reported shock was death of household member (30.4 percent) followed by widespread death or loss of livestock (23.5 percent) and serious illness or injury. The last two columns show the monetary impact of these shocks. In the fourth column we report the average once-off payment associated with these shocks, and in the last column we present the total cost, which comprises the once-off cost and additional costs such as loss or reduction in income attributable to the shock and additional expenses incurred to cope with the shock. According to the research design, death of a household member, from whatever cause, has a once-off expense, in contrast to most of the other commonly occurring shocks, which have both once-off expenses

Table 3.2   Incidence of negative economic shocks in rural Malawi

Event/shock	Frequency	Percentage	Once-off expense (MKwacha)	Total expenses (MKwacha)
Death of relative or family member	189	30.4	985	985
Widespread death of livestock	146	23.5	850	1,961
Serious illness or injury	113	18.2	1,805	3,509
Major crop failure	95	15.3	101	3,375
Theft, fire, or destruction of property	36	5.8	200	9,596
Bankruptcy	23	3.7	5,739	7,170
Abandonment/divorce	13	2.1	0.0	234
Other	5	0.8	0.0	1,200
Total	622	100		

Table 3.3   Coping mechanisms to shocks among rural households in Malawi

	Percentage of households that			
Event/Shock	Sold assets	Borrowed	Were assisted by community	Used insurance
Death of relative or family member	24.46	20.11	29.57	0.00
Widespread death of livestock	0.00	1.40	3.47	0.00
Serious illness or injury	33.63	14.16	21.24	0.00
Major crop failure	7.45	10.64	17.20	2.17
Theft, fire, or destruction of property	2.78	2.78	13.89	0.00
Bankruptcy	18.18	18.18	9.09	0.00
Abandonment/divorce	0.00	7.69	15.38	0.00

and protracted coping expenses. Bankruptcy has the largest once-off expense, and loss of property (mostly tobacco) to fire or theft was the costliest.

As might be expected, households' coping strategies and the nature of social support tend to be functions of the shock. Table 3.3 shows that whereas in the case of death of a family member, 24 percent of affected households used up savings they had previously accumulated, and 20 percent entered into fresh debt, the single most important coping mechanism was community assistance (30 percent). In contrast, following serious illness or injury, the largest number of households used up savings, and relatively lower proportions got community assistance or sank into debt. The data show that social support systems in rural Malawi generally give priority to health-related human misfortunes but much less emphasis on bailing out those afflicted by economic or nature-induced shocks. This has to be understood in the context of covariance of risk in the rural setting. For instance, in the case of widespread death of animals, there is virtually nothing the household and society did other than sympathize. Similarly, in the case of major crop failure, everyone was facing the same predicament, and therefore no one stood ready to assist another. The last column shows the total absence of rural financial markets for insurance against these shocks.

Empirical Estimation and Results

Because hysteresis is very important in subsistence economies, current-period livelihood outcomes (whether incomes or expenditures) invariably depend on past-period realizations. To implement this notion of state dependence, let the income for household i in period $t - 1$ be $Y_{i,t-1}$, and other household characteristics $X_{i,t}$, map into income in period t through an income transformation function given by

$$Y_{i,t} = f(Y_{i,t-1}, X_{i,t}) \qquad (4.1)$$

An equilibrium in this model is a steady-state solution that varies with $X_{i,t}$ such that $Y = f(Y, X_{i,t})$. If there is more than one solution, the notion of multiple equilibria requires the existence of at least one unstable equilibrium and thus of increasing returns for a lower range of Y. A poverty trap occurs if there exists a low-level attractor in the growth process so that a group of households converges to a lower equilibrium. The challenge then is to find a functional form for the production function that gives a smooth nonlinear relationship between $Y_{i,t}$ and $Y_{i,t-1}$ and also allows for multiple equilibria. Following Lokshin and Ravallion (2004), we use a partial adjustment model with a cubic function of the form

$$\ln(Y_{i,t}) = \gamma_0 + \gamma t + \sum_{m=1}^{3} \ln(Y_{i,t-1}) + \beta \ln(X_{i,t}) + \varepsilon_{i,t} \qquad (4.2)$$

To understand the implication of this functional form, notice that a shock to household income in time $t-1$ transmits to household income in time t through the derivative $\partial Y_t / \partial Y_{t-1}$. Moreover, for any equilibrium (e) defined by $Y_t = Y_{t-1}$, that equilibrium is unstable if $\partial Y_t / \partial Y_{t-1}(e) > 1$. Third, the speed of recovery (i.e., the extent to which a shock is not passed on) can be captured by $1 - \partial Y_t / \partial Y_{t-1}$.

Table 3.4 reports regression results manifesting the differential impacts of economics shocks to rural households, again distinguishing between HIV-affected households and those not directly affected. Although all variables included in the model are considered important, our analysis will concentrate only on the evidence for persistence of shocks and poverty traps. To that end, we must first establish whether expenditures and income in 2002 depend on income in 1998. Results in columns b and c suggest that past incomes have no impact on subsequent period expenditures in either type of household. In fact, of all household controls, only three are statistically significant. In AIDS-affected households, household expenditures seem to increase with the age of the household head, whereas economic shocks and the per capita amount of land cultivated seem to have a significant negative effect on expenditure. We hypothesize that there is a negative impact on expenditure/consumption because AIDS necessitates changes in household consumption and investment behavior. HIV/AIDS reduces food availability (through falling production and loss of family labor), reduces access to food (through declining income for food purchases), and reduces the stability and quality of food supply through shifts in labor to less labor-intensive production (Topouzis 2003). The fact that economic shocks have a negative impact on consumption/expenditure in AIDS-affected households seems to validate our null hypothesis. This is principally because HIV/AIDS-affected households are less able to adjust to shocks that require labor time to

Table 3.4 Determinants of household income and welfare in rural Malawi

	Per capita total expenditure		Per capita total income	
Variables (a)	Households with AIDS death (b)	Nonaffected households (c)	Households with AIDS death (d)	Nonaffected households (e)
Constant	−1.414	3.469	7.001	−1.310
	(2.2624)	(1.568)	(7.206)	(3.452)
Lagged income	−0.236%	−0.601	−17.119*	2.669
	(3.366)	(1.797)	(9.245)	(3.956)
Lagged income squared	0.350	0.165	7.615*	−1.085
	1.516)	(0.748)	(4.164)	1.647)
Cube of lagged income	−0.049	−0.007	0.958	0.163
	(0.215)	(0.099)	(0.590)	(0.217)
Economic shock	−0.535**	0.252	0.376	0.791***
	(0.265)	(0.389)	(0.727)	(0.302)
Female-headed household	0.054	0.144	−1.742	−0.913
	(0.479)	(0.205)	(1.316)	(0.451)
Age of household	0.973**	(0.229)	0.821	−0.031
	(0.389)	−0.104	(1.068)	(0.503)
Dependency ratio	−0.332	−0.249	3.197*	−1.154*
	(0.663)	(0.299)	(1.820)	(0.659)
Per capita acreage cultivated	−0.381**	0.143	−0.491	−0.446**
	(0.192)	(0.099)	(0.528)	(0.219)
Value of livestock per capita	−0.018	0.078***	−0.401***	−0.131**
	(0.047)	(0.024)	(0.128)	(0.052)
H/hold head is employed	−0.471	−0.067	2.278	3.172***
	(0.697)	(0.270)	(1.913)	(0.594)
H/hold head is self-employed	−0.559	−0.099	0.181	0.829
	(0.730)	(0.290)	(2.006)	(0.637)
Household grows tobacco	0.186	−0.407**	0.309	0.690*
	(0.332)	(0.169)	(0.912)	(0.372)
Adj. R^2	0.277	0.211	0.484	0.395

Notes: Standard errors in parentheses. ***, **, and * indicate statistical significance at the 1, 5, and 10 percent levels, respectively.

be switched between different activities. In addition, this may also reflect the fact that, because of underdeveloped or nonexistent formal credit markets, the loss of family and friends may also spell the end of access to informal, affordable credit and hence higher vulnerability.

Among households not directly affected by AIDS, per capita expenditure is a positive function of the value of livestock and a negative function of participation in tobacco. Livestock has a positive impact on nonaffected households because in the absence of death and illness, rural households can kill or sell livestock to bridge any financing gaps and smooth expenditure and consumption. In contrast, tobacco has a negative impact on consumption and expenditure because tobacco season takes some 9 months, and the income is lumpy and comes with considerable time lag. Thus, for much of the cropping season, tobacco households tie up their capital and are unable to smooth expenditure and consumption.

However, the last two columns show more interesting results. Column *d* presents evidence of possible existence of poverty traps among households that experienced an AIDS death. The coefficient on lagged income is negative and statistically significant (albeit at the 10 percent level) and suggests path dependence between current income and lagged income. In addition, there is a significant positive relationship between current income and the square of past income. However, the choice of the cubic specification of the production function is rejected because the polynomial variable in the third degree is not significant. The results would yield the following empirical version of the partial adjustment model:

$$Y_t = -17.119 Y_{i,t-1} + 7.615 Y^2_{i,t-1} - 79.855 \qquad (4.3)$$

where the additional variables have been set at their respective means.

Three aspects of these results are important. First, equation 4.3 yields an equilibrium income per capita per month at $Y_t = Y_{-1} = MK92.75$, which is equivalent to half the AIDS-affected households mean per capita income absent any negative shocks (MK184.01). The equilibrium income is also lower than the mean income in the entire sample, even that among nonaffected households. Second, because a shock to income in the previous period transmits to current income through $\partial Y_t / \partial Y_{t-1}$, the equation implies that following a shock to income, AIDS-affected households may take up to 18.12 months to fully adjust before finally settling at the lower equilibrium. In contrast, results in column *e* show no evidence of path dependence among households that were not affected by HIV/AIDS-related death. Neither the coefficient on lagged income, its square, nor its cube is statistically significant. In fact, per capita incomes for nonaffected households are a negative function of economic shocks, dependency ratio, the per capita amount of land cultivated, and the value of livestock. Per capita income is likely to increase if the head of the household is employed or if the household is engaged in cash cropping, such as tobacco.

Conclusion

This chapter set out to investigate the existence of poverty traps among households that experienced an AIDS death. Specifically, we sought to examine whether AIDS-affected households respond differently to negative economic shock from nonaffected household. In other words, does AIDS increase a household's vulnerability to the extent that a negative shock to income could throw previously non-poor households into perpetual destitution? Our most significant finding is that in households that were affected by AIDS, a shock to income will last about 18 months and take the affected household to a lower-than-average equilibrium monthly income of MK92.75. However, it remains unclear if these responses and adjustments after a shock are better or worse than for nonaffected households because there is no evidence of path dependence and poverty traps among the nonaffected households.

Our results have both normative and positive policy analytic implications. At the positive level, we now have an idea regarding the nature of commonly occurring shocks and how they affect the households' livelihood outcomes and strategies. In addition, we also know the transitional dynamics of both income and expenditure in affected and nonaffected households following a negative shock. At the normative level, a proper understanding of the link between the AIDS epidemic and poverty traps is important because poverty traps may help explain why the poor remain so even when historical structural impediments to their advancement are attenuated and long after the playing field has been leveled. Second, large policy interventions may have long-lasting impacts, whereas the impact of small interventions may quickly die out. A policymaker designing a program on poverty reduction needs to recognize that HIV/AIDS-related illness and death is a shock like no other. Besides being a shock in itself, it also creates conditions that heighten household vulnerability, causing previously nonpoor households to become poor and stay poor indefinitely or cause moderately poor households to fall into persistent destitution. As a result, to lever AIDS-affected households from poverty might require some adjustment to a poverty reduction model principally designed for all households.

Two caveats are in order. First, the survey years for the IHS, 1997/98 and the CPS 2000/02 included years of plenty (1998) and famine (2001/02). Although the measures of welfare were temporally and spatially adjusted to control for differences in prices, adjustment were not made for nonnormal weather conditions. It is very likely that our results are also capturing income and expenditure patterns that are more reflective of coping and survival behavior than steady-state expenditure and consumption behavior. Second, there is a nonnegligible possibility of attrition bias in the sample. Because by design the respondent was usually the household head, households where the respondent died from AIDS or any other disease would automatically be removed from the survey. Thus, the so-called AIDS-affected households in the sample are those where someone other than the respondent died. This likely introduced downward bias in the measured impact and may explain why the average numbers seem to suggest that AIDS-affected households were not only well off but also better able to cope with shocks than average households in the sample. The most ideal approach would have been one that, rather than use all households affected by HIV, purposively select and compare those households where the breadwinner died with the other HIV/AIDS-affected and nonaffected households.

References

Ainsworth, M., and M. Over. 1992. *The economic impact of AIDS.* Technical working paper, Population, Health and Nutrition Division, Washington, D.C.: World Bank.

Arndt, C., and J. D. Lewis. 2001. The HIV/AIDS pandemic in South Africa: Sectoral impacts and unemployment. *Journal of International Development* 13 (4): 427–449.

Azariadis, C. 1996. The economics of poverty traps, part one: Complete markets. *Journal of Economic Growth* I: 449–486.

Bloom, D. E., and A. Mahal. 1997. Does the AIDS epidemic threaten economic growth? *Journal of Econometrics* 77 (1): 105–124.

Bollinger, L., J. Stover, R. Kerkhoven, G. Mutangadura, and D. Mukurazita. 1999. *The economic impact of AIDS in Zimbabwe.* Washington, D.C.: Futures Group/RTI/CEDPA.

Bryceson, D. F., and J. Fonseca. 2005. *An enduring or dying peasantry? Interactive impact of famine and HIV/AIDS in rural Malawi.* Paper presented at International Conference on HIV/AIDS, Food and Nutrition Security, Durban, South Africa.

Bryceson, D. F., J. Fonseca, and J. Kadzandira. 2004. *Social Pathways from the Deadlock of Disease, Denial and Desperation in Rural Malawi.* Lilongwe, Malawi: RENEWAL/CARE Malawi.

Crafts, N., and M. Haacker. 2003. *Welfare implications of HIV/AIDS.* IMF Working Paper 03/118. Washington, D.C.: International Monetary Fund.

Cuddington, J. T. 1993. Modeling the macroeconomic effects of AIDS, with an application to Tanzania. *World Bank Economic Review* 7 (2): 173–189.

Cuddington, J. T., and J. D. Hancock. 1994. Assessing the impact of AIDS on the growth path of the Malawian economy. *Journal of Development Economics* 43: 363–368.

Desbarats, J. 2002. *HIV/AIDS and poverty: The impact of HIV/AIDS in the ESCAP region.* Paper presented at the Fifth Asian and Pacific Population Conference (E/ESCAP/PRUD/SAPPC/9).

De Waal, A., and A. Whiteside. 2003. New variant famine: AIDS and food crisis in southern Africa. *Lancet* 362 (9391): 1234–1237.

Diagne, A., and M. Zeller. 2001. *Access to credit and its impact on welfare in Malawi.* IFRPI Research Report No. 116. Washington, D.C.: IFPRI.

Floyd, S., A. C. Crampin, J. R. Glynn, N. Madise, A. Nyondo, M. M. Khondowe, C. L. Njok, H. Kanyongoloka, B. Ngwire, B. Zaba, and P. E. M. Pine. 2003. *The impact of HIV on household structure in rural Malawi.* Paper presented at the Scientific Meeting on the Empirical Evidence for the Demographic and Socioeconomic Impact of AIDS, Durban, South Africa.

Gillespie, S. R., and S. Kadiyala. 2005. *HIV/AIDS and food and nutrition security: From evidence to action.* Food Policy Review, 7. Washington, D.C.: IFPRI.

GOM (Government of Malawi). 1995. *Malawi Policy Framework Paper, 1995/96–1997/98.* Lilongwe: GOM.

————. 2000. Profile of poverty in Malawi: Poverty analysis of the Integrated Household Survey 1998. Lilongwe: GOM.

Greener, R., K. Jefferis, and H. Siphambe. 2000. The macroeconomic impact of HIV/AIDS in Botswana. *South African Journal of Economics* 65 (8): 888–915.

Haacker, M. 2002. *The economic consequences of HIV/AIDS in southern Africa.* IMF Working Paper 02/38. Washington, D.C.: International Monetary Fund.

Haddad, L., and S. R. Gillespie. 2001. Effective food and nutrition policy responses to HIV/AIDS: What we know and what we need to know. *Journal of International Development* 13 (4): 487–511.

Harvey, P. 2004. *HIV/AIDS and Humanitarian Action?* Humanitarian Policy Group, Report 16. London: ODI.

Kydd, J. G., and R. E. Christiansen. 1982. Structural change in Malawi since independence: Consequences of a development strategy based on large-scale agriculture. *World Development* 10 (5): 355–375.

Loevinsohn, M., and S. R Gillespie. 2003. *Food security and rural livelihoods: Understanding and responding.* Food Consumption and Nutrition Division Discussion Paper 157. Washington, D.C.: IFPRI.

Lokshin, M., and M. Ravallion. 2004. Household income dynamics in two transition economies. *Studies in Nonlinear Dynamics and Econometrics* 8 (3): Article 4. http://www.bepress.com/snde/vol8/iss3/art4.

Mkandawire, M. L. C. 1999. *Poverty and macro economic management in Malawi.* Harare, Zimbabwe: Sapes Books.

Mkandawire, T. 1999. *Agriculture, poverty and employment in Malawi.* ILO/SAMAT Working Papers No 9. Harare, Zimbabwe.

National AIDS Commission of Malawi. 2001. *National HIV/AIDS Policy.* Lilongwe.

Orr, A., and S. Orr. 2002. *Agriculture and micro enterprise in Malawi's rural South.* Agricultural Research and Extension Network, Paper No. 119. London: ODI.

Pryor, F. L. 1990. The political economy of poverty, equity and growth in Malawi and Madagascar. New York: Oxford University Press.

Serpell, N. 1999. Children orphaned by HIV/AIDS in Zambia: Risk factors from premature parental death and policy implications. PhD dissertation, University of Maryland.

Topouzis, D. 2003. Addressing the impact of HIV/AIDS on ministries of agriculture and their work. Rome: Joint FAO/UNAIDS publication, FAO/UNAIDS Best Practice Collection.

UNAIDS. 2002. Report on the global HIV/AIDS epidemic. Geneva: UNAIDS.

UNAIDS/WHO. 2004. *AIDS epidemic update.* Geneva: WHO.

UNFPA. 2002. State of the world population, 2002: People, poverty, and possibilities. http://www.unfpa.org/swp/2002/.

World Bank. 1994. *Malawi agricultural sector credit,* 2 vols., Project completion report, Cr. 2121-MAI. Washington, D.C.: World Bank.

Chapter 4

Labor Market and Wage Impacts of HIV/AIDS in Rural Malawi

Andrew R. Dorward and Idrissa M. Mwale

Introduction and Objectives

There is a limited but growing literature on direct impacts of HIV/AIDS morbidity and mortality on the livelihoods of poor rural people. Less is known, however, about indirect impacts of the HIV/AIDS epidemic on the livelihoods of rural communities, allowing for market interactions between households. These are difficult to study, but unskilled wages and food prices are critically important to the welfare of poor people, whether directly affected by HIV/AIDS or not: If the HIV/AIDS epidemic depresses labor demands more than it contracts labor supply, this could lower wage rates in affected communities, damaging the livelihoods of poor households. Promotion of laborsaving enterprises and technologies under such circumstances could have disastrous consequences for the healthy poor.

In this chapter we report preliminary work investigating these issues with household and rural economy (meso) models describing livelihoods and livelihood interactions in Malawi. After this introduction, we briefly review possible livelihood and rural economy impacts of HIV/AIDS and the issues investigated in the chapter. We then describe the models used in the chapter and the different scenarios we investigate. Succeeding sections present the results of modeling these scenarios. This leads on to discussion of the robustness of the findings and their implications for policy and further research.

Potential Livelihood and Rural Economy Impacts of HIV/AIDS

A total of 900,000 adults and children are estimated to be living with HIV in Malawi, which has an adult HIV prevalence (15–49 years) of 14.2 percent, although

Figure 4.1   Livelihoods in markets framework

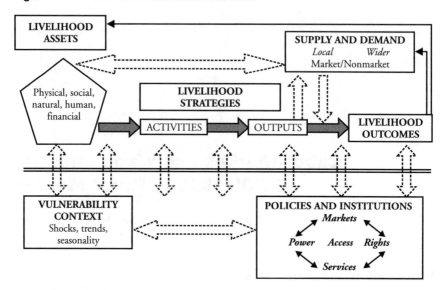

this varies between, for example, urban and rural areas, men and women, and people with different occupations (National AIDS Commission 2003): There tend, for example, to be higher rates of male infection among more wealthy men but higher rates of female infection among the poor. These varying infection rates affect the demographic structure and growth of the population and labor force, but labor is further affected by culturally determined responsibilities, such as women's common responsibilities to care for the sick.

Mwale (2004) reviews literature on the economic and livelihood impacts of HIV/AIDS in Malawi and more generally in Africa. In this, a "livelihoods in markets" framework modified from Dorward et al. (2003) is helpful in identifying the major direct and indirect, individual and systemic impacts of HIV/AIDS on rural livelihoods (see Fig. 4.1).

Direct impacts arise first through reductions in HIV/AIDS-affected households' human capital (labor time, strength, and skills/knowledge) as a result of morbidity and mortality of infected individuals. Further human capital effects arise from direct reductions in the productivity of caregivers and withdrawal of children (particularly girls) from education. These effects are associated with reduced enterprise and household income and increased expenditure demands for treatment and funerals. These losses and expenditures have further long-term impacts on affected households' ownership of and access to physical, human, social, financial, and natural capital. Indirect changes arise in affected households' livelihoods as they change their livelihood strategies and activities to try to respond to all these effects of sickness. Changes in crop and other enterprises are common (with a shift toward less labor- and cash-demanding activities and increased fallow areas), and these may depend on who within the household is infected. Reduced asset holdings also make affected households more vulnerable to shocks.

Figure 4.1 also assists in the identification of wider system effects when significant numbers of households in a rural community or economy experience and react to the direct and indirect household-level impacts of HIV/AIDS morbidity and mortality discussed above. These system effects occur mainly through changes in policies and institutions and in local and wider demand for resources, goods, and services affecting market and nonmarket exchange. Systemic changes that have been observed in policies and institutions include, for example, changes in land tenure systems, family structures, age and gender roles, funeral responsibilities, and social safety net systems. Widespread shifts in consumption, in asset use and ownership, and in productive and welfare activities may also lead to changes in prices. Wages and food prices are particularly important to the poor because they respectively account for very significant parts of their incomes and expenditures, and they affect both those households directly affected by HIV/AIDS morbidity or mortality and those without any sick or deceased members.

Critical though they may be to people's welfare, the impacts of widespread HIV/AIDS and mortality on wages and food prices are not easy to study or to predict. Difficulties in studying them are common to most of the possible systemic effects of high rates of HIV/AIDS in rural communities. Although some of these changes may be obviously related to the HIV/AIDS epidemic (for example, switches in government and private expenditure into health care or changes in marriage customs), for most of them HIV/AIDS may be only one possible factor among many affecting change, and it is not possible to empirically observe and identify the specific impacts of HIV/AIDS. Even where HIV/AIDS is likely to be a major determinant of change (as in the example of health care expenditure), the rate and course of that change will be strongly moderated by other factors (such as general economic performance, political leadership, social attitudes, availability and cost of treatments, treatment delivery capacity, external support), and these factors themselves are subject to uncertainty, change, and complex interactions.

The effects of HIV/AIDS on wages and food prices, and indeed on general price levels, are particularly difficult to observe as the effects of HIV/AIDS may be dominated by other more proximate factors such as weather, macroeconomic policies and performance, international trade relations and prices, other economic or natural shocks, government policies, and so on. The interactions among these factors are complex and often poorly understood, and HIV/AIDS may have ambiguous direct price effects (as described below) as well as modifying the wage or price impacts of changes in other factors (for example by undermining people's capital, it may make people's livelihoods and local markets more vulnerable and sensitive to shocks). HIV/AIDS may also increase social and economic inequality in rural economies and communities, with far-reaching effects on social and economic processes. These difficulties in teasing out the systemic impacts of HIV/AIDS are well illustrated by the debate around the impacts of HIV/AIDS on the recent Southern Africa crisis (see, for example, De Waal and Whiteside 2003).

Unfortunately, as already suggested, HIV/AIDS impacts on wages and food prices are also difficult to predict from theory. HIV/AIDS is likely to lead to local contractions in both production and demand of food. Net price effects will then depend on the balance between these changes, links to wider markets, and uncertain government and donor actions to promote food security. Furthermore, in the longer term, prices themselves influence production decisions, incomes, and demand.

Food prices and production also influence, and are influenced by, labor markets and wages. It is commonly suggested that HIV/AIDS-induced contractions in the labor force will generally increase wages. There is, however, an alternative set of hypotheses:

- Problems in raising cash to meet immediate AIDS-related expenses cause poor households to hire out more labor (at the expense of own farm production) so that, paradoxically, HIV/AIDS leads to an increase in labor supply in the market.

- There is reduced demand for unskilled on-farm labor among less-poor HIV/AIDS-affected households because (1) they are unable to finance labor hire from savings, from semiskilled or skilled employment earnings, or from remittances if the individuals generating these earnings are hit by AIDS, and (2) reductions in family labor and in capital shortages lead to a shift out of generally more labor-demanding cash crops (see, for example, Yamano and Jayne 2004).

- Wider nonfarm labor demand also falls as local demand for nontradable goods and services is reduced by depressed incomes (first of HIV/AIDS-affected households but ultimately of most households as these processes depress the general economy), with further depression from multiplier effects (Arndt and Lewis 2001).

• Consequent increases in poverty incidence and severity raise unskilled labor supply in the market.

In the remainder of this chapter we investigate these hypotheses and the conditions affecting them using a set of Malawian rural livelihood and economy models.

Methodology

Dorward (2003) describes the development of a set of farm/household models that replicate the behavior of major Malawian farm/household types in response to various exogenous changes and the impact of these changes on their welfare. The essential elements of the approach involved the development of (1) a typology of farm/household types across the country, (2) a set of farm/household models describing the behavior of these different farm/households, and (3) a system for tying these farm/household models into a model of the informal rural economy in which they are located, to capture the partial equilibrium interactions between their behavior and local wage rates and maize prices.

The Farm Household Typology

The development of the typology is described in detail by Dorward (2002). With data from the 1997/98 Integrated Household Survey (IFPRI and NSO 2002), cluster analysis was used to identify seven types of households within the mid-altitude areas that hold 60 percent of rural households. Details of these household types are given in Table 4.1. Apart from households with members in formal employment, the data from which the cluster analysis was developed did not

Table 4.1   Farm household classification for plateau zone

Household type label	Rural household Local (%)	Rural household National (%)	Area (ha/ household member)	Assets (MK/ household)	Kept maize (kg/member)	Consumption (MK/day)	Poverty count (%)
"Larger farmers"	4	2	0.86	165	315	16	29
"Medium assets"	18	10	0.36	975	203	10.3	49
"Borrowers"	9	5	0.28	695	107	9.2	57
"Poor male-headed"	34	18	0.20	208	50	6.6	72
"Poor female-headed"	18	10	0.22	105	50	6.6	75
"Employed"	13	7	0.18	360	81	9.8	53
"Remittance"	4	2	0.31	540	128	11.2	49
All	100	53	0.28	240	83	8.4	62

Note: MK = Malawi Kwacha (in 1997/98 approx. MK 25 equivalent to US$1.00).

contain information about skilled employment opportunities. However, in operationalizing the household composition for the livelihood modeling, male members of the "larger farmer" and "medium assets" household types also had access to skilled wage rates.

The Farm/Household Model

A nonlinear programming farm/household model was developed using a Stone-Geary utility function with a linear expenditure system as shown below (see Dorward 2003).

$$MaxE(U) = \sum_s P_s \prod_{j*m} (C_{jm} - \gamma_{jm})^{\beta_{jm}} \tag{4.1}$$

such that, for m = 1 to 2,

$$-t_{jm} + t_{j(m+1)} + \sum_{ij} e_{ijm} x_i + C_{jm} \leq B_{jm} \tag{4.2}$$

for m = 3 to 4,

$$-t_{jms} + t_{j(m+1)s} + \sum_{ij} e_{ijms} x_{is} + C_{jms} \leq B_{jm} \tag{4.3}$$

and for m = 4,

$$-t_{j(m+1)s} = t_{j(m=1)} \tag{4.4}$$

where

m are periods within a year: $m = 1$ describes the "cropping period" (November to January); $m = 2$ the "preharvest period" (February and March); $m = 3$ the "harvest period" (April to June); and $m = 4$ the "postharvest period" (July to October)

s are alternative market conditions (end-of-season maize prices) in periods m = 3 and m = 4

P_s are subjective probabilities of alternative market conditions s

C_{jm} represent total consumption of commodity or resource j in period m

γ_{jm} are minimum consumption requirements for commodity or resource j in period m

β_{jm} are the marginal propensities to consume commodity or resource j in period m

t_{jms} represent transfers of commodity or resource j from periods m to $m+1$ in market condition s

e_{ijms} are technical and price coefficients of use or production of resource or commodity j by activity x_{is} in period m under market condition s

x_{is} are activities undertaken by the household. These include cropping activities, buying and selling of stocks and labor, and stock transfers between periods. For those activities that take place wholly in periods 3 or 4, these are distinguished according to the market condition s under which they are followed.

B_{jm} are supply constraints on commodity or resource j in period m

$j*m$ is the subset of commodities or resources directly consumed by the household and for which consumption is included in the objective function: cash consumption by period, consumption of maize (or calorific equivalents from other crops) by period, leisure ("slack" labor) by period, and end-of-season cash savings

Commodity or resource j includes land, labor, cash stocks, maize stocks, purchased crop inputs, and postharvest cash crop stocks.

Equation 4.1 maximizes expected utility using a linear expenditure system (LES). Equations 4.2 and 4.3 describe constrained resource use and production opportunities in different periods, with buying and selling of those commodities and resources for which there is a market, stock transfers between periods where appropriate, and household consumption where appropriate. Equation 4.3 allows for alternative stocking, market, and off-farm employment strategies to be followed under different market conditions (maize price regimes) in the harvest and postharvest periods and to this extent allows for food purchase price risk, which may encourage subsistence maize production. Equation 4.4 ensures that the model maintains the same opening and closing stocks from year to year and does not generate artificial windfall gains by portfolio changes (for example, by replacing maize stocks by cash).

The model also included upper bounds on some activities to represent practical constraints not allowed for in the general formulation, for example, limited maize storage capacity, sequencing of activities within time periods and transport, labor and market constraints on large-scale root crop sales.

This model structure provides the following important features in its description of farm/household opportunities, constraints, and behavior:

- *Seasonal constraints:* The year is divided into four periods (cropping, preharvest, harvest, and postharvest). The first period involves heavy crop labor demands, but there are also potential trade-offs with other non-own farm work generating lower but more immediate returns, which may be important for poorer households needing to sustain minimal levels of consumption before harvest. There is then limited farm labor demand and lower wages in the preharvest period, but then crop prices fall, and both farm labor demand and wage rates rise in the harvest period. Crop prices then rise in the postharvest period, some farm labor is required for land preparation, and nonfarm employment opportunities and wages rise.

- *Varied activities* are modeled, with seasonal crop demands for labor and purchased inputs. The model allows flexibility in linking these to stocking, buying, and selling activities across and within time periods. Non-own-farm activities are described in terms of hiring out of labor. Specific activities describe borrowing, technical change, and the introduction of new opportunities. No attempt is made to model specific nonfarm enterprises (for example, in terms of capital requirements), and all nonfarm activities (skilled or unskilled) earn a wage, recognizing that this might in fact represent self-employment. Households with semiskilled labor could sell it off the farm for a wage above the unskilled wage rate or use it on-farm with identical returns as unskilled labor.

- *Heterogeneity* between households (as discussed earlier) is described by differences in cropping activities in different agroecological areas, in asset holdings (for example, land, seasonal labor, preseasonal holdings of cash, and grain stocks), and in relations between consumption needs and assets.

- *Partial engagement with imperfect markets* is modeled by a "wedge" between market, farm-gate, and local purchase prices while transaction costs in unskilled labor markets include time demands for supervision when hiring labor and search costs (in terms of time) for those seeking *ganyu* (casual off-farm) employment. Complete credit market failure is assumed in the base model: households cannot borrow without special interventions such as credit tied to the provision of tobacco inputs.

- *Food security objectives in uncertain markets:* Food consumption was modeled in terms of calorific requirements. In the crop and preharvest periods these are met by maize consumption from stocks from the previous season or from purchases. In the harvest and postharvest periods, calories could be provided from own-farm production of grain or root crops or from maize purchases. Subsistence production arose as a result of (1) risks of high purchase prices in adverse seasons and (2) the wedge between maize purchase and sales prices.

- *Nonseparability:* The modeling of seasonal constraints, imperfections in maize, labor, and credit markets (see above), and household objectives allows for strong competition and interaction between consumption and production activities.

- *HIV/AIDS morbidity and mortality effects:* Modifications were made to labor supply, cash needs, and composition for each household type, as described later.

Modeling the Informal Rural Economy

A model of income flows and resource allocations within the informal rural economy (IRE) and between the IRE and the rest of the world[1] was then constructed using information from aggregating farm and household model results. First, aggregate income and expenditure flows were estimated by multiplying the model's income estimates for each farm household type by the estimated number of households of each type. The results of this are shown diagrammatically for the base scenario (using 1997/98 prices) in Figure 4.2. This may be considered as a diagrammatic representation of a social accounting matrix (SAM).

The static representation of the rural economy as an aggregation of independently determined livelihood activities was then turned into a partial equilibrium model responding to HIV/AIDS shocks by simulating the way that individual households' behavior and income and expenditure flows are modified through interaction (1) with each other within the informal economy (as shown by the arrows within the informal rural economy in Fig. 4.2) and (2) with the rest of the world (as shown by the arrows leaving or entering the informal rural economy in Fig. 4.2). In this it was assumed that prices of cash crops and farm inputs are largely determined by world markets (and hence are unaffected by rural Malawi's supply and demand) but that national unskilled wage rates are likely to be affected by supply and demand in rural Malawi and will in turn cause changes in wage rates within the rural economy. The farm household models were therefore run with parameters representing different HIV/AIDS morbidity and mortality scenarios (as described later) and then rerun with wage rates modified so that they gave a partial equilibrium solution[2] with aggregate labor balances consistent with assumptions about elasticities of demand for labor exports from the area.

Figure 4.2   The informal rural economy (income flows in million MK and in percentages of total income)

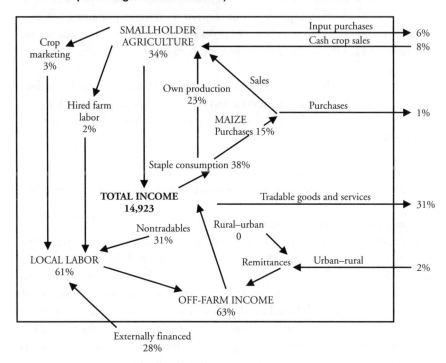

HIV/AIDS Morbidity and Mortality Scenarios

As a preliminary investigation of the plausibility of and influences on the hypotheses outlined above, the study does not use detailed epidemiologic information as a basis for scenario construction. Instead, scenarios allow for plausible and workable variation in mortality and morbidity and in their effects.

To allow simple comparison of the direct impacts of a range of different intensities of a common shock on different individual households, morbidity was initially simulated by varying proportionate loss of (1) labor standardized in terms of the proportion of an unskilled woman's seasonal labor supply, and (2) MK 1,600 cash expenditure (on treatment, etc.) spread across the year. Differential effects of morbidity of skilled household members were investigated for those households that contained these members by varying proportionate loss of such member's labor together with the same proportionate increase in MK 1,600 consumption or expenditure. The effects of mortality were represented by the loss of one (unskilled female or skilled male) adult's labor from a household, a matching reduction of

Table 4.2   Incidence of sick and bereaved households in different IRE scenarios

IRE scenario	"Healthy" households (%)	"Sick" households (%)	"Bereaved" households (%)
Base	100	0	0
A	90	10	0
B	80	20	0
C	70	20	10
D	60	20	20

household consumption and expenditure needs, and an MK 800 reduction in cash stocks at the start of the season.[3]

The IRE model scenarios described a range of morbidity and mortality rates in the population by varying the proportions of "healthy," "sick," and "bereaved" households. "Healthy" households were unchanged from the base, but "sick" households were without 40 percent of the labor of one unskilled female adult (or one skilled male adult) but incurred an extra MK 640 expenditure spread across the year. The characteristics of bereaved households were unchanged from those described in the previous paragraph. Rates of sickness and bereavement in different scenarios are shown in Table 4.2.

Results

Table 4.3 presents estimated impacts of varying morbidity and of mortality on different households' cropping activities, labor use, and net income.

Increasingly severe morbidity leads to declining net income per capita; this is particularly severe for the two poorest household types, poor male-headed and female-headed households (households 4 and 5), and indeed, poor female-headed households where the adult woman becomes sick will not be able to maintain even a greatly reduced minimum consumption level. Poor male-headed households with a sick adult female may be able to survive for longer, but erosion of seasonal capital will fairly quickly become unsustainable. As would be expected, for those households with skilled members, the loss of a skilled member has a greater impact on income per capital than the loss of an unskilled member.

Increasingly severe morbidity also leads to changing cropping patterns as labor and seasonal capital constraints become tighter, with a shift out of hybrid maize and/or tobacco by those (less poor) households initially able to grow these crops.[4] This means that increasing morbidity leads most households to increase areas under low-input maize. For those households that are initially too poor to be able to grow the more capital- and labor-demanding hybrid maize or tobacco, increasing morbidity leads to their increasing inability to cultivate even low-input maize, and they

Table 4.3 Individual household type responses to AIDS morbidity

Household type	AIDS severity	Base consumption	Crop area	Local maize	Hybrid maize	Tobacco	Farm labor (Nov–Jan)	Hire out (in) unskilled (Nov–Jan)	Skilled labor out	Net income per capita (MK)
1. Sk	Base: 0	100%	1.5	0.73	0.75	0.02	1,036	(848)	1,355	5,420
	30%	100%	100%	100%	89%	500%	100%	96%	70%	79%
	60%	100%	100%	126%	53%	900%	94%	85%	40%	58%
	90%	60%	100%	156%	9%	1450%	87%	75%	10%	32%
	Bereaved	100%	99%	145%	36%	800%	89%	80%	0%	70%
2. Sk	Base: 0	100%	1.31	0.75	0.29	0.27	831	(288)	1,936	3,210
	30%	100%	100%	100%	100%	100%	100%	87%	70%	85%
	60%	100%	100%	100%	100%	100%	99%	74%	40%	70%
	90%	75%	100%	100%	59%	100%	107%	94%	10%	51%
	Bereaved	100%	100%	100%	100%	100%	99%	78%	0%	74%
3. UnSk	Base: 0	100%	1.3	0.81	0.49	0	769	458	0	2,374
	30%	100%	100%	117%	71%	NA	94%	83%	NA	89%
	60%	100%	100%	136%	33%	NA	90%	66%	NA	77%
	90%	80%	100%	131%	29%	NA	94%	27%	NA	63%
	Bereaved	100%	100%	144%	24%	NA	86%	53%	NA	94%
4. UnSk	Base: 0	100%	0.56	0.51	0	0	262	921	0	2,219
	30%	100%	57%	61%	NA	NA	57%	99%	NA	87%
	60%	95%	29%	25%	NA	NA	27%	93%	NA	74%
	90%	80%	27%	24%	NA	NA	25%	80%	NA	59%
	Bereaved	85%	54%	47%	NA	NA	59%	74%	NA	88%

5. UnSk	Base: 0	100%	0.39	0.34	0	178	0	673	1,969
	30%	100%	33%	38%	NA	35%	NA	97%	81%
	60%	75%	28%	32%	NA	30%	NA	77%	60%
	90%	66%	54%	62%	NA	56%	NA	76%	44%
	Bereaved	70%	46%	41%	NA	52%	NA	61%	81%
6. Sk	Base: 0	100%	0.8	0.18	0.55	575	0.07	34	3,849
	30%	100%	100%	167%	91%	93%	0%	509%	83%
	60%	85%	100%	217%	75%	88%	0%	733%	63%
	90%	60%	100%	128%	24%	120%	0%	233%	41%
	Bereaved	70%	100%	344%	24%	77%	71%	939%	51%
7. UnSk	Base: 0	100%	1.2	0.32	0.88	840	0	77	3,854
	30%	100%	100%	122%	92%	98%	NA	10%	93%
	60%	100%	101%	178%	69%	92%	NA	-47%	85%
	90%	100%	100%	238%	44%	85%	NA	-111%	77%
	Bereaved	100%	100%	194%	66%	91%	NA!	-204%	106%

Notes: Household type: Results are presented for the seven household types outlined in Table 4.1 with mortality and varying severity of morbidity in skilled (Sk) or unskilled (UnSk) labor. AIDS severity: Percentage of labor time lost and of MK1,600 extra expenditure incurred. Base consumption: Percentage of base consumption needs met; if substantially less than 100% (with strikethrough) the household cannot survive. Crops (local and hybrid maize, tobacco) indicate area cropped in hectares. Unskilled and farm labor is shown for November to January (the peak farm labor demand period) in hours. Percentages indicate percentage of base (no morbidity or mortality).

are forced to decrease the area under this and leave an increasing amount of fallow while maintaining a small area of cassava.

In regard to the effects of morbidity on labor use and markets, morbidity of unskilled labor leads to a reduction in on-farm labor use in almost all households, but only for the two poorest households is this reduction very substantial. Increasing morbidity leads most households who hire out labor in the base scenario to reduce the labor offered into the market, by varying amounts—in some cases turning to hire in labor if this could be financed from skilled labor or remittances. Households who hire in labor in the base scenario increase their labor hire if an unskilled household member becomes sick but decrease labor hire if a skilled member becomes sick.

Bereaved households show patterns of change in net income per person, in cropping patterns, and in labor use and hire broadly similar to those found with increasing morbidity.

Table 4.4 presents results for different morbidity and mortality scenarios in the informal rural economy (IRE), as described earlier. Four sets of scenarios are examined, one in which only unskilled household members are affected by HIV/AIDS, the second in which skilled members are affected in those households in which they are found, and the third and fourth, as for the second, but with unskilled wage rates reduced to 95 percent and 90 percent of their base level, respectively.

In the first scenario set (where AIDS morbidity and mortality is concentrated among unskilled household members and there are no wage changes), increasing morbidity and mortality in the population lead to declining real incomes of affected households (with poorer households affected disproportionately, with increasing inequity), increasing land left under fallow (from a low base), and declining areas under local and hybrid maize and tobacco. There is a slight increase in surplus skilled labor for sale outside the IRE, but a tightening of the unskilled labor market as less unskilled labor is offered for sale outside the IRE.

In the second scenario set, three households now have AIDS morbidity and mortality affecting their skilled rather than unskilled members, and the other households are the same as in the previous scenario set. Wage rates and prices are fixed at base levels. Some results are markedly different; for example, average household income for affected households with skilled labor now falls more than the average income of the poorest households, hybrid maize area falls more, but the tobacco area holds up. The most marked difference, however, is in the surplus labor for sale, as the skilled labor market has dramatically contracted, whereas the unskilled labor market has loosened not just in comparison with the previous scenario set but in comparison with the base situation.[5] This suggests that unskilled wages should fall but that skilled wages should rise. The extent of wage changes will depend on elasticities of skilled and unskilled labor demand outside the IRE, the proportions of skilled and unskilled labor sales outside the IRE, and the ways that this demand may be affected by AIDS. In the final two scenario sets, we therefore simulate the impact of 5 percent and 10 percent reductions in unskilled wage rates. As expected, results in the lower part of Table 4.4 show that a fall in unskilled wages depresses the incomes of all poorer households (including "healthy" households without sickness or bereavement). However, healthy households that normally hire in labor benefit from these lower wages. Lower wages also increase the area under fallow (by squeezing sick and bereaved households harder). Local maize and hybrid areas are similarly depressed, but tobacco areas are stimulated by lower wages.

Discussion

This chapter set out to investigate four hypotheses outlined above. The results presented do not support two of these hypotheses (1 and 4): there is no evidence that impoverishment of households through AIDS leads to an increase in the supply of labor in the unskilled labor market. There is, however, some support for the hypotheses that morbidity and mortality among skilled members of the community can lead to reduced demand for both on-farm labor and unskilled labor providing nontradable goods and services within the local economy (hypotheses 2 and 3). Furthermore, under the particular circumstances described by these models, this reduction in labor demand more than outweighs the small reduction in supply in the unskilled labor market, leading to an overall loosening of the labor market and hence a fall in unskilled wages.

How robust are these findings? Ignizio (1982) identifies four criteria for model validation: logical consistency in model construction; reliability of the data on which the model is based; logical consistency of model responses to simple stimuli; and correspondence of model outputs with reality. The models used in this study do suffer from a number of limitations (Dorward 2003). These include (in the household models) dividing the year into only four seasons; using a unitary household model with limited gender divisions of labor; the rudimentary treatment of risk and of transaction costs; the omission of dry season *dimba* production (growing of crops in irrigated swampy land in valley bottoms) and of horticultural crops and livestock keeping; limited data on labor supply, use, and wages; treating all nonfarm activities as hiring out of skilled or unskilled labor; and not capturing the full extent of inherent variability and heterogeneity in Malawian livelihood systems. The IRE model does not allow for different parts of the country with similar

Table 4.4 IRE responses to and household welfare impacts of AIDS morbidity and mortality

	Base (%)	Scenario (%) Only unskilled — 100%				Scenario (%) Skilled and unskilled — 100%			
		A	B	C	D	A	B	C	D
Morbidity/mortality effects									
Wage rate (% of base)									
All households' real income									
All	100	98	97	94	91	98	96	91	87
"Healthy"	100	100	100	100	100	100	100	100	100
"Sick"		84	84	84	84	79	79	79	79
"Bereaved"				69	69			56	56
Poor male- and female-headed households' real income									
All	100	98	96	93	89	98	96	93	89
"Healthy"	100	100	100	100	100	100	100	100	100
"Sick"		79	79	79	79	79	79	79	79
"Bereaved"				68	68			68	68
Fallow area	100	195	291	367	443	195	291	367	443
Local maize area	100	98	96	94	91	98	97	95	94
Hybrid area	100	99	98	95	92	98	96	90	83
Tobacco area	100	98	97	91	84	99	98	98	98
Skilled labor exports (value)	100	101	102	103	104	94	88	74	59
Unskilled labor exports (value)	100	98	96	89	82	103	105	107	109

Morbidity/mortality effects		Skilled and unskilled							
		95%				90%			
Wage rate (% of base)	100								
All households' real income									
All	100	97	95	91	86	96	94	90	85
"Healthy"	100	99	99	99	99	98	98	98	98
"Sick"		78	78	78	78	78	78	78	78
"Bereaved"				54	54			54	54
Poor male- and female-headed households' real income									
All	100	95	93	89	86	92	90	87	84
"Healthy"	100	97	97	97	97	94	94	94	94
"Sick"		75	75	75	75	74	74	74	74
"Bereaved"				65	65			65	65
Fallow area	100	256	345	415	485	279	346	404	462
Local maize area	100	96	94	93	92	93	93	91	90
Hybrid area	100	90	89	83	77	73	72	67	62
Tobacco area	100	108	106	106	105	107	106	102	98
Skilled labor exports (value)	100	95	90	75	61	130	122	102	82
Unskilled labor exports (value)	100	90	92	95	97	58	60	62	63

agroecology having different land pressure (with smaller or larger holding sizes affecting local labor demand and wages) nor variations in market access. It is also a partial equilibrium model, without allowance for more general changes in the wider economy, involving, for example, changes in demand for labor, in general price levels, in government expenditures, and, as applied in this chapter, not allowing for changes in maize prices. The IRE model as applied here also assumes uniform price changes across the year, whereas prices are likely to change differently at different times of year. Nevertheless, despite these weaknesses, Dorward (2003) argues that the livelihood and IRE models perform sufficiently well on Ignizio's criteria to provide useful insights into the general behavior of individual households and of the IRE and to pose serious and insightful questions about this behavior. The model is also a significant advance on other available formal or informal models of household and IRE behavior.

The validity of the modeling of HIV/AIDS morbidity and mortality in this chapter can also be judged against the four criteria set out above and, for a preliminary study, performs well. We therefore conclude that the possibility of HIV/AIDS leading to falling wages for unskilled labor is very real. The scale and seriousness of this effect is, however, not clear. The results reported here suggest a relatively mild loosening of the market in that the highest incidence of morbidity and mortality modeled leads to a relatively small (probably around 5 percent) fall in wages. This is, however, sensitive to the particular scenarios that were modeled and to the accuracy of the models' descriptions of individual household behavior and of the interactions within the IRE and between the IRE and the rest of the Malawian economy. These effects would be higher with larger cash costs of morbidity or mortality, with allowance for the double burden of rural households' lost remittances and extra costs in caring for sick family members previously working in towns, with allowance for general depression of the national economy, with more inelastic demand for unskilled labor in the rest of the economy or with a less open economy (with less trade and greater relative importance of nontradables in production and consumption). Allowance for the development of land rental markets would probably lead to a loosening of the labor market as compared with model results presented here. It is unclear how the results would be affected by more sophisticated scenarios allowing for different morbidity and mortality rates among male and female adults in the different household types, for loss of labor by caregivers, for seasonal differences in morbidity and in wages, and for household disintegration and its impact on other households. The effects on model results of changing morbidity and mortality rates in line with epidemiologic models would depend on the nature and scale of specific morbidity and mortality rate changes.

Conclusions

This chapter has put forward and tested hypotheses that HIV/AIDS can lead to falling unskilled rural wages, a particularly worrying possibility given the dependence on unskilled labor markets of poor people in Malawi and more widely in Africa. The preliminary analysis presented here suggests

- There is a serious danger of this being the case in some circumstances as a result of reduced on-farm and off-farm demand for unskilled labor.

- The extent to which HIV/AIDS will depress wages is not clear but will depend on the extent of morbidity and mortality, on the morbidity and mortality distribution among skilled and unskilled men and women, and on impacts on skilled labor earnings and remittances.

- Segmentation and other aspects of labor market behavior, land rental markets, the openness of the local economy, and elasticities of labor demand outside the informal rural economy will also be important determinants of wage sensitivity to HIV.

- Where HIV/AIDS does depress unskilled wages, this is likely to increase inequality within rural communities and impose further pressures on poor people and their livelihoods.

- The introduction of laborsaving technologies to assist labor-constrained AIDS-affected households may have very negative impacts in areas where wages are already falling. Indeed, more conventional "labor-demanding" crop technologies may offer the best opportunities for both AIDS-affected and "healthy" poor households, where labor-demanding technologies are defined as increasing both labor and land productivity, but with greater increases in the latter. This leads to both increased returns to labor and increased labor demand, supporting rather than depressing wages. Emphasis may need to be placed on other ways of assisting labor-constrained AIDS-affected households, such as cash transfers to help them with labor hire as well as antiretroviral treatment.

These results should not be generalized: the impact of HIV/AIDS on rural livelihoods is highly context-dependent (see, e.g., Yamano and Jayne 2004; Tumushabe 2005). It is, however, clear that this is an issue that needs further attention in research and policy, first to establish the extent of the problem (how widespread it is, how serious it is when it occurs) and then to determine appropriate responses. An immediate and fairly simple aid in this would be the identification of risk factors predisposing areas to higher risk of depressed wages from HIV/AIDS and the construction of a typology of characteristics of high-risk areas and of appropriate interventions to address this.

Notes

1. The "informal rural economy" is distinguished from large commercial agriculture and from business, government, or NGO operations in rural areas. It includes all the activities of the rural households described by the household models and allows for interactions between the informal economy (these households) and the rest of the world (other agents or activities not explicitly allowed for in the household models, whether located physically in rural space, in other parts of Malawi, or abroad).

2. This is a partial equilibrium because equilibria are allowed for in only two markets. Dorward et al. (2004) describe general equilibrium models linked to the informal rural economy and household models described in this chapter. Dorward (2003) also allows for maize price changes in the IRE, but changes in the maize balance did not appear to be significant with the scenarios modeled in this chapter.

3. Cash expenditures associated with morbidity and mortality were derived from Shah et al. (2002).

4. There is some variation between households with varying balances in their access to labor and capital. Also, with very high morbidity of its skilled member, household 6 puts some land into groundnuts because of their lower capital requirements as compared with tobacco and hybrid maize.

5. These results assume strong segmentation between the skilled and unskilled labor markets.

References

Arndt, C., and J. Lewis. 2001. The HIV/AIDS pandemic in South Africa: Sectoral impact and unemployment. *Journal of International Development* 13 (4): 427–449.

De Waal, A., and A. Whiteside. 2003. New variant famine: AIDS and the food crisis in Southern Africa. *The Lancet* 362: 1234–1237.

Dorward, A. R. 2002. *A typology of Malawian rural households.* Working paper: Institutions and economic policies for pro-poor agricultural growth, July 2002. Wye: Imperial College, London, Wye Campus.

———. 2003. *Modelling poor farm-household livelihoods in Malawi: Lessons for pro-poor policy.* Wye, Ashford, U.K.: Centre for Development and Poverty Reduction, Department of Agricultural Sciences, Imperial College London.

Dorward, A. R., N. D. Poole, J. A. Morrison, J. G. Kydd, and I. Urey. 2003. Markets, institutions and technology: Missing links in livelihoods analysis. *Development Policy Review* 21 (3): 319–332.

Dorward, A., S. Fan, J. Kydd, H. Lofgren, J. Morrison, C. Poulton, N. Rao, L. Smith, H. Tchale, S. Thorat, I. Urey, and P. Wobst. 2004. *Institutions and economic policies for pro-poor agricultural growth.* IFPRI Discussion Paper DSG 15. Washington, D.C.: IFPRI.

IFPRI and NSO. 2002. Integrated household survey, Malawi, 1997–98, Data CD. Washington D.C.: IFPRI; Malawi: National Statistical Office.

Ignizio, J. P. 1982. *Linear progamming in single and multiple objective systems.* Upper Saddle River, N.J.: Prentice Hall.

Mwale, I. 2004. *The impact of HIV/AIDS on rural livelihoods taking into account the labour markets in Malawi.* M.Sc. thesis, Department of Agricultural Sciences, Imperial College London. Wye, U.K.

National AIDS Commission. 2003. *HIV/AIDS in Malawi: Estimates of the prevalence of infection and the implications.* Malawi: National AIDS Commission, Malawi.

Shah, M. K., N. Osborne, T. Mbilize, and G. Vilili. 2002. *Impact of HIV/AIDS on agricultural productivity and rural livelihoods in the Central Region of Malawi.* Lilongwe: CARE International in Malawi.

Tumushabe, J. 2005. *HIV/AIDS and changing vulnerability to crisis in Tanzania: Implications for food security and poverty reduction.* Paper presented at HIV/AIDS and Food and Nutrition Security: From Evidence to Action, April 14–16, 2005, Durban, South Africa.

Yamano, T., and T. S. Jayne. 2004. Measuring impacts of prime-age adult death on rural households in Kenya. *World Development* 32 (1): 91–114.

Chapter 5

An Enduring or Dying Peasantry? Interactive Impact of Famine and HIV/AIDS in Rural Malawi

Deborah Fahy Bryceson and Jodie Fonseca

B etween 2001 and 2003 the rural population of Malawi experienced widespread hunger. During the same time period, Malawi's HIV prevalence was the eighth highest in the world (UNAIDS 2004). Speculation about the links between famine and the HIV/AIDS epidemic followed. De Waal and Whiteside (2003) postulated that a "new variant famine" had arisen among a rural population made more vulnerable to food insecurity by AIDS-related morbidity and mortality. The declining welfare of the Malawian rural population in the context of rising HIV prevalence before the famine was readily apparent (e.g., Ngwira, Bota, and Loevinsohn 2001; Frankenberger et al. 2003).

This chapter concentrates on the material conditions and attitudinal perspectives of local villagers, drawing primarily on transcripts of key informant interviews and focus group discussions from three villages to examine the interactions between HIV/AIDS and famine in rural Malawi. Our investigations were part of a CARE International/RENEWAL study carried out between December 2003 and March 2004 in Lilongwe rural district, Central Region.[1] The chapter focuses on the response of Malawian peasant farmers to the combined threats of famine and HIV/AIDS and quotes extensively from our interviews and discussions in order to convey how rural peasant farmers perceive the challenges they face. The first section provides background on rural livelihoods in Malawi and various historical influences shaping the peasantry over time, followed by a consideration of changing famine coping strategies.

The Malawian Peasantry

Both the colonial and the postcolonial government under Hastings Kamuzu Banda[2] prioritized plantation cultivation of tea and tobacco over smallholder household production, leaving peasant households to rely first on subsistence production and secondarily on migrant labor to Malawi's plantations, the mines of South Africa, or other employment in the surrounding regions. Thus, Malawi's peasant household production units have, for many decades, not been strictly agrarian or self-sufficient in food production. Physical separation of household family members became a norm as a result of male labor migration. Left in the hands of women and older men, the farming household survived largely on subsistence food production and cash remittances from male migrants. The government's indifference to food crops and agricultural extension for female farmers, together with women's lack of money to purchase agricultural inputs, has resulted in a legacy of "female farming" of subsistence crops (Boserup 1970; Bryceson 1995) in addition to exceptionally low levels of agricultural productivity compared to neighboring countries (Ellis and Freeman 2005).[3] Moreover, an overreliance on maize limiting the variety of the country's food crops has magnified the risk of harvest failure.

According to recent estimates, over half of Malawi's smallholder farmers have less than 1 hectare of cultivable land and are unable to produce enough food to feed themselves (Malawi 2002). Because of the changing economic and political dynamics of the region, opportunities for male labor migration to other locations in southern Africa have been mostly eliminated, and wage labor on Malawian plantations has also been diminishing. At the same time, tobacco production by Malawian smallholders has stagnated (Frankenberger et al. 2003).

Malawian villages are remote and insulated in many ways. Typically, traditional authorities at village level are male elders with little formal education. The villagers' worldview is generally restricted to local events and concerns. For the most part, welfare and property rights are determined by sustaining good relations with relatives in one's area of birth. The pervasive low educational attainment of rural adults, which stems from the very late introduction of universal primary education after Banda left the presidency in 1994, reinforces the sense of traditionalism. Throughout the nearly 30 years of Banda's rule, lack of investment in rural areas resulted in a peasantry strikingly lacking in access to agricultural, health, and education services in comparison to surrounding countries. Parastatal market controls hampered rural markets, and road building in rural areas was not prioritized. The 2001–02 famine struck within this economic and cultural setting.

Contrasting Peasants' Age-Old and
Current Responses to Famine

Food security for Malawian peasants is affected by wide variation in rainfall from year to year. In contexts like these, farmers have long been known to be risk-averse in their farming practices and to prioritize food self-sufficiency at the household level (Allan 1965). Paradoxically, the poor harvest and severe food shortages of 2001–02 were preceded by a bumper harvest. Some observers have remarked that the level of famine Malawi experienced was unwarranted by the harvest shortfall in those years, claiming that the Agricultural Development and Marketing Corporation's (ADMARC) decision to export grain stocks was poorly timed and edged the country toward famine (Bookstein and Lawson 2002; Frankenberger et al. 2003).

Despite the extreme duress they faced during the recent famine, only 15 percent of households received food-based assistance from extended family members, and only 19 percent obtained food aid from outside sources such as nongovernmental organizations (NGOs).[4] Most households were forced to fend for themselves. In contrast to the 1949 famine, in 2001–02 the mitigating benefits of migrant labor were mostly lacking. Those with family members in urban areas had some recourse, but most rural households could not rely on kin in cities and towns because of the very low levels of urbanization that define Malawi. Instead, their central means of coping was *ganyu* labor.

Characterized by the exchange of labor for goods, services, or cash, *ganyu* has long been an important form of labor transaction between peasant households (Englund 1999; Bryceson 2006). By definition, *ganyu* is a system in which a household of any socioeconomic status that lacks adequate labor can access additional labor on a seasonal basis, but it is typically associated with the sale of labor by people from poorer households to wealthier households in exchange for cash or goods. During peak agricultural seasons, *ganyu* labor increases and often causes disadvantaged casual wage laborers to divert work from their own fields when they can least afford it. Traditionally, a *ganyu* contract between people with family ties was more balanced and reciprocal. Our oral interviews suggest, however, that this reciprocity degraded under the prolonged stress of hunger, and *ganyu* wages generally declined, as was also the case during the 1992 famine (Peters 1996).

Among peasant farmers elsewhere in Sub-Saharan Africa, the need for alternative off-farm income has been somewhat mitigated by households' ability to fall back on subsistence activities. Most rural households in Malawi, however, have no consistent year-round subsistence fallback. Increasingly, they have been forced to provision their needs one day at a time, operating within the shortest of time horizons.

We rely on *ganyu* and cannot carry out income-generating activities because we have no capital since the little we earn from *ganyu* must be spent on food. (Women's FGD in matrilineal village Chitukula TA, December 3, 2004)

The paradoxical situation of unused labor and land within peasant households, as observed by Ellis, Kutengule, and Nyasulu (2003), has resulted from their increasing reliance on off-farm *ganyu* to meet their urgent need for food. In addition to the growing reliance on *ganyu* with remarkably unfavorable bargaining terms, rural people are also disadvantaged in newly appearing factor markets by their lack of literacy, numeracy, and understanding of the market. To obtain cash to buy food or fertilizers, male farmers are entering into word-of-mouth agreements for share-cropping, land-leasing, and labor arrangements with urban and other patrons. On terms determined by the patron, they receive immediate cash and/or agricultural inputs in exchange for the promised delivery of harvested crops later. These factor markets are poorly documented in the literature on the Malawian agrarian sector to date, but it is readily evident that asset-poor rural households' access to crop harvests, land, and means of livelihood are being further eroded as they rent out acreage to better-off farmers or outsiders.

The rural population's faith in smallholder farming as a way of life seems to have badly eroded. One reason for this may be that they had always supported their rural households through something that is no longer viable: heavy dependence on migrant labor. Another explanation may be the deteriorating yields that have plagued them since the elimination of the fertilizer subsidy (Edriss, Tchale, and Wobst 2004). Moreover, the effect of AIDS on the household labor force may also be a significant blow to their faith in farming. Most likely, the confluence of all these factors has led to a state of heightened vulnerability, demoralization, and defeatism.

Villagers have reached a turning point in agricultural asset management. With the removal of the fertilizer subsidy and the diminished crop-marketing role of ADMARC, rural dwellers are prioritizing casual labor to address the routine hunger they face. In the matrilineal village women's focus group discussion, for example, the harvest was approaching, and near-ripe crops surrounded them, but, in a growing trend, many of these crops were not theirs. The women told us that they devoted all their productive hours to "looking for food," a euphemism for *ganyu*. No one viewed *ganyu* as a sustainable solution, however, and even the village headman stated that he discouraged *ganyu* because he felt it sacrificed long-term viability for short-term gains.

Accordingly, the villagers did not have sufficient recourse to assistance from either external agencies or extended family, nor could they fall back on at-home subsistence food production. The women were exchanging their labor on highly unequal terms, and the men were renting out their land for quick income, leading to a precarious hand-to-mouth lifestyle. Households had also reached a highly individualized state in which they were afraid or unable to seek help from neighbors. Their self-reliance had the unfortunate net effect of overwhelming the local labor and factor markets, driving down wages and fueling impoverishment. Only a small segment of local farmers with the means to hire labor benefited from these circumstances. *Ganyu* laborers sought to sell their labor to those with salaried income such as local teachers or health service personnel, or they journeyed outside their local area to towns in search of short-term contract work (Bryceson 2006).

In so many places around the world through the millennia, the longevity and viability of peasant household production has hinged on the production of subsistence food and agricultural commodities in combination. This strategy helped households use commodity or labor market sales to counter the negative effects of poor food harvests. Conversely, peasants could respond to adverse commodity and labor markets by upping their subsistence production. At present, the land and capital constraints Malawian peasants face offer limited commodity production choices in addition to setting severe constraints on any increase of subsistence production. The long-standing, two-pronged strategy to minimize risk is slipping away.

HIV/AIDS: The New Challenge to Peasant Survival

HIV/AIDS, unlike famine, is a relatively new menace for rural Malawian households. As a "long-wave" phenomenon, the AIDS pandemic in Sub-Saharan Africa has been unfolding for only 25 years. In 1985, estimated HIV prevalence was 2 percent (Taha et al. 1998), rising to 14.2 percent among adults 15–49 years of age at the time of our study (Malawi and NAC 2003). The adult prevalence in urban areas of 23 percent contrasts with a prevalence of 12.4 percent in rural Malawi, although the gap between urban and rural prevalence narrowed from a factor of 5 to 2 during the 1990s. HIV-positive rural dwellers now exceed their urban counterparts by approximately three to one.

Malawians have had very little time to develop coping mechanisms in response to this burgeoning epidemic. Over the past decade, HIV/AIDS has spread against a backdrop of depeasantization and food shortages, traumatizing communities and overwhelming local economies. Given the suddenness and extent of the sickness and death experienced, these initial years of coping have been accompanied by denial and fatalism.

Sex was traditionally perceived as a joyful activity in Malawi (Kadzandira 2002; Matinga and McConville 2003). Men and women were responsible for maximizing sexual pleasure for their partner and themselves. To this end, several ritualized, extramarital events were scheduled throughout one's lifetime to help enhance sexual performance. *Chidzeranu,* or the exchange of wives, was prevalent in some areas. Young male and female virgins were traditionally coached in having sex by a trainer (*fisi*) of the opposite sex. Males would undergo circumcision, although, because of pressure from Christian churches, perhaps not as commonly as in many other African countries. Additionally, adolescents underwent initiation ceremonies with the local chief playing an important role. These rituals also included the sexual cleansing of women after initiation ceremonies and funerals by a *namandwa,* and many patrilineal groups practiced *chokolo,* widow inheritance, expecting the wife of the deceased man to marry one of his brothers. These practices were more closely linked to norms of inheritance than to sexual pleasure, however.

The National AIDS Commission (NAC) has been training traditional counselors in villages to help them reduce risk by altering cultural practices. As a result of the NAC's efforts and public campaigns, villagers are for the most part more aware of the dangers of sexual cleansers and trainers, widow inheritance, and used razor blades in circumcision ceremonies. Chiefs are increasingly mindful of safety measures, and traditional health procedures such as circumcision are now far more likely to be performed with clean blades. There is also evidence that traditional sexual rituals may be performed with condoms or are becoming less frequent in some areas (Shah 2002; Matinga and McConville 2003).

Although some chiefs and other traditional figures are increasingly promulgating safer practices, different media outlets are prescribing conflicting sexual behavior. Under Christian discourse, sexual relationships outside of marriage are socially unacceptable. Because of their perceived role as devices facilitating extramarital sex, condoms are seen as immoral, a viewpoint that contradicts the efforts of the government and donors to make condom usage more widespread. In our study villages at present, the majority of adults view condoms as either abnormal or immoral.

For our study populations, extramarital sex within the village embodied both traditional and new elements. In connection with their market activities and recreational drinking habits, men frequented pubs and in many cases engaged in sexual liaisons fueled by the disinhibition of alcohol.

> Generally, people like having extra- and premarital affairs in the village. It is an old culture that looks normal, and other people are used to it. (Men's FGD in patrilineal village, Khongoni Tribal Authority, August 12, 2003)

> There is a bad system of sleeping with each other's wives in this village. Mostly it is the rich men who do this to poor men's wives because it

offers them money. The women don't refuse due to their poverty. This is spreading HIV. (Men's FGD in patrilineal village, Chitukula TA, April 12, 2003)

Men . . . go to pubs, where they sleep with prostitutes who infect them. (Women's FGD in patrilineal village, Chitukula TA, April 12, 2003)

Both men and women in these villages were increasingly concerned about *kusokola* (looking for food), a practice seen as a famine coping mechanism that exposes women to compromise in the form of transactional sex. During the 2001–02 famine, without commodities or services to sell, women resorted to exchanging sex for food, earning cash or in-kind payment by traveling to trading centers, Lilongwe and other nearby towns (Shah 2002). Sexual activity was being progressively incorporated into women's *ganyu* contracts, a practice that worsened with deepening household impoverishment. In the patrilineal village we sampled closest to Lilongwe, for example, the women had been making frequent trips to the grain mill in a nearby semiurban area out of desperation, collecting the leftover maize bran from the milling process. Staying overnight was often required to gain favored access to the bran. Men working at the mill offered *ganyu* contracts to the women, capitalizing on their vulnerability. In one of the patrilineal village FGDs, the women's husbands relating the situation explained their reaction: "The men [at the mill] offer them the *ganyu* but also entice them to sleep with them. Since the women are bringing food [maize bran home], we cannot object [as husbands]."

"Transactional sex" is not the same thing as "prostitution," which involves earning a livelihood through the solicitation of sex. Prostitutes are part of a service market and create various rules for economic and physical survival in their line of work. Women prostitutes have a professional interest in safe sex and are in a far stronger position to insist on safe sex practices as a condition of service to their clients (Campbell 2003). Thus, it is important to distinguish prostitutes from women who engage in occasional transactional sex. The latter are not professionals selling sex as an occupation. They happen into chance sexual encounters, compromised by their impoverished circumstances and their household's need for food, and are ill-equipped to bargain the terms of the transaction. Given this disempowerment, and the unpredictable nature of transactional sex, the adoption of safe sex practices is problematic.

As deaths from AIDS have increased, villagers have become more and more aware that they face an escalating problem. When discussing causality, villagers tend to blame particular categories of people whom they believe are responsible for the spread of HIV. Women fault the extramarital sex that often accompanies men's heavy drinking (Bryceson 2002c; van Dijk 2002). Men are increasingly vocal about the role of women's *ganyu* earning activities in fueling growing HIV prevalence in the village. Adults complain that young people are especially promiscuous these days, in part because of increasing alcohol consumption. While admitting that they are taking part in these activities, youth blame the poor example that adults set in their social and sexual behavior. The allocation of blame still takes place amid a general consensus that poverty is the root cause of their predicament. Men who have withstood the injury of lost income-earning opportunities over the last few decades now face the embarrassment of their wives' desperation-driven sexual activities. Up until recently, men were accustomed to earning the household's cash income while women were preoccupied with subsistence farming. It would be difficult for men to avoid conflicting emotions about their wives' food-procuring activities.

Conclusion

The last 25 years have been challenging for rural smallholders throughout Sub-Saharan Africa, but this has been particularly true in Malawi over the past half-decade when the impacts of HIV/AIDS and famine in combination have relentlessly undermined household welfare. The peasant household's strength as a unit of production is collapsing as household assets and livelihood portfolios have simultaneously veered, first, from self-sufficient unpaid labor performed within the household, particularly by women and children, toward *ganyu;* second, from agriculture toward nonagriculture with income earning shifting increasingly to trade and services, including sexual services; and, third, from household toward individualized labor, in which every able-bodied person, including women and youth, works to earn cash for subsistence needs. These are fundamental changes to peasant household labor patterns reflective of deagrarianization and depeasantization trends (Bryceson 2000, 2002a, b). Women and girls are now finding *ganyu* outside of their villages. In view of the shortfalls in household food provisioning, their menfolk are acquiescent.

Depeasantization in Malawi differs from the situations in many other parts of Sub-Saharan Africa. Rural income diversification, a significant aspect of the depeasantization process, is proceeding in Malawi unaccompanied by the relatively secure subsistence fallback that smallholder households have relied on so heavily in other African countries (Bryceson 2002a). Rural Malawians face acute food insecurity because of very low agricultural productivity in combination with relatively high rural population density and land shortage. The cessation of the fertilizer subsidy threatened peasant households' subsistence food production even further. The majority of households no longer have access to adequate land and/or agricultural output to guarantee basic household food needs throughout the year.

In his insightful book, *Famine that Kills,* de Waal (1989, p. 227) argued that during the Sudanese famine of 1984/85, farmers in Darfur preferred to go hungry rather than sell off the livestock that they knew would ensure their long-term survival. In doing so, they preserved a material foundation for continuing to work as agrarian producers. Furthermore, they endeavored to preserve social cohesion in their communities. In Malawi, this knee-jerk response by smallholder peasants was not prominent. Most had little if any livestock to sell.[5] Instead, they prioritized off-farm *ganyu* casual labor to address their immediate food needs over longer-term staple food planting and harvesting cycles on their own household landholdings, causing seasonal underutilization of household land and labor. A vicious cycle of impoverishment is in progress, propelling more and more into abject poverty, undermining smallholders as viable agricultural producers, and eroding their well-being and solidarity as peasant communities.

Most rural dwellers view food insecurity as the most important indicator of poverty (Malawi and NEC 2002, p. 15). Village leaders estimated that the upper stratum of farmers, constituting a small proportion of households, is food self-sufficient year-round. Middle-stratum households have sufficient maize to last 5 to 6 months after harvests, but poor households may only have a month's worth or less of food supplies each year. The extent of the shortfall in food supply and the year-by-year repetition of this shortfall erode household self-esteem.

Famine threatens peasant households and villages in the immediate term, while HIV/AIDS menaces individuals and the peasant population in a more insidious longer-term way. Famine safeguards have been integrated into the cultural fabric of the peasant society, in contrast to the more recent threat of AIDS, which people have yet to come to terms with. In our interviews and group discussions, we were told repeatedly that hunger was the most fundamental problem for individual and household survival.

> HIV/AIDS is not very threatening compared to the hunger which most households face. In fact it is hunger, which is contributing to the rise in HIV infections in the area. (Religious leader in patrilineal village, Khongoni TA, August 12, 2003)

Risk assessment involves gaining knowledge on which one weighs the odds and chooses the best course of action to minimize adversity. In this case, the Malawian peasantry, specifically peasant women, are successfully addressing the immediate food shortfall. However, with the increasing frequency of food shortages[6] and declining assets and income, they are in effect forestalling death by engaging in what could be termed the most essential exchange: sex for food.

Notes

This is an edited and condensed version of a more detailed paper (Bryceson and Fonseca 2006). We are grateful to CARE International and the Regional Network on HIV/AIDS, Rural Livelihoods and Food Security (RENEWAL), facilitated by IFPRI, who sponsored the study on which this chapter is based. Special thanks go to the CARE Malawi staff and John Kadzandira of the University of Malawi for their contribution to the data collection and analysis.

1. The three villages surveyed were: Dzama in Chitukula Tribal Authority (TA), 29 kilometers from Lilongwe, Vizimba in Khongoni TA, located 60 kilometers from Lilongwe, both of which were primarily patrilineal villages, and the matrilineal village of Chimponda (Chitukula TA, 30 kilometers distance from Lilongwe). Our field methodology began with gender- and age-segregated focus group discussions and key informant interviews. Village heads were contacted a few days in advance to arrange times for our focus group discussions and key informant interviews. A random sample survey of 141 households was conducted between February 27 and March 3, 2004, with the aim of providing background demographic data. At the time of our investigations, more than a year after the famine, there were still people on food-for-work programs and roughly 600 chronically ill receiving direct food transfers in the two tribal authorities where we conducted interviews.

2. Banda became Malawi's first prime minister on February 1, 1963, after the end of British rule and became president in 1966 when Malawi was declared a one-party republic. He declared himself president for life in 1971 but was defeated in the country's first multiparty elections in 1994.

3. Ellis and Freeman's (2005, p. 43) four-country comparative study recorded net average agricultural outputs per hectare (US$/ha): Kenya 297, Uganda 282, Tanzania 182, and Malawi 64. "Net agricultural output" refers to the gross output produced per hectare, multiplied by farm-gate sales prices minus purchased inputs and labor costs, then converted to US$ at the current prevailing exchange rate for purposes of comparison of mixed product outputs.

4. Data from our survey of 141 households, which included questions on famine coping strategies.

5. This was because of the lack of recovery of household livestock assets arising from their sale during the 1992 famine as well as a widespread problem of rural livestock theft during the post-Banda era.

6. At the time of writing (February 2006), severe food shortages were again being experienced in rural Malawi, putting an estimated 5 million people at risk (approximately 40 percent of the total population), reported by the Famine Early Warning Systems Network (http://www.fews.net/centers/innerSections.aspx?f=mw&m=1001810&pageID=monthliesDoc).

References

Allan, W. 1965. *The African husbandman.* London: Oliver & Boyd.

Bookstein, A., and M. Lawson. 2002. Briefing: Famine in southern Africa. *African Affairs* 101: 635–641.

Boserup, E. 1970 (reprinted 1989). *Woman's role in economic development.* London: Earthscan Publications.

Bryceson, D. F. 1995. *Women wielding the hoe.* Oxford: Berg Publishers.

————. 2000. African peasants' centrality and marginality: Rural labor transformations. In *Disappearing peasantries: Rural labor in Africa, Asia and Latin America,* eds. D. F. Bryceson, C. Kay, and J. Mooij. London: Intermediate Technology Publications.

————. 2002a. The scramble in Africa: Reorienting rural livelihoods. *World Development* 30 (5): 725–739.

————. 2002b. Multiplex livelihoods in rural Africa: Recasting the terms and conditions of gainful employment. *Journal of Modern African Studies* 40 (1): 1–28.

————. 2002c. Pleasure and pain: The ambiguity of alcohol in Africa. In *Alcohol in Africa: Mixing business, pleasure and politics,* ed. D. F. Bryceson. Portsmouth, N.H.: Heinemann.

————. 2006. *Ganyu* casual labour, famine and HIV/AIDS in rural Malawi: Causality and casualty. *Journal of Modern African Studies* 44 (2): 1–30.

Bryceson, D. F., and J. Fonseca. 2006. Risking death for survival: Peasant responses to hunger and HIV/AIDS in Malawi. *World Development* 34 (9) (forthcoming).

Campbell, C. 2003. *Letting them die: Why HIV/AIDS prevention programmes fail.* Oxford: James Currey.

de Waal, A. 1989. *Famine that kills: Darfur, Sudan, 1984–85.* Oxford: Clarendon Press.

de Waal, A., and A. Whiteside. 2003. New variant famine: AIDS and food crisis in southern Africa. *Lancet* 362: 1234–1237.

Edriss, A., H. Tchale, and P. Wobst. 2004. *The impact of labour market liberalization on maize productivity and rural poverty in Malawi.* Robert Bosch Foundation, Policy Analysis for Sustainable Agricultural Development (PASAD) Project, University of Bonn, Germany, <http:// www.pasad.unibonn.de/pasadJournalpaper.pdf>.

Ellis, F., and H. A. Freeman. 2005. Comparative evidence from four African countries. In *Rural livelihoods and poverty reduction policies,* eds. F. Ellis and H. A. Freeman. London: Routledge, p. 31–47.

Ellis, F., M. Kutengule, and A. Nyasulu. 2003. Livelihoods and rural poverty reduction in Malawi. *World Development* 31 (9): 1495–1510.

Englund, H. 1999. The self in self-interest: Land, labor and temporalities in Malawi's agrarian change. *Africa* 69 (1): 139–159.

Frankenberger, T., K. Luther, K. Fox, and J. Mazzeo. 2003. *Livelihood erosion through time: Macro and micro factors that influenced livelihood trends in Malawi over the last 30 years.* TANGO International, Inc., CARE Southern and Western Africa Regional Management Unit (SWARMU), March 2003.

Kadzandira, J. M. 2002. *Sources of risks and vulnerability for Malawian households and communities.* Centre for Social Research, University of Malawi, background paper for the World Bank 2002 Poverty Reduction study.

Malawi, Government of. 2002. *Malawi national land policy.* Lilongwe: Ministry of Lands, Physical Planning and Survey.

Malawi and NEC. 2002. *Qualitative impact monitoring (QIM) of the poverty alleviation policies and programmes in Malawi, Volume 1: Survey findings.* Lilongwe: National Economic Council.

Malawi National AIDS Commission. 2003. *HIV prevalence and AIDS mortality statistics.* Lilongwe: Malawi National AIDS Commission.

Matinga, P., and F. McConville. 2003. *A review of cultural beliefs and practices influencing sexual and reproductive health, and health-seeking behaviour, in Malawi.* Lilongwe: DFID.

Ngwira, N., S. Bota, and M. Loevinsohn. 2001. *HIV/AIDS, Agriculture and food security in Malawi.* Lilongwe and The Hague: Regional Network on HIV/AIDS Rural Livelihoods and Food Insecurity (RENEWAL) Working Paper 1.

Peters, P. E. 1996. *Failed magic or social context? Market liberalization and the rural poor in Malawi.* Cambridge, Mass.: HIID Development Discussion Paper.

Shah, M. K. 2002. *Buying sex for three sweet potatoes: Participatory assessment of adolescent sexual and reproductive health in Makala village.* Lilongwe: CARE International Consultancy Report.

Taha, T. E., G. Dallabeta, J. D. Chiphangwi, L. A. R. Mtimavalye, N. G. Liomba, N. Kumwenda, D. Hoover, and P. Miotti. 1998. *Trends of HIV-1 and sexually transmitted diseases among pregnant and postpartum women in urban Malawi.* Unpublished MS, copy at College of Medicine Library, Blantyre.

UNAIDS. 2004. http://www.unaids.org/Unaids/EN/Geographical+area/ByCountry/Malawi.asp.

van Dijk, R. 2002. Modernity's limits: Pentecostalism and the moral rejection of alcohol in Malawi. In *Alcohol in Africa: Mixing business, pleasure and politics,* ed. D. F. Bryceson. Portsmouth, N.H.: Heinemann.

Chapter 6

Understanding Rwandan Agricultural Households' Strategies to Deal with Prime-Age Illness and Death: A Propensity Score Matching Approach

Cynthia Donovan and Linda A. Bailey

Objectives

The increasing prevalence of HIV in Rwanda, along with the likelihood of continued effects of the genocide of 1994, suggests that many rural households may be facing extreme stress, and their agricultural production may be changing. Policymakers and development practitioners seek to understand how Rwandan households are affected and how they are reacting to the stress so that development policies can best support improvements in rural livelihoods under this changing environment. If production systems are shifting to less nutritious crop mixtures or ones that increase the potential for soil erosion on the hillsides, measures may be needed to counterbalance the negative effects.

This research seeks to evaluate the agricultural strategies used by households in dealing with morbidity and mortality and to determine differences in crop production between households that have experienced a recent adult illness or death from illness and those without adult morbidity or mortality. With 90 percent of the population living in rural and semirural settings and engaged in agriculture, the consequences of illness and death may be reflected in agricultural production, particularly because of a declining labor supply, as suggested by Gillespie (1989).

Several characteristics of rural Rwanda might tend to dampen the potential negative effect on agricultural production of labor lost through adult morbidity and mortality. Given high land scarcity in rural areas, high population densities, population growth, and relatively few off-farm income opportunities, farmers may not be faced with the kind of labor difficulties predicted, even in the face of HIV/AIDS. In addition, Gillespie did not allow for potential household responses to loss of adult labor, such as obtaining additional labor through social networks, attracting new household members, and hiring labor, as found in other studies (Yamano and Jayne 2004; Mather et al. 2004a).

One of the key analytic challenges to understanding possible changes and differences is that of determining what the households affected by death and illness would have been doing if they had not had such traumatic events, to thereby understand the impact of the events. The chapter provides insight on both the research question and the use of a specific research methodology, propensity score matching (PSM), applied in the context of adult mortality and morbidity.

This chapter provides several contributions to the research. It takes earlier theoretical literature about potential effects and empirically tests some of the effects. It uses a nationally representative cross-sectional survey that also has a limited panel set to quantitatively assess impacts. This combination is a relatively low-cost method where annual agricultural surveys are already being conducted. Propensity score matching has been used in the program evaluation literature when experimental design was not possible, but there have been few applications in a development context. This combination of data allows application of PSM to difference in difference estimations in an effort to control for the unobserved differences between households.

This research is also one of the few that looks separately at the effects of HIV/AIDS during the period of adult illness and after an adult death has occurred. As will be noted, the relatively small death effects found in this work may be a reflection that predeath measurements occurred during the illness period, when the household was already adjusting to HIV/AIDS. If the "predeath" measurement of outcome is taken after adult illness has ensued, the households may have already adjusted household assets, crop production, and so on, in which case the "death effect" would underestimate the extent to which the household was initially affected and had to change because adjustments during illness may be later compensated through demographic or other changes in the households. The periods just before and after death may be when some households are feeling and trying to deal with the worst of the shocks and may undertake strategies that lead into a poverty trap. This research demonstrates that measuring the average effects of adult illness and death separately provides a test of how illness and death effects compare and provides insight into the possible need for interventions during illness to mitigate the most severe effects, which cause permanent livelihood declines.

Background

In the early years of the HIV/AIDS epidemic, researchers relied on economic logic to understand the potential impacts of the disease on household structure, production, and livelihoods. In the agricultural sector, major labor scarcities were predicted, both because of the lack of labor contribution by those with AIDS and also because of the need to care for the ill and the pressure to sell production assets to cover medical and burial costs. The loss of skills of the person with AIDS and loss of time for skill transfer to children were all predicted to contribute to severe labor shortages and knowledge loss, which would result in cropping shifts and declines in agricultural production (Topouzis and du Guerny 1999).

Over time, the empirical base to evaluate the morbidity and mortality impacts and the strategies used to minimize them is improving. The early studies were generally of specific locations with high prevalence (e.g., Ainsworth, Ghosh, and Semali 1995), but broad studies over entire countries have also been conducted (Shisana and Simbayi 2002). Qualitative studies that focused on stated adjustment strategies of households are now being complemented by more quantitative studies that seek to measure impact. Longitudinal studies compare households in two or more periods of time (Beegle 2003; Yamano and Jayne 2004). One of the patterns emerging from the literature is the heterogeneity of household response strategies and the impacts of adult mortality, such that the impacts of adult mortality appear to be conditioned by household characteristics such as the gender and role of the deceased, predeath asset levels, and postdeath household composition and community characteristics such as population density and cropping systems (Mather et al. 2004b).

Research in Kenya indicates that the demographics of the household and the gender and role in the household of the person who is ill or had died strongly condition the outcome (Yamano and Jayne 2004). Tanzanian research demonstrates that households change their labor allocations to adapt to illness and death in different ways, and the overall effect on agricultural production will vary (Beegle 2003).[1] In Mozambique, households in the south are larger and less dedicated to agriculture, such that agricultural impacts are thought to be low, whereas in the north with more nuclear-households and a focus on agriculture, the overall agricultural impact may be significant, if the epidemic continues to rise (Mather et al. 2004b).

Understanding Adjustment Strategies of Households

Assessing how households deal with the stress related to HIV/AIDS in rural areas has required new research tools and a multidisciplinary approach. For example, because of the costs and technical demands of assessing HIV status of populations, earlier research in Rwanda and elsewhere has used adults between the ages of 15 and 60 as "prime-age" (PA) adults because they are in sexually active years as well as in their most productive working years. It is this age group that tends to suffer from premature death and that is most likely to be associated with HIV/AIDS, particularly if murder and accidents can be removed as a cause of death.

Donovan et al. (2003) presented the preliminary results from the household survey of 1,520 rural Rwandan households that is analyzed here. During that survey, respondents were asked about what strategies they pursued to respond to the stress of a current PA adult with chronic illness or the death of a PA adult from January 1998 through early 2002. They were also asked about the major impacts the stress had on their agricultural activities. In cases of both illness and death, and regardless of the gender of the person involved, the majority of households cited a loss of farm labor. Among the agricultural strategies, it was logical to find that the strategies cited involved trying to replace lost labor, bringing in new family members or hiring in labor. The declared strategies varied depending on the gender and role of the person who was ill or died. However, there were very few households indicating a shift in cropping mix, although this is often cited in HIV/AIDS literature as a likely strategy (Topouzis and du Guerny 1999).[2]

Simple comparisons of crop production and area in different crops between affected and unaffected households suggested that there had been shifts in production or that there are characteristics of households with PA illness or death that make them more likely to cultivate more sweet potatoes or less coffee, for instance. There may be an underreporting of cropping shifts in the strategy responses, but the stated strategies indicate attempts to maintain agricultural labor supplies. The ex post comparisons of households also showed that the households affected by illness or death did tend to be ex post in the lower two expenditure quartiles (Donovan et al. 2003). One of the concerns raised by the previous work (Donovan et al. 2003) is that some of the shifts may entail more erosive cropping or cropping patterns that suggest substantially lower income generation by affected households. For intervention programs, it will be important to assess this more thoroughly.

Methodology

There is a large body of literature that seeks to understand how programs or events affect people or households. Rosenbaum and Rubin (1983) proposed an evaluation technique called propensity score matching (PSM). The method has seen a recent surge in use, and we employ this method here. Propensity score matching provides an alternative to experimental methods to evaluate program or event effects.[3] To get the true effect of illness or death, we need two things: the outcome of a household with an illness or death (hereafter, an "affected" household) and the outcome of that same household under the same conditions but without illness or death. Because the latter is unobservable, we need to construct a proxy for the missing counterfactual data. Information on each affected household is matched to that of "similar" unaffected households for the same two periods. To determine which households to match, the PSM method evaluates the predicted probability of experiencing an illness or death on the basis of household and local area characteristics. PSM matches each affected household with "similar" unaffected households and uses the outcome of the unaffected households as a proxy for the outcome of the affected household if it had not had an illness or death.

The identification of "similar" is a key feature. There are two aspects to the similarity. First, there may be something about the affected households and why they have a member infected with the HIV virus that makes them different from the general set of households. For example, if a household with a head who has higher than average education is more likely to have a member with HIV, we would want to consider the education of the head (before the trauma) in matching the households. Secondly, if education of the head tends to be a factor determining the outcome, in this case crop production, clearly we would want to compare the outcomes of households with similarly educated heads. Thus, matching entails identifying a set of characteristics that are associated with an increased propensity to have a member with HIV and are likely to influence the outcome, crop production. The better the set of characteristics in accounting for outcome differences in the absence of treatment, the better the chance of eliminating confounding factors that affect the outcome (Becker and Ichino 2002).

Unlike regression approaches using instrumental variables (IV), PSM uses characteristics that have not been affected by the event under study but that are correlated with both the outcome and the event. With HIV/AIDS, it is often difficult to find an appropriate instrument that is unrelated to the outcome of interest. Another benefit of PSM over the IV approaches is that no functional form must be assumed for the relationship between the outcome and the characteristics.[4] However, it is assumed that those characteristics can be mapped into a single number, the propensity score. Rosenbaum and Rubin (1983) show that if the expected outcome in the counterfactual state for an affected household is equal to the expected outcome for an unaffected household, conditional on a set of characteristics, then the expected counterfactual outcome for the affected household is equal to expected outcome for the unaffected household, conditional on that single number, the propensity score.

We estimate the effect of the illness or death on household outcomes for the cases of affected households, not for all households in the general population. This is known in the literature as the average treatment effect on the treated (ATT). For this, we will estimate the counterfactual of what crop production for affected households would have been if no prime-age adult had became ill or died in these households. The estimation of death effects and illness effects will be done separately, so hereafter the estimation strategy will be discussed in terms of the "affected households." Death and illness refer only to those of prime-age adults. Also, the outcome variables to be evaluated are the crop production in 2001/02 (ex post) and the change in crop production from 1999/2000 to 2001/02 for specific crops.

We use a probit model to estimate the propensity score for each household. The dependent variable is an indicator of prime-age death or illness in a household, with separate probit regressions for each type of stress. Recognizing that our estimate of the propensity score is imperfect and that idiosyncratic factors will affect the individual unaffected household outcomes, we estimate the counterfactual outcomes by averaging outcomes across households that come within a set distance of the predicted propensity score for an ill household. This averaging over many similar unaffected households should provide a better estimate of the counterfactual by averaging out unobservable factors affecting both the probability of death and production outcomes (assuming the unobservable factors are not systematically related to the probability of death or illness). This method of estimating the counterfactual is known as radius matching. An additional effort to control for household unobservables is made by calculating the difference in crop production from 2000 to 2002 and then estimating the effects on those differences, as suggested in the work of Smith and Todd (2005) and Wooldridge (2002).[5]

Data

The Department of Agricultural Statistics (DSA) at the Rwandan Ministry of Agriculture, beginning in 1999/2000 and through 2001/02, visited a set of 1,584 Rwandan agricultural households during each of the two main agricultural seasons to detail their crop production and land use during the season. In early 2001, a demographic survey was conducted with these households, including information on age, sex, education, and work activities. In early 2002, the households were again asked about their members, including new members, members who were no longer with the households, and currently ill members. There was no medical testing conducted to determine HIV status. Instead, the chronic illness or death from illness by adults in their prime ages (15–60 years of age) was used to proxy for probable HIV/AIDS presence among ill members (Donovan et al. 2003).

For this analysis, households with a current prime-age adult who was chronically ill (at the time of the FSRP interview in 2002) or those who experienced a prime-age adult death in the previous four years will be compared to households without prime-age adult illness or death ("unaffected households"). Three years of production data are available for the households to capture the main period of effects of illness and at least part of the period of effects of a death. The 1999/2000 crop year had periods of drought and so was not a very good crop year for most households in Rwanda. We expect that production for most crops by households in 2001/02 would have increased because of better rainfall, even if land area dedicated to the crop remained constant. It is how affected households compare to unaffected that will be of interest.

For a variety of reasons, some households were no longer in the sample in 2002, so only 1,520 households were included. To understand the reasons for attrition of households, neighbors and relatives were asked to indicate why a household could no longer be interviewed. In most cases, the informants indicated that people had left to find new land or look for work, but there were a few households that had left because of a death.[6] Additionally, households with incomplete information had to be dropped from the sample. Thus, there remain 1,168 households in the analysis, of which 65 experienced a PA death. In estimating the PSM for illness, households with a death are dropped from the control, and vice versa, to avoid confounding cases.

Propensity Score Estimation Results

The results of the propensity score estimation are presented in Table 6.1 both for the cases of households with a PA illness and for those with a PA death and are based on STATA (2004) programming by Becker and Ichino (2002). Characteristics in each of the probit regressions between death and illness vary (see Annex 6.2). A key reason for exclusion of some variables was the belief that they might not have been measured before the death. Because deaths go back four years and illness goes back only 12 months (with most cases less than that), there are aspects recorded in 2000 that should not be considered "pre-event." Balancing property requirements, based on statistical tests of differences in means between matched and control households, ensure that when groups are matched based on the propensity score, the average characteristics within a group are not significantly different.

As can be seen in Table 6.1, almost the full set of available households was matched with death households. In the case of illness, the common support region (CSR) is narrower, and 30 percent of the unaffected households are excluded from the control group.[7] The characteristics used in the probits are expected to be useful in predicting probability of having a member with AIDS (i.e., being an affected household). As noted earlier, unlike instrumental variables estimations, those characteristics can also be associated with crop production outcomes. For example,

Table 6.1 Coefficients from probit estimates of propensity scores: Propensity to have a PA illness in household or a PA death in household

Characteristics	Prime-age illness in household				Prime-age death in household			
	Coefficient	SE	z	P > |z|	Coefficient	SE	z	P > |z|
Central agricultural zone	0.484	0.193	2.51	0.01	-0.298	0.142	-2.10	0.04
Eastern agricultural zone	0.904	0.221	4.10	0.00	-0.317	0.176	-1.80	0.07
Cellule population (log)	-0.169	0.148	-1.15	0.25	0.144	0.129	1.11	0.27
Cellule with departures greater than arrivals (1 = yes)	0.016	0.155	0.11	0.92	-0.044	0.136	-0.32	0.75
Regular market in cellule (1 = yes)	0.424	0.178	2.39	0.02	0.203	0.158	1.29	0.20
Newly forested areas in last 12 months (1 = yes)	0.203	0.141	1.43	0.15	-0.220	0.131	-1.67	0.10
Access to primary market good more than 4 km	0.561	0.227	2.47	0.01	0.148	0.200	0.74	0.46
Health center (1 = yes)	-0.030	0.170	-0.18	0.86	0.222	0.134	1.66	0.10
Churches (number)	-0.208	0.122	-1.70	0.09	-0.140	0.091	-1.54	0.12
Access to rural credit in cellule (1 = yes)	-0.172	0.170	-1.01	0.31	0.065	0.141	0.46	0.64
Access to farmer association in cellule (1 = yes)	0.196	0.215	0.91	0.36	0.049	0.181	0.27	0.79
Use of fertilizers and pesticides in cellule (1 = yes)	0.502	0.167	3.01	0.00	-0.149	0.137	-1.09	0.28
Sex of household imputed head in 1999 (1 = male; 2 = female)	0.284	0.167	1.70	0.09	0.200	0.137	1.46	0.14
Age of head in 1999	-0.003	0.005	-0.65	0.52	-0.001	0.004	-0.15	0.88
Head completed primary school in 1999 (1 = yes)	0.021	0.171	0.12	0.90	-0.144	0.164	-0.88	0.38
Head is either married or separated (1999)	0.454	0.156	2.91	0.00	-0.400	0.148	-2.69	0.01
Household uses manure/pesticides	-0.102	0.182	-0.56	0.58	na			
Number of rooms in house > 4 (1 = yes)	0.104	0.188	0.55	0.58	0.216	0.153	1.41	0.16
Total income in 2000 (log)	-0.105	0.058	-1.79	0.07	na			
Residence in cellule for more than 8 years (1 = yes)	-0.395	0.157	-2.52	0.01	0.147	0.132	1.12	0.26
Household member has received remittances (1 = yes)	-0.056	0.137	-0.41	0.68	na			
Household has paid for transport (1 = yes)	0.567	0.186	3.05	0.00	na			
Constant	-0.632	1.252	-0.50	0.61	-2.466	0.931	-2.65	0.01
Number of observations	1,129				1,168			
Log likelihood	-210.98				-265.135			
LR chi^2 (22)	75.33				42.59			
Probability > chi^2	0				0.0009			
Pseudo R^2	0.1515				0.0743			

having a regular market in the community may be related to higher contacts outside the home and also might be associated with higher incentives for agricultural production for surplus sales. Those households that have lived in the area since before the genocide in 1994 may have greater stability in both land and household members. One of the puzzling results is that households in central and eastern zones tend to have higher illness prevalence but lower death prevalence than those households in western zones.

Estimated Effects of Illness for Households Experiencing Illness

The PSM of affected households with unaffected control households within the common support region identified significant differences for the total crop production in 2001/02 of selected main crops and for the change in crop production of those crops from 1999/2000 to 2001/02. The ex post total production helps us to understand if the households are significantly different after the effects of illness or death are felt. We look at production changes over time to allow for the possibility that ill households had different starting points of production. As suggested earlier, if ill and nonill households differed in their initial production levels (on average), we would mistakenly attribute this difference to having an ill prime-age adult if we looked only at the ex post results.

Ex Post Level of Crop Production

Table 6.2 shows that for beans, peas, maize, cassava, Irish potatoes, cooking bananas, fruit bananas, and coffee, there were no significant estimated effects of illness on production in 2001/02. However, beer bananas (a cash crop) showed a significantly lower total production amount for households with illness compared to households without illness. Beer bananas require processing generally completed by women, so as the labor demands on women to care for the ill increase and labor declines because of illness among women, this would be expected.

Sweet potato production for households experiencing illness was significantly higher than production for households without illness. Sweet potatoes play a key role in consumption in Rwanda (Tardiff-Douglin 1991), and they have a labor advantage in production. The labor demands for sweet potatoes are not necessarily lower than those for other crops, but the timing of labor is more flexible, as harvesting can take place over time, and planting can be timed outside the main planting period for other crops. That flexibility makes it an important food security crop, and households with an illness are cropping up to an average of 531 kilograms more than comparable households.

Table 6.2 Matching estimates of the effects on production in 2002 for selected crops: Average treatment effect (ATT) on households with a prime-age adult illness (in kilograms)

Crop	Beans	Peas	Maize	Cassava	Irish potato	Sweet potato	Cooking banana	Beer banana	Fruit banana	Coffee
ATT	30.25	−0.05	−16.80	−2.61	26.73	531.18	−118.42	−64.64	71.59	−0.32
t-statistic	0.83	−0.02	−0.69	−0.02	0.11	2.54***	−1.43	−1.78*	1.63	−0.05
Households with illness	64	64	64	64	64	64	64	64	64	64
Control households	753	753	753	753	753	753	753	753	753	753
Average control production	161.26	8.19	81.50	507.39	251.81	905.53	520.50	281.57	118.01	17.88

Source: DSA data, 2002. Estimates based on propensity score specification found in Table 6.1.

Notes: Controls refers to the number of households without prime-age illness who form the basis for the counterfactuals. Radius of 0.01 was used for matching. Significance of t: *, **, *** indicate 0.10, 0.05, and 0.01 significance levels, respectively.

Changes in Crop Production

The changes in crop production from one period to the next reflect a difference-in-differences approach, for the changes are contrasted between the affected and unaffected households (Table 6.3). As expected with the improved climatic condition in 2001/02, the control households increased their production of all the major commodities. The effect of illness on beer banana and sweet potato production remains strong. Households with an illness experienced higher growth in sweet potato production and much lower growth/recuperation in production of beer bananas. In general, illness households increased sweet potato production by more than 450 kilograms over the increase experienced by similar unaffected households. Beer bananas increased only 43 percent of the increase experienced by the control households. Because beer bananas have been a major source of income for women (Kangasniemi 1998), this result implies a relative decline in women's income-earning potential in the affected households compared to the control households. Additionally, coffee production declined significantly among households with illness over the period.

Estimated Effects of Death on Crop Production for Households Experiencing Death

Households experiencing a death show few significant differences in crop production as compared to matched nonaffected households without a death or illness. This tends to follow the descriptive analysis in Donovan et al. (2003), indicating that households with a death appear to be quite similar to those without a death in the period after a death.

Ex Post Level of Crop Production

Table 6.4 shows the results of evaluating the difference in levels of production in 2001/02 between those households with and without a death. All crops show lower production amounts for households with a death, but with variability between households, significant differences are found only for beans, beer bananas, and fruit bananas. The difference in bean production might be important for beans are a key food security crop for Rwandan households, and the average household production per control household for 2002 was 150 kilograms of beans (Table 6.4), so this reflects 18 percent lower production levels in affected households. The banana shifts indicate lower income potential with the lower production for beer bananas of 31 percent, and there is a strong 38 percent difference in fruit bananas, compared to control households. Again, if production shifts occur in years of illness, before death, our analysis does not capture that effect.

Table 6.3 Matching estimates of the effects on change in production from 1999 to 2002 for selected crops: Average treatment effect (ATT) on households with a prime-age adult illness (in kilograms)

Crop	Beans	Peas	Maize	Cassava	Irish potato	Sweet potato	Cooking banana	Beer banana	Fruit banana	Coffee
ATT	20.99	0.74	−21.19	101.12	−72.23	467.88	−102.65	−205.40	−35.81	−9.31
t-statistic	0.60	0.24	−0.79	0.73	−0.96	2.45***	−1.57	−1.82*	−0.87	−1.79*
Households with illness	64	64	64	64	64	64	64	64	64	64
Control households	753	753	753	753	753	753	753	753	753	753
Average control production change	41.93	2.33	43.38	10.20	84.46	243.14	307.00	361.17	58.85	9.25

Source: DSA data, 2002. Estimates based on propensity score specification found in Table 6.1.

Notes: Controls refers to the number of households without prime-age illness who form the basis for the counterfactuals. Radius of 0.01 was used for matching. Significance of t: *, **, *** indicate 0.10, 0.05, and 0.01 significance levels, respectively.

Table 6.4 Matching estimates of the effects on production in 2002 for selected crops: Average treatment effect (ATT) on households with a death (in kilograms)

Crop	Beans	Peas	Maize	Cassava	Irish potato	Sweet potato	Cooking banana	Beer banana	Fruit banana	Coffee
ATT	−27.62	−2.60	−10.79	−108.46	−45.71	−75.83	−112.53	−88.06	−40.204	−5.42
t-statistic	−1.87*	−1.29	−0.67	−1.43	−0.34	−0.55	−0.89	−3.10***	−2.648***	−0.83
Households with a death	77	77	77	77	77	77	77	77	77	77
Control households	1,046	1,046	1,046	1,046	1,046	1,046	1,046	1,046	1,046	1,046
Average control production	150.38	9.50	86.13	506.40	262.06	830.42	443.86	282.07	106.75	19.44

Source: DSA data, 2002. Estimates based on propensity score specification found in Table 6.1.

Notes: Controls refers to the number of households without prime-age death who form the basis for the counterfactuals. Radius of 0.01 was used for matching. Significance of t: *, **, *** indicate 0.10, 0.05, and 0.01 significance levels, respectively.

Crop Production Changes

Table 6.5 presents the results of analysis on the changes in production quantities from 1999/2000 to 2001/02. As expected because of the improved climatic conditions between the two years, the control households increased their production of both bananas along with sweet potatoes and the other crops. The affected households showed significant differences only in beer and fruit bananas. Those bananas do not show the production growth found in other households. For erosion, this is not a good sign, and there is no indication that less erosive crops supplanted the bananas, although income potential clearly declines as fewer of these types of bananas are produced. Contrary to conventional expectation that affected households shift into labor-flexible or laborsaving crops such as cassava and sweet potato, we do not find an increase in cassava and sweet potato production among affected households.

Implications and Conclusions

This chapter presents an application of PSM to the measurement of the impacts of adult illness and death on crop production in Rwanda. We use a combination of cross-sectional and panel data to construct the counterfactual required to estimate these impacts. This application demonstrates that, given appropriate variables and sample size, PSM enables analysts to estimate the impacts of adult illness and death using cross-sectional data with recall complemented with a small amount of panel information. Although panel data are preferred for the econometric estimation of impacts, governments and development practitioners cannot always wait for the ideal data to inform local policy decisions.

Given the small subsample size of illness and death, we did not differentiate impacts conditional on gender or household position of the deceased, as has been done elsewhere (Yamano and Jayne 2004). Yet this research highlights an important differentiation that has not received much attention to date in the quantitative impact literature, the distinction between production impacts during the illness period as compared with those in the postdeath period.

These results suggest that accurate measurement of the impact of adult death depends on when measurements are taken. Although there have been a few studies that look at different periods after death, the impacts for the illness period have rarely been evaluated. If major shifts occur during the period of illness that are difficult to reverse, such as removal of tree crops, intervention strategies may need to be designed with this specifically in mind. Other research is needed to see if changes during illness also involve asset sales that could lead to permanent changes. If irreversible changes tend to occur during the illness period, it is extremely important

Table 6.5 Matching estimates of the effects on change in production from 1999 to 2002 for selected crops: Average treatment effect (ATT) on households with a death (in kilograms)

Crop	Beans	Peas	Maize	Cassava	Irish potato	Sweet potato	Cooking banana	Beer banana	Fruit banana	Coffee
ATT	−6.89	−1.72	−0.83	8.81	48.25	−209.96	−78.58	−198.91	−41.17	−4.97
t-statistic	−0.51	−0.94	−0.04	0.10	0.38	−1.26	−0.75	−3.01***	−2.49***	−0.94
Households with a death	77	77	77	77	77	77	77	77	77	77
Control households	1,046	1,046	1,046	1,046	1,046	1,046	1,046	1,046	1,046	1,046
Average control production change	40.65	3.76	36.82	38.73	73.21	172.70	267.50	361.74	55.69	7.79

Source: DSA data, 2002. Estimates based on propensity score specification found in Table 6.1.

Notes: Controls refers to the number of households without prime-age death who form the basis for the counterfactuals. Radius of 0.01 was used for matching. Significance of *t*: *, **, *** indicate 0.10, 0.05, and 0.01 significance levels, respectively.

for intervention strategies to be designed for this period. This may also point to the important role that antiretroviral drugs may play in giving households greater time to adjust, potentially diminishing the irreversible loss of assets.

Regarding the measured impacts, over the illness period, we find relative increases in sweet potato production for ill households and shifts out of beer bananas and coffee. The latter imply lower cash income, and the sweet potato spreads labor demand and provides subsistence production. If banana and coffee trees are replaced with annual crops, that will increase soil erosion problems over time. Investments in sweet potato productivity, however, would have positive results for the affected households while at the same time contributing to welfare across Rwandan rural households, a clear case for increased agricultural research and extension.

Death appears to induce shifts out of beer and fruit bananas only, indicating the possible longer-term shift out of tree crops when households are under stress and the consequent reduction in cash income and in erosion protection. We did not find significant effects on other crops. This suggests that labor shortages among affected households looking over time are not as great as suggested by some of the theoretical literature because households adjust their labor demands and supplies. With a larger sample, effects conditional on gender and/or household position might be found, for other research indicates that some households are less likely to bring in replacement labor or recuperate from crises. The high population density and land scarcity in Rwanda may be one of the factors conditioning how households respond, limiting their flexibility in agriculture and thus resulting in relatively lower cropping impacts after a death than have been found in other regions.

Annex 6.1 Special Issues in Data for Propensity Score Matching

This data set lends itself to using the PSM and difference-in-differences estimation for several reasons. First, the households were derived from a random sample with clustering, and so both affected and unaffected come from the same population. Second, because the households were all asked the same questions during the same period, we do not experience some of the difficulties found in the traditional matching literature where different sampling and surveys are used for households that participated in training and those that did not (e.g., Smith and Todd 2001). Finally, although the panel on production is brief, it still provides a basis for controlling for household-level time-invariant characteristics. The dataset also includes a fairly rich set of variables on which to match households, including community-level variables, important to achieve unbiased results (Diaz and Handa 2004).

There are some challenges in using these data. A key difficulty is that the number of cases of affected households is relatively small (65 cases of illness and 78 cases of death). Bryson, Dorsett, and Purdon (2002) looked at various studies with small treatment samples and suggested that the method is still valuable when sample numbers are low, although the matching is more difficult. In this case, the radius matching used a radius of 0.01, a fairly broad band. In addition, matching with replacement enabled unaffected households to be matched with more than one affected household if its propensity score was within the bounds.

Estimating the ATT rather than the average treatment effect (ATE) for all households was selected to respond to another potentially difficult issue. PSM is based on the mean stable unit treatment value assumption, in which "the impact of the program on one person does not depend on whom else, or how many others are in the programme" (Bryson, Dorsett, and Purdon 2002, p. 11). In the case of HIV/AIDS in highly affected communities, this would not be true, and looking at the general effects with ATE is clearly not justified.

Another issue is that of the common support region (CSR). Basically, the analysis matches affected households to unaffected households within the ranges of overlap between the predicted propensity scores of the treated and untreated households. Unaffected households with values of the matching characteristics that are much higher or lower than that observed within the affected households are excluded from the analysis. The same is true for affected households. In small datasets, this can mean a fairly restricted number of matches. It also means that interpretation of the results is confined to households within the CSR. If income is one of the characteristics and all the affected households have total incomes below 500,000 Rwandan francs, then the CSR will not extend to higher-income households if their probability of being affected lies outside the range (Bryson, Dorsett, and Purdon, 2002).

PSM relies on having pre-event variables or characteristics that are unaffected by the event under study on which to match the households. In the case of illness in these data, 82 percent of the cases of illness were ill for less than 25 weeks of the previous year (as measured in 2002), such that the production data from 1999/2000 would be from before the onset of severe illness. In the case of a death from illness, using the 1999/2000 production and other data is more tenuous, for the onset of illness would be before 2000, and effects of the illness may already be reflected in those early estimates. This is a common problem for HIV/AIDS researchers because the time span involved can be long, and the effects are felt throughout illness and after death. Given these caveats, the results of the PSM for households with illness and death are reported below.

Annex 6.2

Table 6.6   Mean characteristics by household type for households in the common support region for characteristics included in the propensity score

	Households with death	Control households	Households with illness	Control households
Community-level variables				
Central agricultural zone	0.32	0.39	0.38	0.44
Eastern agricultural zone	0.17	0.23	0.46	0.32
Cellule departures greater than arrivals (1 = yes)	0.37	0.40	0.51	0.44
Regular market in cellule (1 = yes)	0.21	0.18	0.25	0.21
Newly forested areas in last 12 months (1 = yes)	0.31	0.38	0.49	0.39
Health center (1 = yes)	0.46	0.34	0.35	0.29
Access to rural credit in cellule (1 = yes)	0.26	0.28	0.25	0.26
Access to farmer association in cellule (1 = yes)	0.87	0.84	0.88	0.85
Use of fertilizers/pesticides in cellule (1 = yes)	0.40	0.45	0.52	0.52
Cellule population (log)	6.81	6.75	6.74	6.71
Churches in cellule (number)	0.51	0.54	0.37	0.40
Characteristics of head before event[a]				
Proportion female	0.50	0.31	0.29	0.31
Completed primary school (1 = yes)	0.17	0.22	0.25	0.24
Head is either married or separated (1999)	0.23	0.42	0.60	0.47
Age of pretreatment head in 1999	43	42	41	43
Household level variables before event				
Household uses manure/pesticides	na	na	0.18	0.18
Household has received remittances	na	na	0.60	0.57
Household has paid for transport (1 = yes)	na	na	0.22	0.10
Distance to primary market (km)	1.83	1.71	2.40	1.77
Number of rooms in house	3.60	3.58	3.77	3.54
Total income in 2000	na	na	141,058	159,603
Length of residence in cellule	10.44	9.40	7.83	8.27
N	78	1,051	65	761

Notes: [a]Some data imputed. Control households represent only those households from the nonillness, nondeath households in the full sample that were matched using propensity score matching, radius of 0.01. "na" indicates variables not included in death estimates.

Notes

This research has been funded through USAID/Rwanda Mission and USAID/Bureau for Africa and the Bureau of Economic Growth, Agriculture and Trade. For more information on this research and other MSU research on adult mortality in Sub-Saharan Africa, see the website http://www.aec.msu.edu/fs2/adult_death/index.htm.

1. Beegle's (2003) research in Tanzania is one of the few studies that looks at households with a view to separating effects evidenced recently after a death as compared to longer (more than six

months) after a death. It also looks at labor allocation, a key aspect, infrequently addressed in the research.

2. For further evaluation of strategies and ex post household characteristics, see Donovan et al. (2003).

3. Bryson, Dorsett, and Purdon (2002) provides an excellent review of the use of propensity scores, and Wooldridge (2002) gives the econometric details of the method, as well as additional insights on its use and limitations. Jalan and Ravallion (2003) apply the method in a developing country context.

4. DiPrete and Gangl (2004) provide a valuable comparison between PSM and IV estimations and ways to evaluate each. They are seen as complementary analyses, not necessarily substitutes.

5. Annex 6.1 presents some special data considerations for propensity score matching, as used with these data.

6. See Donovan et al. (2003) for further information on sampling and sample attrition.

7. Annex 6.2, Table 6.6 presents the information on values of the characteristics for the affected and control households, based on those within the CSR.

References

Ainsworth, M., S. Ghosh, and I. Semali. 1995. *The impact of adult deaths on household composition in Kagera Region, Tanzania.* Unpublished manuscript, Policy Research Department. Washington, D.C.: World Bank.

Becker, S. O., and A. Ichino. 2002. Estimation of average treatment effects based on propensity scores. *STATA Journal* 2 (4): 358–377.

Beegle, K. 2003. *Labor effects of adult mortality in Tanzanian households.* World Bank Policy Research Working Paper 3062. Washington, D.C.: World Bank.

Bryson, A., R. Dorsett, and S. Purdon. 2002. *The use of propensity score matching in the evaluation of active labour market policies. A study carried out on behalf of the Department for Work and Pensions.* London: Policy Studies Institute and National Centre for Social Research.

Diaz, J. J., and S. Handa. 2004. *An assessment of propensity score matching as a non experimental impact estimator: Evidence from a Mexican poverty program.* Draft available at http://www.unc.edu/%7Eshanda/research/diaz_handa_matching.pdf.

DiPrete, T. A., and M. Gangl. 2004. Assessing bias in the estimation of causal effects: Rosenbaum bounds on matching estimators and instrumental variables estimation with imperfect instruments. *Sociological Methodology* 34 (1): 277–310.

Donovan, C., L. Bailey, E. Mpyisi, and M. Weber. 2003. *Prime-age adult morbidity and mortality in rural Rwanda: Effects on household income, agricultural production, and food security strategies.* Kigali: Food Security Research Project/MINAGRI.

Gillespie, S. 1989. Potential impacts of AIDS on farming systems: A case study from Rwanda. *Land Use Policy* 4 (October): 301–312. Available at www.fao.org/sd/PE1101_en.html.

Jalan, J., and M. Ravallion. 2003. Does piped water reduce diarrhea for children in rural India? *Journal of Econometrics* 112: 153–173.

Kangasniemi, J. 1998. *People and bananas on steep slopes: Agricultural intensification and food security under demographic pressure and environmental degradation in Rwanda.* Unpublished dissertation, Michigan State University.

Mather, D., C. Donovan, T. Jayne, M. Weber, E. Mazhangara, L. Bailey, K. Yoo, T. Yamano, and E. Mghenyi. 2004a. *A cross-country analysis of household responses to adult mortality in rural Sub-Saharan Africa.* MSU International Development Working Paper No. 82, Draft for Review. East Lansing, Mich.: Department of Agricultural Economics, MSU.

Mather, D., H. Marrule, C. Donovan, M. Weber, and A. Alage. 2004b. *Analysis of adult mortality within rural households in Mozambique and implications for policy.* Research Report 58E. Maputo: Department of Policy Analysis, Directorate of Economics, MADER.

Rosenbaum, P., and D. Rubin. 1983. The central role of the propensity score in observational studies for causal effect. *Biometrika* 7 (1): 41–55.

Shisana, O., and L. Simbayi. 2002. *Nelson Mandela/HSRC study of HIV/AIDS: South African national HIV prevalence, behavioral risks and mass media, household survey 2002.* Johannesburg: Nelson Mandela Foundation and Human Sciences Research Council.

Smith, J., and P. Todd. 2001. Reconciling conflicting evidence on the performance of propensity-score matching methods. *American Economic Review* 91 (2): 112–118.

———. 2005. Does matching overcome Lalonde's critique of nonexperimental estimators? *Journal of Econometrics* 125 (1-2): 305–353.

STATA Corporation. 2004. STATA version 8.2 software. College Station, Tex.: STATA.

Tardiff-Douglin, D. 1991. *The role of sweet potato in Rwanda's food system: The transition from subsistence orientation to market orientation.* Bethesda, Md.: Developmental Alternatives Incorporated (DAI).

Topouzis, D., and J. du Guerny. 1999. *Sustainable agricultural/rural development and vulnerability to the AIDS epidemic.* FAO and UNAIDS joint publication. UNAIDS Best Practice Collection. Rome: FAO. December.

Wooldridge, J. 2002. *Econometric analysis of cross-section and panel data.* Cambridge, Mass.: MIT Press.

Yamano, T., and T. S. Jayne. 2004. Measuring the impacts of working-age adult mortality on small-scale farm households in Kenya. *World Development* 32 (1): 91–119.

Chapter 7

Chronically Ill Households, Food Security, and Coping Strategies in Rural Zimbabwe

Shannon Senefeld and Ken Polsky

Introduction

The more we learn about the interaction between HIV/AIDS and livelihoods, the more complex the picture seems to become. Although we must avoid paralysis in the face of such complexity, we must also be humble about our perceptions. We must look closely at the local context and the diverse external factors in addition to HIV and AIDS that constrain households and livelihoods at any given time.

Limited information exists on the actual impacts of HIV/AIDS on coping strategies and how to operationalize programming to respond to any impacts that do exist. This research aimed to identify how HIV/AIDS impacts coping strategies in rural Zimbabwe and how these impacts could be factored into the design of humanitarian programs. To further our understanding of the relationships between HIV/AIDS and livelihood security in rural Zimbabwe, we isolated and analyzed a number of different variables.

Methodology and Design

The data in this study, collected in April 2003 in rural Zimbabwe as part of an emergency response project, C-SAFE,[1] are from the project baseline survey and were used for secondary data analysis in this study. C-SAFE and the United Nations World Food Programme collaborated on the design and implementation of the study and related tools.

Data Collection

One comprehensive survey was used for all sampled households. The survey was a self-report measure that included basic demographic data, the number of household members, presence of chronically ill people, number of orphans within the household, and other basic data regarding the household as well as information on each household's assets. An asset wealth variable was created within quartiles within the respondent population. In addition, a coping strategies index (CSI) was adapted for use within the survey.

Coping Strategies Index

Developed by CARE and field tested by the World Food Programme (WFP) and CARE, the CSI has been used for early warning and food security assessments in eight African countries and has proven to be an accurate index of food security (Maxwell et al. 1999; Christiansen and Boisvert 2000). The CSI provides a quantitative score for each household that is a cumulative measure of the degree of coping and, thus, a measure of food insecurity. In similar studies in six countries in the Greater Horn of Africa, the CSI has been found to be an accurate indicator of household food security. The CSI has been used to monitor household food security in emergencies as well as to assess the impact of various food aid interventions.

The CSI measures frequency and severity of a household's coping strategies for dealing with shortfalls in food supply. Data are weighted according to frequency and perceived severity of behavior, determined by community members in focus groups. Weighted scores are combined into an index that reflects current and perceived future food security status. Comparison of scores and averages provides a summary of overall household food security and establishes a baseline for monitoring drought trends and impact of interventions (Maxwell et al. 1999).

The coping strategies index includes four categories of strategies: consumption, expenditure, income, and migration. Consumption strategies include buying food on credit, relying on less-preferred maize substitutes, reducing the number of meals eaten per day, regularly skipping food for an entire day, eating meals comprised solely of vegetables, eating unusual wild foods, restricting consumption of adults so children can eat normally, and feeding working members at the expense of nonworking members. Expenditure strategies include avoiding health care or education costs in order to buy food. Income strategies include selling household and livelihood assets such as livestock. Migration strategies include sending children to relatives' or friends' homes or migrating to find work.

The CSI is an inverse measure. Increased use of coping strategies indicates a decrease in food security. Likewise, a decrease in food security results in increased frequency and severity of coping strategies. Thus, an analysis of coping strategies indicates a decreasing food security situation when coping strategies accelerate from temporary measures (e.g., reduction in number or quality of meals for a brief, defined time period) from which a household can recover to measures that undermine future lives and livelihoods and damage social, financial, physical, or natural assets irreversibly.

Sample Frame

The study employed a two-stage random sampling methodology, selecting a total of 1,625 rural households in Zimbabwe. Several strata were considered, including districts and types of households based on livelihoods (TANGO 2003). Because prior information was not available on all strata, the design and sampling frames were based on administrative boundaries. Sampling frames were derived from current household lists. All households residing in rural areas were eligible to be sampled. Urban areas were excluded because they were not targeted for C-SAFE interventions.

First-stage selection focused on wards within districts proportional to population; the second stage involved random selection of households within wards (TANGO 2003).

The sample size was calculated using the following formula:

$$n = \frac{z^2 pq}{d^2} \qquad (7.1)$$

where n = sample size, z = statistical certainty desired, p = estimated prevalence rate, $q = 1 - p$ (proportion without the attribute of interest), and d = degree of precision. The desired precision (d) was set at 8 percent (0.08), and the statistical certainty was set at 95 percent ($z = 1.96$). Because the general prevalence rate of key variables was not known, the value of p was set at 50 percent (0.5) to maximize the impact of this variable on sample size. Thus, the resulting sample size per district (n) was 180, and the overall resulting sample size was 1,620 (TANGO 2003).

Analysis

The survey specifically requested information on the presence of chronically ill individuals within the household. Chronically ill households are defined as households with at least one family member of any age who had been ill for more than 3 months during the 12 months preceding the survey.

The survey results were analyzed using SPSS. Basic demographics are reported for all survey respondents. Bivariate correlations were conducted on several variables. In addition, multivariate analyses were used to determine predictive relationships, and t-tests, ANOVA, and chi-square tests were conducted to determine differences between groups.

Results

A total of 1,625 households were surveyed in rural Zimbabwe. Of the participating households, 73.5 percent were headed by men, and 26.5 percent were female-headed. Approximately 6.5 percent of elderly-headed households reported no other adult members within the household. Only 21 (1.3 percent) of the 1,625 households reported a head of household under 19 years of age, with only one of these households with the head under 15 years of age. The majority of the households were headed by someone aged 40 to 59 years, and the majority of heads of household were married (72.5 percent). Approximately 20 percent of the heads of household reported being widowed. More than 68 percent of respondents reported having between four and eight household members. Slightly less than two-thirds of households reported having at least one child under 5 years of age, and approximately 83 percent of households reported having at least one child aged 6 to 18. Male adults were more noticeably absent from households than female adults, as 33.9 percent of respondents reported no adult men aged 20–59 in the household, whereas only 13.8 percent of these households reported no female adults in the same age category. Approximately 35 percent of the households reported at least one orphan under the age of 15 was living in the household at the time of the survey. Nearly 95 percent of the surveyed households reported having lived in their current communities for at least one year before the survey.

Chronically Ill Households versus Nonaffected Households

Surprisingly, there was no significant difference between chronically ill (CI) households and non-CI households in gender of household head. Chronically ill households were positively correlated with larger families ($r = 0.11$, $P\ 0.01$) and having children aged 5–14 drop out of school ($r = 0.11$, $P\ 0.001$). CI households were also more likely to have experienced the death of a child under 5 during the last 12 months, $\chi^2(2, N = 1,622) = 34.3$, $P < 0.001$, as well as the death of an adult household member, $\chi^2(3, N = 1,619) = 127$, $P < 0.001$. Households that reported the head of household dying within the last 12 months were also positively correlated with sending children away to friends and/or relatives ($r = 0.23$, $P < 0.05$).

On coping, overall, there was a significant difference between CI and non-CI households. The presence of chronically ill persons in the household was a significant predictor of the overall coping strategies sum, $\beta = 0.057$, $t(1,611) = 2.3$,

$P < 0.05$. To repeat, there is an inverse relationship between use of coping strategies and food security. Coping strategies were also dependent on asset wealth of the household, $\beta = -0.135$, $t(1,611) = -5.48$, $P < 0.001$. Surprisingly, however, there was no significant difference between CI and non-CI households in terms of overall asset wealth. However, because this was a one-time survey, it does not capture previous declines in asset wealth, which may have occurred within CI households.

Chronically ill households were more likely to report an avoidance of education costs [$\chi^2(2, N = 1,624) = 17.4$, $P < 0.001$], a reduction of spending on healthcare costs in order to purchase food [$\chi^2(2, N = 1,624) = 12.17$, $P < 0.01$], and a reduction of spending on agricultural and livestock inputs [$\chi^2(2, N = 1,624) = 19.85$, $P < 0.001$]. There was a near-significant correlation between CI households and whether household crops or livestock had been stolen ($P = 0.08$).

Households with at least one chronically ill member living in the household were more likely than other households to skip days without eating [$t(1,623) = -2.44$, $P < 0.05$], eat less preferred foods [$t(1,622) = -2.02$, $P < 0.05$], rely on wild foods for meals [$t(1,617) = -2.87$, $P < 0.01$], reduce adult consumption of food so children could eat [$t(1,620) = -2.25$, $P < 0.05$], and prioritize food within the household for working household members rather than nonworking members [$t(1,623) = 2.87$, $P < 0.01$].

Demographic Analysis of Chronically Ill Households

Of the 1,625 households surveyed, 27 percent (440) were chronically ill, affected households, having at least one CI, of any age, present in the household. The majority of households ($n = 395$) reported adult CI, but an additional 91 households reported a child CI. Of the 91 households with a child CI, approximately half ($n = 45$) were in households where no adult CI was present.

Of these chronically ill, affected households, approximately 72 percent had a male head of household. Mean household size was 7.2 members, and 40.5 percent reported household members older than 60 years of age. However, only 7.5 percent were headed by someone older than 60 with no additional household members aged 18–59. CI households included a mean of 1.1 children under 5 years of age (SD = 1.19) and 2.2 children aged 5–14 (SD = 1.55). Forty-two percent of households hosted at least one orphan under the age of 15, and approximately 20 percent of households supported more than one orphan.

Approximately 20 percent of households reported children aged 5–14 dropping out of school, with the most commonly cited reason being inability to pay school fees (72 percent). Nearly 40 percent of households cultivated less land than they did in the previous growing season. Reasons included lack of labor (16.4 percent), lack of rainfall (62.9 percent), lack of draft power (52 percent), lack of fertilizer (19.5 percent), and lack of seed (52.9 percent).

More than three-quarters (79 percent) of households reported skipping meals at least one day a week as a means to deal with their food shortages. More than half (55 percent) reported restricting adult consumption so that children could eat normally. More than one-quarter (25.3 percent) reported eating wild foods at least one time per week. More than half (58 percent) of households reported spending less money on educational costs. A small portion of households (12 percent) reported prioritizing household consumption for working household members.

Of these chronically ill households, 35.5 percent were categorized as asset very poor, and 42.3 percent were asset poor. Only 4.8 percent were asset rich, and 17.5 percent were asset intermediate. In order to understand the differences among these chronically ill affected households, analyses of variance were conducted among the asset wealth range to determine differences among the households and their wealth ranking. There was a significant relationship between the gender of the head of household and asset wealth, with female-headed households more likely to be asset poor or very poor, $F(3,436) = 6.26$, $P < 0.001$. Asset wealth also related to children aged 5–14 leaving school, with lower-asset households more likely to report children dropping out of school, $F(3,436) = 6.11$, $P < 0.001$. Households that were asset poor or asset very poor were also significantly related to a lack of draft power ($P < 0.001$) and lack of fertilizer, $F(3,344) = 5.55$, $P < 0.001$, as main reasons for uncultivated land.

In terms of coping strategies, asset-poor and asset–very poor households were significantly correlated with eating less preferred foods ($P < 0.05$), skipping days without eating ($P < 0.05$), eating wild foods ($P < 0.05$), and eating vegetables only ($P < 0.05$). There was also a significant relationship between poor households and the presence of a household member who had been ill within the past two weeks ($P < 0.05$).

Surprisingly, there was no direct, significant relationship between asset wealth and presence of orphans or elderly-headed households.

Limitations

One of the main limitations for research focusing on HIV/AIDS is the inability to identify people living with HIV or AIDS. Thus, most research now uses "chronically ill" as a proxy indicator for HIV infection. Initial analyses indicate that this overestimates incidence of HIV infection. Barrère (2005) examined the use of this proxy indicator and found that, based on national infection rates, only 54 percent of a chronically ill sample in Malawi were likely to have HIV or AIDS.

However, given that 24 percent of households responded that there was in fact chronic illness in the household, and the estimated prevalence rate in Zimbabwe was 24.6 percent (UNAIDS 2004), we can assume that CI is an appropriate proxy indicator for this Zimbabwe sample.

The data analyzed here were collected for an emergency project intervention, which was designed to respond to the emergent needs of the affected population. The collection of the data, therefore, was designed to yield relevant information for programmers to design appropriate interventions for the affected population while also allowing the project implementers to track changes within the targeted population. Because the primary objective of the data collection was to inform programming priorities, the data collected may be somewhat different from data collected for an academic exercise.

For example, because this information was collected for an emergency project intervention, only certain geographic areas of Zimbabwe were represented in the sample. These data cannot be considered representative of urban populations, for example, nor perhaps of those pockets of vulnerable households in the better-off districts. They are representative, however, of those areas of the country most affected by food insecurity.

Moreover, because these data were intended to be used as a monitoring tool for an emergency development project, respondents were interviewed only once. However, a longitudinal study would have served as a better design for understanding the impact of chronic illness on household food security and coping strategies. Although the same areas of the country were revisited for additional annual interviews, the same respondents were not tracked over time. The results of such a longitudinal design may yield even greater descriptive data on the impact of HIV/ AIDS within the household over time.

Under an emergency program, there are additional constraints on data collection and analysis. In addition to the sampling constraints and data collection methods, project implementers are also bound by budgetary and time constraints. Within an emergency response project, program implementers are required to move at a rapid pace and within accepted budgetary parameters, often prioritizing existing funds to program activities rather than larger data collection designs. This, in turn, affects the analyses that can be performed on the resulting data set.

Finally, although the use of CSI and total physical assets makes the data set sensitive to short-term adaptations to stress, our understanding of the long-term impacts of HIV and AIDS on livelihood strategies, as well as the impact of those livelihood strategies on HIV and AIDS, will be aided by tools derived from the CRS Integral Human Development Framework.

Discussion

This analysis of the coping strategies employed by chronically ill households adds a foundation of evidence to many of the hypotheses regarding the livelihood impacts of HIV and AIDS but challenges others. The resulting recommendations are primarily in the areas of targeting, program design, and directions for subsequent research.

First of all, the presence of chronic illness or orphans at the household level has been found to be insufficient as a targeting criterion, as these factors were not found to correlate with asset wealth. Furthermore, these results show the need for a specific vulnerability scale within chronically ill, affected households. If the CSI is used as a selection criterion for all food security interventions, these households could easily be identified. However, often a large project cannot administer such tools to all potential beneficiaries. Instead, there is a need to look at appropriate indicators that will highlight vulnerability and respond accordingly. In this research, these factors clearly emerged. Among CI households, these vulnerability factors included larger households, recent death of an adult or child family member, and the avoidance of education costs, as well as poor asset wealth.

Furthermore, the level of food insecurity has been found to be insufficient to determine the kind of support required, as research has shown that among households within the same asset wealth category, the chronically ill households show a greater increase in the use of harmful coping strategies. With this in mind, the research reveals trends as to which of the many negative impacts of HIV and AIDS on livelihoods are the priorities to address with project interventions for households with chronically ill members in food-insecure environments.

CI households were more likely to have their children drop out of school, indicating a need for education assistance projects. CI households were also more likely to use migration strategies, which supports a growing effective dependency ratio among other family members and indicates a need for projects to target these host households before they also begin employing more damaging coping strategies.

Furthermore, because CI households were more likely to modify diets to less nutritious alternatives, their coping strategies are particularly dangerous for HIV or AIDS individuals, as proper nutrition is critical for prolonging life and productive life. There is a need to target asset-poor CI households with increased nutritional interventions to prolong the HIV window of the seropositive family members. The tendency to reduce spending on health care for food purchases indicates a need to complement health care activities and interventions with appropriate food security interventions. With regard to the design of food distributions, the research demonstrates that CI households are likely to direct food within the household to working members. Therefore, food distributions may be more beneficial with family rations.

With regard to agriculture, the most commonly cited reasons for not cultivating land were lack of fertilizer and draft power, so a clear need emerges for a livelihood security analysis that leads to support for access to financial services, income generation, livelihood inputs, modifications to livelihood strategies to avoid, and water security interventions. With more than 40 percent of CI households reporting loss of cultivated land, CI households are trapped in a vicious cycle of increasing food insecurity. As a result, food security interventions need to be built around supporting the positive coping strategies and discouraging the harmful coping strategies employed by vulnerable households in stress.

However, although the gender of the household head was not found to be correlated with whether or not the household was affected by chronic illness, the research has confirmed the findings of earlier research that woman-headed households are found disproportionately among the most food-insecure wealth categories. Therefore, efforts to improve productivity among food-insecure chronically ill households must take into consideration the entire equation of household labor and not only consider the amount of labor required for the principal household crops.

In the examination of total household labor productivity within an integral human development livelihood framework, additional solutions relating to the labor required for household tasks, and even administrative tasks, may be discovered. So, although the research suggests priority directions for programming, the specific content and design of those programs must still be determined using the best diagnostic and program design methods available to program managers.

Furthermore, additional research may also reveal more about the kinds of programs required. Although the results from this study highlight various coping strategies employed by CI households, there is a need for additional longitudinal data in order to understand causality relationships, the impact on food security, and implications for supporting and collaborating with affected communities and households to decrease vulnerability and manage risk. Ideally, future research would be able to identify the relative importance of various casual factors on coping strategies and food security of CI households.

Notes

1. C-SAFE (Consortium for Southern Africa's Food Emergency) is a jointly planned and implemented response by World Vision, CARE, and CRS to the current food security problems of three southern Africa countries: Malawi, Zambia, and Zimbabwe.

References

Ayieko, M. 1998. *From single parents to child-headed households: The case of children orphaned in Kiumu and Siaya Districts.* HIV and Development Programme Study Paper No. 7. Geneva: UNDP.

Barnett, T., and A. Whiteside. 2002. Poverty and HIV/AIDS: Impact coping and mitigation policy. In *AIDS, public policy and child well-being,* ed. G. A. Cornia. Florence: UNICEF Innocenti Research Center (IRC).

Barrère, B. 2005. *Pre-test of new HIV indicators.* Presentation from ORC Macro, UNICEF, DHS, and USAID. Washington, D.C., January 6, 2005.

Bonnard, P. 2002. HIV/AIDS mitigation, using what we already know. FANTA Technical Note 5. Washington, D.C.: FANTA.

Christiaensen, L., and R. Boisvert. 2000. On measuring household food vulnerability: Case evidence from northern Mali. Working paper, Ithaca, N.Y.: Department of Agricultural, Resource, and Managerial Economics, Cornell University.

De Waal, A. 1989. *Famine that kills.* Oxford: Clarendon Press.

De Waal, A., and A. Whiteside. 2003. New variant famine: AIDS and food crisis in southern Africa. *Lancet* 362: 1234–1237.

FANTA (Food and Nutrition Technical Assistance). 2000. *Potential uses of food aid to support HIV/AIDS mitigation activities in Sub-Saharan Africa.* Washington, D.C.: FANTA.

FAO. 2004. *HIV/AIDS, gender inequality and rural livelihoods: The impact of HIV/AIDS on rural livelihoods in Northern Province, Zambia.* Rome: FAO.

Farming Systems Association of Zambia. 2003. *Interlinkages between HIV/AIDS, agricultural production and food security.* Baseline Survey Report, Southern Province, Zambia. Rome: FAO.

Gillespie, S., and S. Kadiyala. 2004. *Evidence base: HIV/AIDS and food security.* Washington, D.C.: IFPRI.

Haddad, L. J., and S. Gillespie. 2001. *Effective food and nutrition policy responses to HIV/AIDS: What we know and what we need to know.* Washington, D.C.: IFPRI.

Kadiyala, S., and S. Gillespie. 2003. *Rethinking food aid to fight AIDS.* Washington, D.C.: IFPRI.

Mather, D., C. Donovan, T. S. Jayne, M. Weber, E. Mazhangara, L. Bailey, K. Yoo, T. Yamano, and E. Mghenyi. 2004. *A cross-country analysis of household responses to adult mortality in rural Sub-Saharan Africa: Implications for HIV/AIDS mitigation and rural development policies.* East Lansing, Mich.: Michigan State University.

Maxwell, D., C. Ahiadeke, C. Levin, M. Armar-Klemesu, S. Zakariah, and G. M. Lamptey. 1999. Alternative food security indicators: Revisiting the frequency and severity of "coping strategies." *Food Policy* 24 (4): 411–429.

Rugalema, G. H. R. 1999. *Adult mortality as entitlement failure: AIDS and the crisis of rural livelihoods in a Tanzanian village.* Ph.D. thesis, Institute of Social Studies, The Hague.

———. 2002. *Coping or struggling? A journey into the impact of HIV/AIDS on rural livelihoods in southern Africa.* De Nieuwlanden, Wageningen University and Research Centre, Technology and Agrarian Research Group.

SADC FANR (South African Development Community Food, Agriculture, and Natural Resources) Vulnerability Assessment Committee. 2003. *Towards identifying impacts of HIV/AIDS on food insecurity in southern Africa and implications for response: Findings from Malawi, Zambia, and Zimbabwe.* Harare, Zimbabwe.

Stokes, S. 2003. *Measuring impacts of HIV/AIDS on rural livelihoods and food security.* Rome: FAO.

TANGO (Technical Assistance to Nongovernmental Organizations). 2003. *C-SAFE Zimbabwe baseline survey report of findings.* Tucson, Ariz.: TANGO.

UNAIDS. 2004. *Report on the global AIDS epidemic.* Geneva: UNAIDS.

White, J. 2002. *Facing the challenge: NGO experiences of mitigating the impacts of HIV/AIDS in Sub-Saharan Africa.* Natural Resources Institute, Greenwich University, Greenwich, U.K.

Zambia VAC (Vulnerability Assessment Committee). 2003. *Livelihood and vulnerability assessment, final report.* Lusaka.

Chapter 8

HIV/AIDS and the Agricultural Sector in Eastern and Southern Africa: Anticipating the Consequences

Thomas S. Jayne, Marcela Villarreal, Prabhu Pingali, and Guenter Hemrich

Background

There is now widespread recognition that HIV/AIDS is not simply a health issue. Effectively combating the pandemic will require a coordinated multisectoral approach. Although many in the agricultural sector embrace the idea of playing a role in combating HIV/AIDS, there has been very little analysis by agricultural policy analysts to guide them. Despite the fact that the pandemic is now in its third decade in Africa, available analysis to date provides a very murky picture of how HIV/AIDS is affecting the agricultural sector: its structure, cropping systems, relative costs of inputs and factors of production, technological and institutional changes, and supply and demand for agricultural products. Until these issues are clarified, policymakers will be inadequately prepared to forecast anticipated changes to the agricultural sector and respond proactively.

This chapter is intended to respond to the need to better understand the implications of the AIDS pandemic for the agricultural sectors in the hardest-hit countries of eastern and southern Africa. The six countries of the world with estimated HIV prevalence rates exceeding 20 percent[1] are all in southern Africa: Botswana, Lesotho, Namibia, South Africa, Swaziland, and Zimbabwe (UN Census Bureau 2003). Five other countries, all in southern and eastern Africa (Cameroon, Central African Republic, Malawi, Zambia, and Mozambique), have HIV prevalence rates between 10 and 20 percent. For shorthand, we hereafter refer to these countries as the "hardest hit" countries.

This chapter reviews available empirical evidence of the effects of AIDS on rural household livelihoods and discusses the implications for long-term processes of demographic and economic structural transformation. We highlight four processes that have been underemphasized in previous analyses: (1) the momentum of long-term population growth rates; (2) substantial underemployment in these countries' informal sectors; (3) sectoral declines in farm sizes and land/labor ratios in the smallholder farming sectors; and (4) effects of food and input marketing reforms on shifts in cropping patterns. Understanding these trends is necessary to anticipate the consequences of the HIV/AIDS epidemic for the agricultural sector and to consider the implications for agricultural policy.

Figure 8.1a Population in the medium variant ("with AIDS") and in the no-AIDS scenario ("without AIDS"), by sex and age group, seven most highly affected countries, 2000

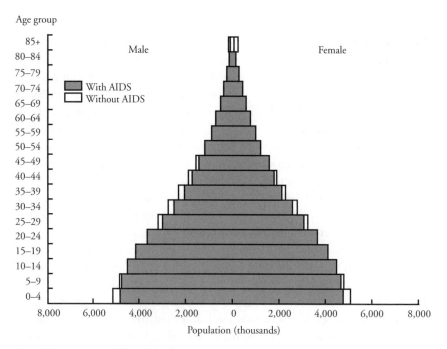

Source: U.S. Census Bureau (2003).

Effects of AIDS on Future Demographic Changes

In most of eastern and southern Africa, where HIV prevalence rates generally exceed 10 percent, there will be many fewer adults in the coming decades compared to a "no-AIDS" scenario (U.S. Census Bureau 2003). By the year 2010, five countries in the region will be experiencing negative population growth rates: Botswana (–2.1 percent per year), Mozambique (–0.2 percent), Lesotho (–0.2 percent), Swaziland (–0.4 percent), and South Africa (–1.4 percent) (U.S. Census Bureau 2003). By 2020, AIDS mortality will produce population pyramids in these countries never seen before (Fig. 8.1).

By 2025, among the seven countries where HIV prevalence exceeds 20 percent, there will be roughly 20 million men in the working age years between 20 and 59 years as opposed to 31.5 million if AIDS had not existed. By contrast, there

Figure 8.1b Projected population in the medium variant ("with AIDS") and in the no-AIDS scenario ("without AIDS"), by sex and age group, seven most highly affected countries, 2025

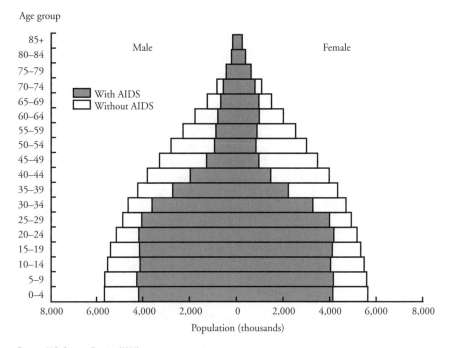

Source: U.S. Census Bureau (2003).

Table 8.1   Comparison of total population size for the seven hardest-hit countries, 2000 versus 2025[a]

		Population projections (millions)		
Sex/age categories		2000 estimate	2025 forecast "no-AIDS" scenario	2025 forecast "with AIDS"
Male	< 20 years	18.6	22.9	16.8
	20–59 years	17.5	32.1	18.6
	> 59 years	2.1	4.7	3.2
Female	< 20 years	18.9	23.0	16.4
	20–59 years	17.7	32.6	17.8
	> 59 years	2.3	5.4	3.5

[a] Botswana, Lesotho, Namibia, South Africa, Swaziland, Zambia, and Zimbabwe.
Source: U.S. Census Bureau (2003).

will be only 18 million women in the 20 to 59 year age range as opposed to 32 million in the "no-AIDS" case. And because of the early death of so many adults of reproductive age, there will also be many fewer children born, also indicated in Figure 8.1. Population pyramids in five or six other countries will have similar shapes, though less extreme than those shown in Figure 8.1.[2]

However, it is also important to compare future projected population to current population. Notwithstanding the catastrophic death toll that is projected to occur over time in these countries, the absolute number of adults projected to be alive in 2025 is roughly similar to what it is today. This is because the momentum of population growth, in the absence of AIDS, would have produced much greater population sizes in the coming decades. Although AIDS is projected to erode population growth to roughly zero in the seven hardest-hit countries, the net result is a roughly stable number of working-age adults over time. Table 8.1 compares population estimates in 2000 and projected estimates for 2025 by age and sex categories in the seven countries where HIV prevalence is estimated to exceed 20 percent.

According to these demographic projections, there will be a slight increase in the number of men between 20 and 59 years of age between 2000 and 2025 and virtually no change in the number of women. The projections indicate a decline in the number of men and women below 20 years of age by 2025. Because AIDS will particularly influence the number of people under 20, both through the impact of increased child mortality and fewer adults living long enough to have children, dependency ratios may actually become slightly more favorable over time.

These projections are consistent with those of the United Nations (2003). According to its projections, countries with HIV prevalence above 20 percent will register annual population growth rates of roughly +0.2 percent between 2000 and

2025. Countries with HIV prevalence between 10 and 20 percent (Cameroon, Central African Republic, Kenya, Malawi, and Mozambique) will have population growth rates of +1.33 percent per year.

However, not reflected in the population figures in Table 8.1 is the loss of available labor as a result of periods of sickness, caregiving for those afflicted with the disease, and mourning periods after a death, which can be substantial (Government of Uganda 2003). Thus, the "effective" labor pool in the economy is likely to be overestimated if consideration is given only to changes in the absolute numbers of adults shown in Table 8.1. Moreover, people who survive into adulthood have already received substantial social investments (education, skills, food production), and it can be assumed that, in most cases, their lives enrich the lives of those around them. Their death translates into a loss to society of existing knowledge and skills as well as the transfer of knowledge to succeeding generations.

The Effects of HIV/AIDS on Agriculture and Rural Livelihoods: Current Understanding

Potential Changes in Labor Markets as a Result of AIDS

Understanding the future effects of AIDS on the agricultural sector requires an organizing conceptual framework of how labor is likely to shift between urban and rural areas and between agricultural and nonagricultural activities as the demographic changes shown in Figure 8.1 begin to manifest. The classic theory of rural–urban migration is based on the work of Harris and Todaro (1970). These models start from the observation that labor allocates itself into three broad employment categories: (1) the agricultural sector; (2) the formal sector, mainly in urban areas but also in small towns, commercial farms, mines, and rural civil service (where wages generally exceed those of agriculture); and (3) the "informal" sector. Many people who have migrated to urban areas in search of formal-sector jobs but could not obtain one often find themselves in the informal sector, where jobs and businesses are relatively easy to find but pay relatively little (e.g., petty trading, tailoring, crafts, shoe shining). The informal sector often masks substantial underemployment.

According to the Harris-Todaro model and its extensions, the fractions of the total labor force that reside in each of these three sectors (agriculture, the formal sector, and the informal sector) depend on (1) formal sector wage rates and benefits; (2) the returns to labor in agriculture or agricultural wage rates; and (3) the availability of formal-sector jobs compared to the number of people migrating off the farm to search for them, which influences the probability of actually finding formal employment in urban areas as opposed to generally less lucrative informal sector jobs.

Now, what happens if a sizable fraction of workers in all three sectors are forced to quit working because of illness, subsequent death, and related caregiving functions? According to these economic labor models, the answer depends on the size of the underemployed informal sector. If surplus labor exists in an underemployed informal sector, then rising costs of agricultural labor caused by incipient AIDS-related labor shortages will induce labor migration from the informal sector to agriculture.

Studies reveal that the informal sectors of eastern and southern Africa have swelled massively in recent decades, largely because of inadequate income opportunities in rural areas and the need for rural households to diversify their incomes by engaging in sectors whose returns are not highly correlated with those in agriculture (Bryceson and Potts 2005). Urbanization in these countries generally does not reflect a strong demand for urban labor but, rather, reflects the pushing out of labor from rural areas where population densities are high and where farm sizes have declined to levels inadequate to sustain all the members of succeeding generations. These points, taken together, might indicate that incipient agricultural labor shortages caused by AIDS may induce labor migration out of the urban informal sector into agriculture. In this way, underemployment in the informal sector is likely to act as a shock absorber to buffer the agricultural sector from labor shortages.

What is the evidence of migration of labor to agriculture? A growing number of empirical household-level studies from eastern and southern Africa indicate that family size of afflicted households does not decline by one member after the death of a prime-age adult (e.g., Beegle 2003; Mather et al. 2004; Yamano and Jayne 2004; Chapoto and Jayne 2005). These studies indicate that former resident adults often return to the farm to compensate for the loss of labor caused by the deceased adult. Although not all of these studies are able to determine the location from which new adult members are coming, there are indications that many returning adults are coming from urban and periurban areas.

This picture is supported by 1990 and 2000 national censuses in Zambia, where HIV prevalence is estimated at roughly 20 percent. By comparing the numbers of individuals and households identified as "agricultural" and "nonagricultural" as well as "urban" versus "rural," we can draw inferences about labor migration over the decade of the 1990s. However, Zambia's trends may not be representative of the region, but it is the only intercensus information in southern Africa that we have to draw on. Census figures reported here are prepared by the government Central Statistical Office (CSO). As shown in Table 8.2, the total population of Zambia grew from 7.38 million to 9.89 million people between 1990 and 2000, a 33.8 percent increase. Yet, over the same period, the rural population grew at a much higher rate than the urban population: the rural population grew by 43.6 percent compared to

Table 8.2   National population within households and number of
households, Zambia

Population characteristics	1990	2000
Total population	7,383,097	9,885,591
Rural population	4,497,391	6,458,729
Urban population	2,885,706	3,426,862
Population of agricultural households, total	3,591,588	7,181,807
Population of agricultural households, rural	3,521,498	5,965,504
Population of agricultural households, urban	70,090	1,216,303
Population of nonagricultural households, rural	975,893	493,225

Source: Census 1990 and 2000, CSO, Zambia. The authors acknowledge Dr. Jones Govereh
of the Zambia Food Security Research Project for compiling these numbers.

only 18.8 percent for urban areas, suggesting reverse migration from urban to rural areas. Some of this reverse migration is attributed to the decline of Zambia's copper industry. However, the growth in the number and proportion of Zambian households engaged in agriculture appears to be universal across all provinces and not confined to the Copperbelt Province, where the copper industry is centered (Govereh, Jayne, and Shaffer 2006).

Also according to the 1990 and 2000 censuses, the population of rural households engaged in agriculture grew from 3.521 million to 5.965 million people over the decade, a 69.4 percent increase. And the population of nonagricultural rural households actually declined from 975,893 to 493,225. These figures represent a huge shift in Zambia's labor force from urban to rural areas and from nonagricultural to at least partially agricultural activities. Certainly, a combination of factors have contributed to these trends, including the demise of the copper industry, increasing poverty leading to increased reliance on semisubsistence crop production, and AIDS. Unemployment and underemployment in Zambia's urban and informal sectors appear to have provided a ready labor pool for the agricultural sector over this period.

However, the supply of labor from the urban and informal sectors is not infinite. As the long-term effects of the disease progress through the next several decades, it is unclear whether the demand for agricultural labor will eventually outstrip the supply of underemployed labor in the informal sector. If the agricultural sector continues to absorb labor at a faster rate than the overall population growth rate (which for Zambia is projected to be 1 percent per year over the next decade), then labor shortages may indeed begin to manifest in future decades. However, there is

Table 8.3   Land-to-person ratio (mean 10-year averages) in selected countries

	1960–69	1970–79	1980–89	1990–99
Ethiopia	0.508	0.450	0.363	0.252
Kenya	0.459	0.350	0.280	0.229
Mozambique	0.389	0.367	0.298	0.249
Rwanda	0.215	0.211	0.197	0.161
Zambia	1.367	1.073	0.896	0.779
Zimbabwe	0.726	0.664	0.583	0.525

Sources: Compiled from data on FAOStat web site: http://faostat.fao.org/faostat/default.jsp.

Note: Land-to-person ratio = (land cultivated to annual and permanent crops)/(population in agriculture).

little evidence to date to suggest that labor shortages in Zambian agriculture have been increasing.[3]

In fact, there continues to be strong evidence of increasing land pressures caused by population growth through the end of the 1990s. Data from FAO indicate that mean land-to-person ratios have declined substantially in the past half-century (Table 8.3). The pace of the decline in land-to-person ratios has not slowed during the 1990s, even in the hardest-hit countries. Declining land-to-person ratios are occurring as a result of the past momentum of rural population growth and limited availability of unused arable land. HIV/AIDS may slow down the secular decline in farm size and reduce the rate of rural outmigration in the hardest-hit countries.

Overall, the emerging picture is that, even in the hardest-hit countries of Africa, the labor force is unlikely to grow over the next several decades, but it will not shrink either. The quality of the labor force will be adversely affected by AIDS. The cost of skilled labor may rise if the AIDS disease depletes the ranks of the educated and skilled workers faster than they can be replenished. By contrast, the cost of agricultural labor is unlikely to rise because any upward pressure on agricultural wages is almost certain to induce reverse urban–rural migration from the underemployed informal sector and cross-border migration from regions where HIV prevalence is relatively low and where population pressures are already intense (parts of eastern Africa such as Burundi, Rwanda, and central Kenya). For many decades, excess demand for relatively unskilled labor has been dampened by regional migration. Malawi, for example, has historically served as a labor pool for commercial farms and mines in Zimbabwe and South Africa. Mozambique, Lesotho, and Swaziland have played similar roles for South Africa. Because these countries are all hard hit, excess demand for labor may draw forth different patterns of regional migration, perhaps involving densely populated areas of eastern Africa, though this is somewhat speculative.

Influences of AIDS on the Use of Capital in Agriculture

Agriculture-led structural transformation has almost always involved increased intensification of capital in the farm production process (Johnston and Kilby 1975; Mellor 1976). The main types of capital-led intensification have featured fertilizers, improved hybrid seed, chemicals, and draft power. These technologies have also featured prominently in the brief "smallholder green revolution" successes of eastern and southern Africa (Byerlee and Eicher 1997).

Farm households tend to utilize remittance and off-farm income as a primary means to afford expensive assets such as oxen, plows, and fertilizer, which are used to capitalize farm production (Reardon, Crawford, and Kelly 1995). These sources of income are often jeopardized among AIDS-afflicted households, particularly those that are asset-poor and vulnerable to begin with (e.g., Donovan et al. 2003; FASAZ 2003; Mushati et al. 2003; Yamano and Jayne 2004). Cash constraints on farm intensification are compounded during illness and after a death, when medical and funeral expenses rise and caregiving by other members reduces their income-earning potential as well. Evidence indicates that households attempt to first sell off small animals and other assets with the least impact on long-term production potential. Cattle and productive farm equipment are sold in response to severe cash requirements after a death in the family (Yamano and Jayne 2004). To the extent that afflicted households shed assets and are forced to reduce their use of cash inputs in agriculture, the cumulative effect may be a decline in the proportion of small-scale farmers able to produce a marketable surplus from farming.

Afflicted households face a multifaceted loss of labor, capital, and knowledge. Unlike the loss of labor and knowledge, which represent a loss to entire communities, capital assets lost by afflicted households are generally redistributed within the rural economy rather than lost entirely. This may exacerbate rural inequality over time and, particularly, deplete the productive potential of relatively poor households.

Effects on Land Distribution

Figure 8.1, which shows how the population pyramid of hard-hit countries will change over the long term, holds important implications for land allocation. As shown earlier, by 2025 the number of male and female adults in the age ranges between 40 and 64 years will be less than half of what it would have been in the absence of AIDS. As afflicted households lose productive members of their families, including those possessing the rights to their households' land, conflicts over the inheritance of land may escalate over the coming decades (Barnett and Blaikie 1992).

Poor and disadvantaged households in particular may have difficulty maintaining their rights to land after incurring a death. Widows and orphans are particularly vulnerable to losing access or ownership rights to land after the death of the husband and father. The cumulative effects of loss of land rights may turn out to be an increase in the concentration of land within the small farm sector, with land being reallocated at the margin from poor households to relatively wealthy ones. This is a likely outcome if relatively wealthy households are better able to maintain their control over land after incurring a prime-age death in the family and also if they are able to gain control over land assets shed by poorer households that cannot continue to productively use their land after incurring a death. Land disputes and possible land concentration over time are consistent with broader economy-wide predictions that AIDS is likely to exacerbate income inequality in many countries (Lehutso-Phooko and Naidoo 2002).

Although an important coping strategy for afflicted households may be to rent out land that cannot be productively utilized after incurring a death, Barnett (1994) found that widows especially were reluctant to do this for fear of losing rights to their land. These problems of land tenure overlap with the problem of gender disparities. Much research has documented that widows and their dependents are in a more tenuous position with regard to maintaining control over land (Barnett and Blaikie 1992). When combined with evidence that female-headed households tend to be poorer in general than their male-headed household neighbors, governments and donors face a serious challenge to devise means to protect poor households' (and particularly poor female-headed households') rights to land within future poverty alleviation and rural development strategies.

Influences on Agricultural Production

The microlevel empirical record on the effects of HIV/AIDS on agriculture is still quite limited but is growing rapidly. The time periods over which impacts are measured are mostly short-run, which probably understate the full impact on households and communities over time. Even given this short-run time dimension, the weight of the empirical evidence to date does indicate that AIDS is having a measurably adverse impact on household agricultural production, although these impacts are often mitigated by attracting new household members (or bringing back members residing away from home) to compensate for the lost labor and knowledge of the deceased. Effects appear to be highly sensitive to the age, sex, and position of the deceased, being the greatest in cases where the household head or spouse dies, and the initial level of wealth of the household (Drimie 2002).

For example, a study in Kenya found that rural households suffering a prime-age death between 1997 and 2000 generally incurred a decline in agricultural production relative to nonafflicted households, but the magnitude and statistical significance of this finding depended greatly on the sex, age, and position in the household of the person who died as well as the household's initial (predeath) level of wealth (Yamano and Jayne 2004). The only statistically significant effects were observed in the case of male head-of-household death among households in the bottom half of the wealth distribution, but these effects were very severe. Households in this case suffered a 68 percent reduction in the value of net agricultural output (after deducting costs of inputs). Moreover, these results were robust to the year of death, suggesting that households that suffered a death in 1997 did not show any recovery compared to households that incurred a more recent death such as in 1999 or 2000.

Yamano and Jayne (2004) found that households suffering the death of head of household or spouse were largely unable to replace the labor lost through the death, whereas households suffering the death of another adult (other than the head or spouse) were largely able to attract new household members. This at least partially stabilizes the supply of family labor for agriculture but implies that off-farm and remittance incomes may in some cases be reduced, exacerbating capital constraints in agriculture. By contrast, Beegle (2003), using longitudinal data from the hard-hit Kagera District of Tanzania, found only short-run and temporary effects of AIDS-related mortality on households' agricultural activities, although it should be noted that the study is based on data collected in the early 1990s.

A different set of studies have documented the adverse effects of worker HIV/AIDS on the commercial agricultural sector. For example, Fox et al. (2003) found a significant decline in labor productivity among HIV-positive tea pluckers in Kenya, and Rugalema (1999) found that agricultural companies reliant on hired labor are suffering from rising costs and falling profits as a result of the disease.

Accounting for Differences in Agricultural Systems

Agricultural systems in eastern and southern Africa exhibit considerable heterogeneity. For example, areas of northern Zambia and northern Mozambique have relatively high land-to-labor ratios and use few capital inputs. By contrast, southern Malawi, parts of Rwanda, and the Central Highlands of Kenya are densely populated, have low land-to-labor ratios, and have exhibited substantial out-migration of labor for decades. Many other small-scale farmers in northern Zimbabwe and southern and central Zambia are relatively capitalized, relying on animal draft power for land preparation and inorganic fertilizer. Because of differences in factor endowments between regions, the effects of AIDS-related mortality on agricultural households are likely to vary substantially.

Land-labor-capital ratios also vary greatly within most countries of eastern and southern Africa. For example, nationwide surveys in five countries in the region show that after households are ranked by landholding size per capita, there are

Table 8.4   Smallholder land distribution in selected African countries

Country	(a) Sample households (*n*)	(b) Mean landholding size[a] (hectares)	(c) Farm size ranked by quartile[a] (hectares per person)				
			Mean	Lowest	2nd	3rd	Highest
Kenya, 1997	1,416	2.65	0.41	0.08	0.17	0.31	1.10
Ethiopia, 1995	2,658	1.17	0.24	0.03	0.12	0.22	0.58
Rwanda, 1984	2018	1.20	0.28	0.07	0.15	0.26	0.62
Rwanda, 1990	1,181	0.94	0.17	0.05	0.10	0.16	0.39
Rwanda, 2000	1,584	0.71	0.16	0.02	0.06	0.13	0.43
Malawi, 1998	5,657	0.99	0.22	0.08	0.15	0.25	0.60
Zambia, 2000	6,618	2.76	0.56	0.12	0.26	0.48	1.36
Mozambique, 2000	3,851	2.10	0.48	0.10	0.23	0.40	1.16

Source: Jayne et al. (2003a).

Note: Numbers for Ethiopia, Rwanda, Mozambique, and Zambia, including Gini coefficients, are weighted. Numbers for Kenya are sample statistics.

[a] Landholding size figures include rented land.

huge variations in land-to-person ratios within the small-scale farm sector in each country (Table 8.4). The 25 percent of smallholder households with the smallest farms typically controlled less than 0.1 hectare of land per person. These households are virtually landless, although this same group earns over 50 percent of its income from agriculture, except in the case of Kenya, where the agricultural income share of the bottom land quartile was exactly 50 percent (Jayne et al. 2003a). At least for this stratum of smallholder households, land is likely to remain a primary constraint on income growth, and it is not clear that the loss of a household member would change this much. At the other end of the spectrum, the 25 percent of smallholder households with the largest land-to-labor ratios controlled at least seven times more land per capita, generally in the range of 0.5 to 1.0 hectare per capita. This stratum of better-off farmers generally hire agricultural labor. Also, the death of a family member among these households (where labor-land ratios are relatively low) is likely to induce a search for attracting nonresident members back to the farm. These two processes, attempts to attract nonresident household members back to the farm and demand for hired labor by relatively large smallholder farms and large-scale farms, are likely to provide the incentives for reverse rural migration from the informal sectors in urban areas.

The situation as presented in Table 8.4 indicates that because of the heterogeneity in land-labor ratios within the small-scale sector, the limiting input into agricultural production will certainly differ between households controlling less than 0.1 hectare per capita and those controlling more than 2 hectares per capita. There are strong reasons for anticipating that AIDS will progressively decapitalize highly afflicted rural communities, meaning a loss of savings, cattle assets and draft equipment, and other assets. The loss of capital assets that often substitute for labor in the production process may indeed raise the demand for labor.

Some studies have conjectured that HIV/AIDS is bringing about important changes in farming systems. Particular emphasis has been put on the recent shift in area cultivated from maize to roots and tubers, which has been observed in several countries in the region. For example, the proportion of crop area devoted to cassava and sweet potato in Malawi has risen from 4 percent to 10 percent over the past two decades. In some provinces of Zambia, cassava production has also risen dramatically in recent years (Govereh, Jayne, and Shaffer 2006).

It is possible that AIDS has contributed to these shifts in crop area. However, it is important to acknowledge that other major changes in agricultural policy have occurred in these countries that have also veered some farming systems in the region toward tuber crops. Most notably, many countries in eastern and southern Africa had formerly implemented state-led maize promotion policies featuring panterritorial producer prices, major investments in marketing board buying stations in smallholder farming areas, and subsidies on fertilizer distributed on credit to small farmers along with hybrid maize seed. These maize-marketing policies in Kenya, Malawi, Zambia, and Zimbabwe (among others) were either eliminated or scaled back significantly starting in the early 1990s as part of economy-wide structural adjustment programs. These policy changes clearly reduced the financial profitability of growing maize in the more remote areas, where maize production was formerly buoyed by panterritorial pricing, and has shifted cropping incentives toward other food crops, especially those relatively unresponsive to fertilizer application, such as cassava (Smale and Jayne 2003).

Many areas in southern Africa where cassava production has increased in recent years appear to be those where the profitability of maize production has declined in recent years rather than areas of especially high HIV prevalence. These provinces have faced major declines in the maize-fertilizer price ratios over the past 15 years as a result of changes in agricultural policy. By contrast, several provinces with relatively high HIV prevalence, Central (18.7%), Copperbelt (26.2%), and Lusaka Rural (27.2%), have recorded relatively little increase in the share of cropped area devoted to these roots and tubers (Chapoto and Jayne 2005). There has indeed been a general increase in cassava production over time in many parts of Zambia, but the survey data indicate that nonafflicted and afflicted households are incorporating cassava into their crop mix at similar rates. If afflicted households incurred several labor shocks, one would have expected to find afflicted households devoting a greater proportion of their land to cassava and to other laborsaving crops.

Using data from Kagera District in Tanzania, Beegle (2003) also found that households experiencing a death did not shift cultivation toward subsistence food farming. She concludes that afflicted households were able to maintain their supply of labor by drawing new members to the farm, a finding highlighted in other empirical studies (Ainsworth, Ghosh, and Semali 1995; Menon et al. 1998; Mather et al. 2004). Donovan et al. (2003) also found no distinct gender-based differences in the composition of crops grown after the death of an adult in the household but did find an increase in sweet potato cultivation. They speculate that sweet potato may have become more attractive for households suffering a labor shock because of its more flexible planting and harvesting schedule compared to most other crops. Overall, these results suggest a need for caution in singling out labor as the main factor of production that is affected by rising adult mortality rates.

In summary, the evidence is mixed as to how AIDS is affecting agricultural systems and cropping patterns. There are good reasons to believe that capital constraints will become more binding over time as the number of deaths from the disease rises in the hardest-hit countries, which may force many afflicted households to adopt less capital-intensive technologies and crops. Efforts to better anticipate and respond to the stresses that AIDS will impose on rural communities will benefit from a careful identification of the different agricultural systems found in eastern and southern Africa. Even within a particular agricultural system, there is also great heterogeneity, such that appropriate programmatic responses to AIDS may be household-specific, conditioned by the gender and household position of the deceased individual, initial vulnerability before the onset of illness, and a household's ability to attract new members. If these emerging findings receive further empirical support from ongoing studies, then it will be necessary to move away from generalized conclusions about the main factors constraining afflicted households' ability to recover and begin formulating appropriate policy and programmatic responses based on the specific characteristics of the region, the regional economy, the localized farming system, the profitability and riskiness of alternative crops, and households' characteristics and available resources.

Conclusions and Policy Implications

Governments and international organizations need solid guidance on the cost-effectiveness of alternative kinds of investments to simultaneously defeat the AIDS pandemic and the chronic poverty that characterized the region even before the onset of the disease but has been further exacerbated by it. Because every dollar invested in AIDS prevention, treatment, and mitigation cannot be used to promote basic education, improved agricultural technology, the development of infrastructure and markets, and other long-term investments necessary to raising living standards, it is crucial to achieve an effective balance between investments to prevent and treat HIV/AIDS and investments to promote long-run economic growth.

Effective responses to AIDS also requires an accurate understanding of how rural households respond to illness and death caused by AIDS. Over the past decade, a current orthodoxy has emerged concerning the effects of HIV/AIDS on agriculture. The most commonly cited effects are:

- Reduction in area cultivated

- Shifting area into less labor-intensive crops, such as cassava or sweet potatoes, and away from more labor-intensive (higher-value) cash crops

- Reduction in weeding labor, which contributes to lower yields and thus lower crop value

- Reduction in use of other inputs because of lack of finances resulting from the loss of wage income of the deceased and health/funeral expenses

- Declines in crop production, losses in off-farm income, and increased poverty

Although there are solid a priori reasons underlying these conclusions, many of them are subject to important methodological problems, based on highly qualitative methods that rely on nonverifiable interpretation of data, or are conceptual and speculative in nature.

Most quantitative household-level studies provide a less catastrophic assessment of the impact of rising AIDS-related mortality on the agricultural sector. Despite the conventional wisdom stated above, the limited number of longitudinal studies based on household survey data indicate that the impact of prime-age mortality on household welfare varies greatly, depending on the particular agricultural system and household-specific characteristics such as the age, sex, and position of the deceased in the household, the household's initial level of wealth, and ability to attract new members. Households are sometimes able to vary the proportion of inputs used to produce a given amount of crop output, and they can also vary their crop mix to adjust to shifts in availability of their resources. Examples of this include substituting hired labor for family labor (e.g., sharecropping arrangements), renting animal traction services for land preparation instead of preparing the land with family labor, substituting fertilizer application for labor, or reducing the amount of land cultivated to maintain a similar intensity of labor input on the smaller amount of land under cultivation. Even highly resource-constrained small farmers do not produce agricultural products in fixed input proportions over time. Rather, they respond to changes in relative prices and adjust to other changes in their environment. To the extent that factors are substitutable, households incurring a shock to their own labor supply (for example, because of an AIDS-related death) can and will often vary the proportions of land, labor, and cash or adjust their cropping patterns based on the particular mix of resources that they possess after the death. Hence, the loss of family labor through a death in the household does not mean that labor necessarily becomes the limiting input in agricultural production, and hence, it does not necessarily follow that the appropriate policy response for agricultural research and extension systems is to focus inordinately on laborsaving agricultural technology. Laborsaving technology may indeed be appropriate for many households (those who already face high land-labor ratios and lack other resources that could be substituted for labor, such as cash for hiring labor). The main implication for crop research and extension systems is that a broad range of agricultural production technologies, appropriate for the wide range of land-labor-capital ratios found among small-scale farm households, are needed to respond to the AIDS disease.

However, the household survey analyses generating these findings and policy implications have their own methodological limitations. First, such studies to date have measured the effects of death in their households on household-level outcomes, typically over a 2- to 5-year time frame, compared to nonafflicted households. Yet because nonafflicted households are likely to be indirectly affected by the mortality occurring around them, nonafflicted households may not be a valid control group. A second problem concerns the often careless interpretation of cross-sectional survey data, which have little or no information on households' conditions before they were afflicted by mortality. By definition, cross-sectional data provide a snapshot of household conditions at a certain point in time. Cross-sectional data are capable of providing information on afflicted households' conditions only after a death has occurred, not before. But the study of AIDS is an inherently dynamic analysis that requires an understanding of how household behavior and welfare change over time, from before being afflicted, during the illness phase, the postdeath phase, and, one hopes, in the recovery process. Third, studies covering a relatively short time frame, whether qualitative or quantitative, are likely to fail to detect intergenerational effects such as the inability of deceased adults to pass along accumulated knowledge to future generations and the less tangible benefits that children receive from their parents (Bell, Devarajan, and Gersbach, 2003; Gertler, Levine, and Martinez 2003).

On the basis of available evidence and projections, three trends are likely to emerge. First, as the supply of skilled and semiskilled labor becomes relatively constrained as the disease progresses, the costs of skilled labor in the (mostly non-agricultural) formal sector is likely to rise. This means that knowledge-intensive activities, both in agriculture and nonagriculture, may suffer a decline in competitiveness unless steps are taken to accelerate skill training and general human capital development. However, the increased risks of premature death from HIV/AIDS erode the returns to investing in human capital development. Aggressive public sector initiatives may be necessary to maintain growth in human capital development throughout the economy and in the agricultural sector (e.g., agricultural extension agents) despite the continuous drain on human capital by AIDS. Macroeconomic models that do not account for the complex effects of AIDS on human capital and intergenerational knowledge transfers are probably underestimating the economic and social consequences of the disease.

Second, AIDS may slow the rate of labor migration from rural to urban areas in the hardest-hit countries. Several household-survey analyses have already shown evidence of urban-to-rural labor migration among afflicted households (e.g., Ainsworth, Ghosh, and Semali's [1995] study of Kagera District in Tanzania and Menon et al.'s [1998] study of Rakai District in Uganda). Migration of labor from urban to rural areas may help rural households and communities preserve existing farming systems or slow the transition to less labor-intensive ones. However, the process of urban-to-rural migration as a mitigating effect of the AIDS disease on rural labor depends on the assumption of widespread underemployment in the informal sector, and that the returns to labor in agriculture are enough to induce underemployed urbanites back to the farm.

Third, agricultural systems are likely to become less capital-intensive in hard-hit areas as assets and wealth are depleted. The effects of AIDS on agriculture appear to strike hardest on the poor, and the disease may exacerbate income inequalities as poor households sell off assets and land to those who can afford to buy.

Potential Agricultural Sector Recommendations to Mitigate the Effects of AIDS

This section discusses potential agricultural policies and programmatic responses of four types to mitigate the impacts of HIV/AIDS: (1) factor use and input market; (2) agricultural research and extension systems; (3) commodity markets; and (4) gender-differentiated resource allocation.

Policies and Programs Affecting Factor Use and Input Markets

- *Land Tenure/Security Policies:* Research findings have underscored the need to reduce insecurity of land tenure for women (and their dependents) who lose their husband (father). The limited available evidence indicates that widows and their dependents are most vulnerable to losing their land and becoming substantially poorer after suffering the premature death of the husband. Policies that improved women's rights (e.g., land tenure security for widows) might also reduce the spread of AIDS associated with women resorting to risky behaviors caused by poverty and disenfranchisement.

• *Development of Land Rental Markets:* Relatedly, government efforts to ensure that landowners will not lose their land if they rent it out to others will help in the development of viable land rental markets. Evidence suggests that land rental markets are constrained in many cases by landowners' fears that they will lose their land if they allow others to use it repeatedly. For AIDS-afflicted households that do suffer from a shortage of family labor, their welfare could be enhanced by well-functioning land rental markets that allowed them to earn income from allowing others to make productive use of the land.

• *Strategies to Promote Labor-Saving Modes of Land Preparation and Weeding:* The importance of land preparation and weeding in total labor input to crop cultivation calls for increased public investment to make laborsaving land preparation and weeding technologies more accessible to nonafflicted as well as afflicted farm households. Conservation farming techniques that shift land preparation labor to the dry season may be particularly attractive in many areas. In other areas, strategies to rapidly increase the stock and health of animal assets within the small-scale farm sector as well as the stock of animal and draft equipment such as plows and harrows may be important. Enhancing farmers' incentives and ability to acquire draft animals and equipment will help alleviate the crucial labor burden of land preparation. Moreover, relatively asset-poor households that still cannot afford to buy such assets themselves will nevertheless be in a better position to utilize such services through the increased availability of oxen and equipment through draft rental markets. In short, there may be increasing payoffs to increasing public goods investments in livestock veterinary and extension services and, where feasible, stimulating new investment in private veterinary services. There are some examples, as in Mali, where a successful system of private veterinary drug retailers has developed.

• *Invest in Improving Access to Water and Fuel:* Borehole sinking and agroforestry projects can reduce time spent on these labor-intensive tasks (Gillespie 1989). These may have a high benefit-to-cost ratio in terms of health effects and simultaneously increase the amount of labor that could be freed up for productive income-earning activities. Benefits will be especially high for women, who do most of the water and fuel fetching.

Policies and Programs Affecting Agricultural Research and Extension Systems

- *Agricultural Seed Development and Dissemination:* Given the wide variations in land-to-labor ratios found throughout eastern and southern Africa, labor-saving technologies may not be appropriate for all afflicted households or in all hard-hit communities. Payoffs to research in improved seed technology (generally considered to be land-saving) have historically been very high (Oehmke and Crawford 1996), and it is unlikely that seed research will be any less valuable given the existence of AIDS. In fact, the past record of payoffs to improved seed development may make this one of the most effective means to raise the livelihoods of afflicted and nonafflicted households alike over the longer run.

  Despite the likelihood of more severe capital constraints over time, low-external-input technologies are unlikely to contribute much to AIDS mitigation. It is possible that low-input technologies are appropriate in a limited number of household situations. For the most part, however, low-external-input technologies without soil fertility enhancement mean substantially lower yields and production and lower returns to land and labor.

  It is in this vein that caution is warranted about promoting new crops simply because they are laborsaving or possess important nutritive qualities. Although these are important criteria, the promotion of new crops also needs to be assessed in terms of its effect on returns to land and labor and broader agricultural and rural development objectives. For example, if the promotion of the crop would shift cropping patterns and displace other crops that yield higher production per unit of land and labor input, then there may be adverse effects on agricultural productivity, crop income, and food security. The trade-offs between superior nutritive value of certain crops versus lower overall value of output produced need to be assessed in greater detail to determine whether production of certain crops ought to be promoted.

- *Conservation Agriculture Approaches that Provide Productivity Improvements and Economize on Labor Input:* This proposal also relates to the previous set of proposals affecting agricultural input use. By using labor in the dry season for land preparation, conservation agriculture methods may assist in ameliorating the severe labor constraint at land preparation periods. When the first rains come and planting needs to quickly follow, those farmers practicing conservation agriculture would have been able to spread the work out over time and achieve it (Haggblade and Tembo 2003).

- *Programs to Educate and Change Behaviors of Agricultural Extension Workers:* Agricultural extension systems have been adversely affected by the AIDS epidemic as many workers have died. Agricultural extension workers possess attributes known to be correlated with HIV contraction: mobility, education, and relative affluence. There is a need to focus on attitude and sex behavior change among agricultural extension workers and to utilize them as forces for positive behavior change in the community.

- *Programs to Increase the Number of Trained Agricultural Extension Workers:* As men and women die of AIDS, much of their accumulated knowledge and skill is lost to the succeeding generation. Problems of intergenerational knowledge transfer, if not redressed, will reduce the productivity of labor in agriculture as well as the contribution of people to society and the contribution of society to individuals (Bell, Devarajan, and Gersbach 2003). This highlights the importance of education and skill development, which goes far beyond the ministry of agriculture. However, an important role for the ministry of agriculture is to rehabilitate the agricultural extension system. This means more than reviving the number of extension agents and contacts with farmers but also improving the mode of transmitting information to farmers.

Policies and Programs Affecting Commodity Marketing Systems

- *Improved Input and Commodity Marketing Systems:* Although this issue is important irrespective of its relation to HIV/AIDS, we include it here to highlight the fact that one of the most important ways to reduce the impacts of AIDS is to strengthen the resilience of the rural economy. Efforts to improve the competitiveness and productivity of smallholder agriculture are likely to be among the most important ways to help afflicted households and communities cope with the ravages of AIDS. Agricultural markets for inputs and commodities are central to this process.

    Greater public goods investments in road, rail, and port development, and communications infrastructure, are also crucial. High domestic transportation costs have clearly impeded fertilizer use in the region, as they account for roughly half of the total price borne by farmers and contribute to the fact that fertilizer prices are among the highest in the world (Jayne et al. 2003b).

Policies and Programs Affecting Gender-Differentiated Allocation of Resources

• *Redress Gender Biases in Agricultural Programs:* It is primarily men who receive the specialized crop husbandry and marketing knowledge to grow these crops under out-grower and cooperative arrangements.

    Marked gender inequalities in the access and ownership of productive resources make the whole society more vulnerable in the wake of an external shock such as AIDS. In large parts of Africa, although men traditionally control and own many resources, women gain access and use rights through marriage. When marriage links are broken through the death of the spouse, and women are denied access or use of the resources or lose them through property grabbing, they are frequently left with only their body to gain access to food, money, or rights. Programs that seek to ensure gender equality in participation and access will have a protective effect for the society. In addition, they will have an empowerment effect on women, further protecting them against HIV.

• *Education Campaigns Aimed at Reducing Widow Inheritance:* Studies in Kenya and Uganda indicate that the widespread traditional practice of widows being "inherited" by one of the deceased husband's brothers is no longer mandatory (Rugalema 1999; Government of Uganda 2003). It is now well recognized that this custom has exacerbated the spread of AIDS. Unfortunately, initiatives to stop these practices may leave widows in a weak economic position, which has been observed in some cases to contribute to other types of risky sexual behavior. Alternative approaches to caring for widows and their dependents are necessary to reduce the spread of the disease.

Concluding Remarks

Based on projections of future demographic change in the hardest-hit countries of eastern and southern Africa, the full impacts of HIV/AIDS on the agricultural sector are only just starting to manifest and will intensify over the next several decades. It is critical that agricultural policymakers anticipate the changes that HIV/AIDS will bring to the agricultural and rural sector and proactively respond through the development of policies and programs that factor in these projected impacts of the disease.

    One of the most important ways in which agricultural policy can contribute to reducing the spread and consequences of AIDS is to contribute effectively to poverty reduction. Risky sexual behaviors are at least partially related to limited opportunities to earn a livelihood through other means. Moreover, raising households' and communities' living standards over the long-run through productivity-enhancing investments in agricultural technology generation and diffusion, improved crop marketing systems, basic education, infrastructure, and governance will improve their ability to withstand the social and economic stresses caused by the disease. Greater focus on these productivity-enhancing investments is likely to be a critical part of an effective response to the HIV/AIDS pandemic, and the extent to which progress is made in these areas over the next 20 years is likely to greatly influence living standards in these hardest-hit countries of eastern and southern Africa.

Notes

The authors acknowledge support from the FAO; the Food Security III Cooperative Agreement, funded by USAID; and the Tegemeo Agricultural Monitoring and Policy Analysis Project, funded by USAID/Kenya. This chapter has benefited from the comments of Clare Bishop, Cynthia Donovan, Natasha Mesko, James Shaffer, John Staatz, and Michael Weber. The views expressed in this chapter reflect the views of the authors only.

1. Prevalence rates refer to the estimated percentage of HIV-positive adults between 15 and 49 years of age.

2. This assumes that current projections by UNAIDS and U.S. Census Bureau are correct. These estimates are acknowledged to be potentially overstated because (1) they are based on blood tests of women visiting antenatal clinics located mainly in urban areas, which are considered to have higher prevalence rates than in rural areas; and (2) the antenatal data do not include men, who are likely to have lower rates of HIV infection than women (UNAIDS 2002; Chin 2003).

3. The information available to us from the Zambia census was not disaggregated by gender, and it would be important in a more detailed analysis to consider potential differences in, and implications of, migratory patterns by gender.

References

Ainsworth, M., S. Ghosh, and I. Semali. 1995. The impact of adult deaths on household composition in Kagera Region, Tanzania. Washington, D.C.: Policy Research Department, World Bank. Unpublished manuscript.

Barnett, T. 1994. The effects of HIV/AIDS on farming systems and rural livelihoods in Uganda, Tanzania, and Zambia. Working paper. Norwich, U.K.: University of East Anglia.

Barnett, T., and P. Blaikie. 1992. *AIDS in Africa: Its present and future impact.* London: Belhaven Press.

Beegle, K. 2003. *Labour effects of adult mortality in Tanzanian households,* World Bank Working Paper, Washington, D.C.

Bell, C., S. Devarajan, and H. Gersbach. 2003. *Long run economic costs of AIDS: Theory and applcation to South Africa.* Report posted on Development Gateway, http://www.developmentgateway.org.

Bryceson, D., and D. Potts (eds.). 2005. *African Urban Economies: Viability, Vitality, or Vitiation?* Basingstoke, U.K.: Palgrave Macmillan.

Byerlee, D., and C. K. Eicher, eds. 1997. *Africa's emerging maize revolution.* Boulder, Colo.: Lynne Rienner.

Chapoto, A., and T. S. Jayne. 2005. *Impacts of HIV/AIDS-related mortality on rural farm households in Zambia: Implications for poverty reduction strategies.* Paper presented at the IUSSP Seminar on "Interactions between Poverty and HIV/AIDS," December 12–13, 2005. Capetown, South Africa. *Economic Development and Cultural Change,* forthcoming.

Chin, J. 2003. *Understanding the epidemiology and transmission dynamics of the HIV/AIDS pandemic.* School of Public Health, University of California/Berkeley. Paper presented at USAID, Washington, D.C., October 2003.

Donovan, C., L. Bailey, E. Mpyisi, and M. Weber. 2003. Prime-age adult morbidity and mortality in rural Rwanda: Effects on household income, agricultural production and food security strategies. Research Report, Food Security Research Project, Ministry of Agriculture, Livestock, and Forestry, Kigali.

Drimie, S. 2002. *HIV/AIDS and land: Case studies from Kenya, Lesotho, and South Africa.* Report for Southern Africa Regional Office of the Food and Agricultural Organization of the United Nations (FAO), Human Sciences Research Council, Pretoria, South Africa.

FASAZ (Farming System Association of Zambia). 2003. *Inter-linkages between HIV/AIDS, agricultural production, and food security.* Integrated Support to Sustainable Development and Food Security Programme, Food and Agriculture Organization of the United Nations. Rome: FAO.

Fox, M., S. Rosen, W. MacLeod, M. Wasunna, M. Bii, G. Foglia, and G. Simon. 2003. *The impact of HIV/AIDS on labour productivity in Kenya.* Draft discussion paper, Center for International Health and Development, Boston University, Boston.

Gertler, P., D. Levine, and S. Martinez. 2003. *The presence and presents of parents: Do parents matter for more than their money?* Unpublished manuscript, Berkeley: University of California Berkeley.

Gillespie, S. 1989. Potential impact of AIDS on farming systems: A case study from Rwanda. *Land Use Policy* 6: 301–312.

Govereh, J., T. S. Jayne, and J. Shaffer. 2006. *Trends in Zambian agriculture, 1990–2004.* Working Paper 14, Food Security Research Project, Lusaka.

Government of Uganda. 2003. The impact of HIV/AIDS on agricultural production and mainstreaming HIV/AIDS into agricultural extension in Uganda. Ministry of Agriculture, Animal Industry and Fisheries, Kampala.

Haggblade, S., and G. Tembo, 2003. *Conservation farming in Zambia.* Discussion Paper, Environment, Productivity, and Technology Division, International Food Policy Research Institute, Washington D.C.

Harris, J., and M. Todaro. 1970. Migration, unemployment, and development: A two-sector analysis. *American Economic Review* 40: 126–142.

Jayne, T. S., T. Yamano, M. Weber, D. Tschirley, R. Benfica, A. Chapoto, and B. Zulu. 2003a. Smallholder income and land distribution in Africa: Implications for poverty reduction strategies. *Food Policy* 28 (3): 253–275.

Jayne, T. S., J. Govereh, M. Wanzala, and M. Demeke. 2003b. Fertilizer market development: A comparative analysis of Ethiopia, Kenya, and Zambia. *Food Policy* 28 (4): 293–316.

Johnston, B. F., and P. Kilby. 1975. *Agriculture and structural transformation: Economic strategies in late-developing countries.* New York: Oxford University Press.

Lehutso-Phooko, M., and J. Naidoo. 2002. Income inequality prospects with HIV/AIDS: A social dimension. *Labour Markets and Social Frontiers* 2: 11–16. South Africa Reserve Bank.

Mather, D., C. Donovan, T. S. Jayne, M. Weber, E. Mazhangara, L. Bailey, K. Yoo, T. Yamano, and E. Mghenyi. 2004. A cross-country analysis of household responses to adult mortality in rural Sub-Saharan Africa: Implications for HIV/AIDS mitigation and rural development policies. International Development Working Paper 82, Department of Agricultural Economics, Michigan State University, East Lansing.

Mellor, J. 1976. *The new economics of growth: A strategy for India and the developing world.* Ithaca, N.Y.: Cornell University Press.

Menon, R., M. J. Wawer, J. K. Konde-Lule, N. K. Sewanlambo, and C. Li. 1998. The economic impact of adult mortality on households in Rakai district, Uganda. In *Confronting AIDS: Evidence from the developing world,* eds. M. Ainsworth, L. Fransen, and M. Over. European Commission, Brussels.

Mushati, P., S. Gregson, M. Mlilo, J. Lewis, and C. Zvidzai. 2003. Adult mortality and the economic sustainability of households in towns, estates, and villages in AIDS-affected eastern Zimbabwe. Paper presented at the Scientific Meeting on Empirical Evidence for the Demographic and Socio-Economic Impact of AIDS, Durban, South Africa, March 26–28, 2003, University of Durban.

Oehmke, J., and E. Crawford. 1996. The impact of agricultural technology in Sub-Saharan Africa. *Journal of African Economies* 5 (2): 271–292.

Reardon, T., E. Crawford, and V. Kelly. 1995. *Promoting farm investment for sustainable intensification of agriculture,* International Development Paper 18, Department of Agricultural Economics, Michigan State University, East Lansing.

Rugalema, G. 1999. HIV/AIDS and the commercial agricultural sector of Kenya. Report. FAO/UNDP, Rome.

Smale, M., and T. S. Jayne. 2003. Seeds of success: maize in historical retrospective. In *Successes in African agriculture: Building for the future,* ed. Steven Haggblade. International Food Policy Research Institute, Washington, D.C.

UNAIDS. 2002. Report on the global HIV/AIDS epidemic. UNAIDS, June 2002.

United Nations. 2003. *The impact of HIV/AIDS on mortality.* Population Division, United Nations Secretariat, New York.

U.S. Census Bureau. 2003. *The AIDS pandemic in the 21st century.* Report for XIV International Conference on AIDS, Barcelona, July 2002, International Program Center, U.S. Census Bureau.

Yamano, T., and T. S. Jayne. 2004. Measuring the impacts of working-age adult mortality among small-scale farm households in Kenya. *World Development* 32 (1): 91–119.

Chapter 9

The Ecology of Poverty: Nutrition, Parasites, and Vulnerability to HIV/AIDS

Eileen Stillwaggon

H IV/AIDS continues to spread throughout the developing world, in transition countries, and among poor and marginalized populations in industrialized countries. In its third decade, and even with increased resources, global AIDS policy is still failing to stem the epidemic. HIV prevention fails because it ignores the fundamental causes of the epidemic, it is unscientific, and it attempts to intervene at the last minute with programs limited to behavior change.

The HIV epidemic is not an isolated event. It is the predictable result of declining economies, insecure food systems, and inadequate investment in water, sanitation, health care, and education. The crisis of sustainable agricultural systems, most notably in Sub-Saharan Africa but elsewhere as well, has aggravated the health crisis in developing countries and favored the spread of HIV. The collapse of agricultural economies caused rapid urbanization, unemployment, and increasing inequality. The AIDS literature addresses, to some extent, the effect of economic crisis on behavior through the disruption of relationships and through pressures toward unsafe sex, in particular in the form of commercial sex for survival. Little emphasis, however, has been placed on the direct, biological effects of malnutrition and unsanitary conditions on the vulnerability of individuals and societies to HIV.

The epidemic of HIV cannot be explained by behavioral factors alone, even though a necessary condition is contact through sex, needles or other medical instruments, or mother to child. Scientific evidence demonstrates the role of biological cofactors such as malnutrition and parasitic and infectious diseases in enabling the transmission of HIV. Although AIDS policy organizations use the phrase, "AIDS is a development issue," they do not incorporate scientific information about the diseases and conditions of poverty into their programming for HIV prevention. Consequently, their policies are limited to programs that address only behavioral factors. This chapter integrates analysis of poverty with the epidemiology of infectious and parasitic diseases. Combining medical, economic, and geographical data, it demonstrates the specific disease synergies that promote HIV transmission in poor populations.

How Diseases Spread

An individual's vulnerability to any disease depends on the strength of the immune system, which is affected by nutrition, stress, and the presence of other infections and parasites, as well as other factors. Transmission of a disease also depends on the virulence of the pathogen. HIV has a very low probability of transmission between otherwise healthy adults: one in 1,000 contacts from women to men and one in 500 contacts from men to women (World Bank 1997). The low probability of transmission between healthy adults, however, has little applicability among poor people in Sub-Saharan Africa, Asia, Latin America, and transition countries because they are already immunocompromised as a result of malnutrition, parasites, or other infections. The risk of infection with HIV is greater than that in well-nourished, healthy populations, not only because of higher prevalence of HIV in the population but also because of the prevalence of those cofactor conditions that decrease immune response in HIV-negative persons and increase viral load in HIV-infected persons. Infectious and parasitic diseases and malnutrition create an environment of risk. In a risky environment, the likelihood of infection with HIV is greater with each sexual contact, regardless of the number of contacts.

Malnutrition

Probably the most fundamental cause of the widespread epidemic of HIV, particularly in Sub-Saharan Africa, is the failure of agricultural systems and food supply. Food insecurity has promoted the spread of HIV both indirectly, through migration and the resort to risky behaviors, and directly, through its biological effect. Malnutrition undermines the immune response, directly increasing vulnerability to disease.

Epidemiology has long recognized the importance of adequate nutrition for protection from disease. In the late 1960s, the World Health Organization officially acknowledged the important synergies between malnutrition and infection. With the advances of molecular biology of the past several decades, it is possible to see the specific mechanisms by which overall malnutrition and micronutrient deficiencies weaken the immune system. That weakened immune response makes people more vulnerable to all infectious and parasitic diseases, regardless of whether they are transmitted by water, food, air, soil, or sex.

Increased susceptibility to infection results from both protein and energy malnutrition (macronutrition) and deficiencies of specific micronutrients, such as iron, zinc, and vitamins. Infection and malnutrition are synergistic; minor illnesses can cause lack of appetite, which is very dangerous in a person who is already nutritionally deficient and parasite-laden. Fever increases the demands for energy at the same time that intake decreases. Diarrheal diseases cause a rapid loss of nutrients (Scrimshaw and SanGiovanni 1997).

Both undernutrition and micronutrient deficiency, even in the absence of readily observable symptoms, weaken every component of the immune system, both its adaptive and nonadaptive responses. Numerous studies have demonstrated the effects of even moderate protein-energy malnutrition (PEM) on the physical barriers, epithelial (skin) and mucosal protection (Woodward 1998). The humoral response is also affected through atrophy of the lymph system, and reduction in size and weight of the thymus results, affecting T-cell production (Beisel 1996; Chandra 1997). Children with PEM, regardless of degree or type (stunting or wasting), have reduced cell-mediated adaptive immunity (Chandra 1997; Woodward 1998). Protein is very important in resistance to infection because most elements of the immune system depend on cell replication, which requires protein (Scrimshaw and SanGiovanni 1997). Protein deficiency has been shown to impair resistance to tuberculosis, for example, by preventing containment of the mycobacteria within the primary lesions (McMurray 1998).

Micronutrient deficiencies also weaken every component of the immune system, even when deficiencies are relatively mild (Chandra 1997). Some diseases, such as scurvy (from vitamin C deficiency) and pellagra (from a lack of niacin, a B vitamin), result from specific nutrient deficiencies. Besides their role in deficiency-specific diseases, many nutrients are needed both singly and in conjunction with others to maintain an immune system that can resist the entire array of infectious, parasitic, and even chronic degenerative diseases. Iron-deficiency anemia, for example, is the most widespread nutritional deficiency in the world and is especially common in women and children. Iron is essential in promoting resistance to infection through humoral response (B cells), T cells, and NK cells (Scrimshaw and SanGiovanni 1997).

Even mild zinc deficiency can cause a large decrease in natural killer cell activity and reduced production of thymic hormone, affecting T-cell production (Beisel 1996; Cunningham-Rundles 1998). Zinc deficiency also impedes wound healing, undermines skin integrity as a barrier to infection, and weakens resistance to parasite infection, which aggravates malnutrition (Chandra 1997). Zinc deficiency is a common result of prolonged diarrhea; supplementation reduces diarrhea and is a low-cost way to reduce malnutrition and boost immune response (Ruel et al. 1997).

Vitamin A deficiency reduces the number of natural killer cells, diminishing nonspecific, or natural, defense mechanisms against antigens. Vitamin A also is required for the production of T cells, or specific defenses. Insufficiency of vitamin A is the deficiency that is most synergistic with infectious disease (Semba 1998). Infection increases excretion of vitamin A, producing a deadly synergism of malnutrition, infection, and increased vitamin A deficiency (Stephensen et al. 1994). Even children with subclinical vitamin A deficiency show a reduced immune response and greater vulnerability to infection, particularly of the skin and mucous membranes (Solomons 1998). Subclinical vitamin A deficiency is more likely to occur in children who also show signs of PEM (Khandait et al. 1998).

Vitamin A is particularly important in the promotion of physical barriers to infection. Vitamin A deficiency disturbs the integrity of the skin and mucous membranes and permits the invasion of pathogens in the eyes, the respiratory system, and the genitourinary and digestive systems (Semba 1998). Vitamin A deficiency also impairs iron utilization and so interacts with anemia (Sommer et al. 1996). Supplementation with vitamin A along with iron can eliminate anemia. Supplementation with vitamin A is very low cost, and its cost-effectiveness is enhanced because of its interaction with iron.

Nutritional deficiencies interact with parasite infection to make a combined assault on nutrition and immune support (Friedman et al. 2003). Vitamin A supplementation is an effective low-cost strategy to reduce malarial illness in young children (Shankar et al. 1999). Interventions that address nutritional deficiencies and parasitic infection are important for their own sake and for HIV prevention, especially because blood transfusions are a common therapy for malaria, which is endemic in areas where blood supplies may also be unsafe (Hedberg et al. 1993).

In sum, overall malnutrition combined with micronutrient deficiency is widespread in Sub-Saharan Africa, South Asia, and elsewhere among very poor people and is responsible for suppression of immunity through all three routes: physical barriers, humoral immunity, and cell-mediated immunity. In particular, vitamin A deficiency produces a greater susceptibility to STDs, particularly of the ulcerative type, in malnourished populations in tropical areas. It is important to reiterate that STDs (including HIV) are not a special case; they are infectious bacterial and viral diseases that can most easily be transmitted to a host whose immune system is weakened by malnutrition and by the synergistic effects of other infectious and parasitic diseases. STDs find their most fertile ground in the most nutritionally immunosuppressed population, such as we find in many countries in Africa and Asia. In particular, malnutrition that disturbs epithelial integrity promotes access for any disease, including genital ulcer diseases that provide entry points for HIV.

Maternal malnutrition in general and deficiencies of specific micronutrients, such as vitamin A, are associated with greater risk of vertical (mother to child) transmission of HIV. In Malawi, it was observed that mothers severely deficient in vitamin A had a much higher risk of transmitting HIV to their children, perhaps because of its effect on the vaginal mucosa or the integrity of the placenta (Semba et al. 1994; Nimmagadda, O'Brien, and Goetz 1998). Increased viral load in the mother and decreased maternal antibody protection, both associated with impaired T- and B-cell production from vitamin A deficiency, are also probable causes of greater transmission (Landers 1996). Randomized trials in Tanzania found that multivitamin supplementation decreased fetal deaths and increased T-cell counts in HIV-infected mothers (Fawzi et al. 1998). Nutritional supplementation of mothers was expected to reduce vertical transmission by reducing viral load in secretions in the birth canal and in breast milk (Fawzi and Hunter 1998). Although recent trials of vitamin A supplementation have not yet been successful in reducing vertical transmission, they suggest useful avenues for research. The environment of poverty, malnutrition, and parasitosis in which HIV flourishes provides a complicated laboratory for trials of any single intervention. Complementary interventions in malaria treatment or other nutritional supplements might be necessary in order to detect the effectiveness of vitamin A supplementation for HIV prevention in this multiburdened population.

Systemic maternal virus burden is an important factor in HIV transmission to infants. Local virus burden (in the birth canal), however, may be even greater than systemic viral load, and therefore, measures of systemic viral load might understate the risk of vertical transmission. Anemia is associated with greater viral shedding, with consequent locally higher viral burden in the birth canal, increasing the risk of transmission from mother to child, which could be remedied with nutritional supplementation (John et al. 1997).

Malnutrition in its various forms promotes viral replication and consequently can contribute to greater risk of vertical or sexual transmission (Friis and Michaelsen 1998). Supplementation improves health outcomes for HIV-infected persons, including children. In addition to helping people living with HIV, the reduction in viral load from improved nutrition reduces the risk of transmission for children and adults.

Parasitic Diseases

The economic crisis in developing countries and the austerity policies that were subsequently enforced contributed to the neglect of sanitary infrastructure and programs to eradicate parasitic and infectious diseases. Development policies in most countries ignored the crucial role of good health not only for human development but also for the economic viability of poor countries. Populations burdened by parasites cannot learn or work to their full capacity and are more susceptible to epidemics, such as that of HIV/AIDS.

Parasitic and infectious diseases interact with malnutrition. Malnourished people are more vulnerable to those diseases, and their illnesses are more severe than those of well-nourished people. Parasites also aggravate malnutrition by increasing calorie requirements and draining nutrients. Through their effect on malnutrition and through specific synergies with HIV transmission detailed below, parasitic diseases increase the spread of HIV/AIDS.

Malaria

Malaria is caused by a protozoal parasite spread by mosquitoes. The endemic zone of malaria is increasing as a result of lack of control efforts and perhaps also climate disturbance from global warming. Over 300 million people in Africa suffer from acute malaria each year, and almost one million children in Africa die of malaria annually. Malaria is also implicated in the spread of HIV in Sub-Saharan Africa.

Malaria stimulates HIV replication, and HIV viral loads (the amount of virus in the blood, semen, or other body fluid) are significantly higher in malarial patients than in HIV-infected persons without malaria. The higher HIV viral load in malarial patients, even after four weeks of treatment for malaria, suggests that malaria could cause faster progression of HIV (Whitworth et al. 2000). High viral load as a result of malaria coinfection correlates with risk of HIV transmission through blood, from mother to child, and through sexual contact. In Malawi, men with malaria were found to have seven times the median viral load of HIV-infected men without malaria. The reduction in viral load that results after treatment for malaria indicates that the causation is not from higher viral load to malaria but rather from malaria to higher viral load (Hoffman et al. 1999).

HIV-infected persons also have higher malaria-parasite densities in their blood, which increases the likelihood of malaria transmission in a population with high HIV prevalence (Whitworth et al. 2000; Rowland-Jones and Lohman 2002). The greater prevalence of malaria and the higher parasite loads both mean that HIV also promotes malaria transmission. Malaria is a very serious health problem in the developing world, especially in Sub-Saharan Africa. Malaria control is essential for reducing HIV transmission in children and adults through its effect on viral load for mothers and for sexual partners (Corbett et al. 2002). Controlling malaria would also alleviate one of the world's most devastating health problems.

Helminthic and Filarial Infections

Poor communities lack sanitary facilities for disposal of human waste, which perpetuates the cycle of contamination of soil with numerous kinds of worms. Lack of easy access to clean water makes it difficult to keep hands and food preparation areas clean. Consequently, soil-transmitted helminths are virtually ubiquitous in shantytowns, rural communities, and even among more affluent urban residents in many countries. Nearly 1.5 billion people are infected with ascariasis, 1.3 billion with hookworm, and over 1 billion with trichuriasis (PPC 2002). Worms cause malnutrition, even in adequately fed persons, because they drain the food supply through diarrhea, and they cause anemia from intestinal bleeding. They also weaken immune response because the immune system is exhausted from chronic reaction to the nonself invaders. Helminthic and filarial infections have also been shown to increase susceptibility to HIV acquisition and likelihood of transmitting HIV.

One of the reasons that ubiquitous health conditions, such as worm infection, are overlooked as cofactors is frequently the lack of a control group. In developing countries, virtually everyone harbors at least one parasite, so it is almost impossible to conduct research on a population not affected by endemic parasitic disease. By comparing recent immigrants from Ethiopia with earlier immigrants from Ethiopia and elsewhere, a team of Israeli researchers has shown that immune activation of the host caused by endemic infections, particularly helminthic (worm) infections, makes the host more susceptible to HIV infection and more vulnerable to HIV replication once infected (Bentwich et al. 1999). More than 80 percent of immigrants they studied had at least one helminthic parasite, 40 percent had two parasites, and 3 percent were infected with four different intestinal parasites. Even those who were HIV-negative and TB-negative evidenced broad immune dysregulation (Borkow et al. 2000). Blood cells taken from HIV-negative but helminth-infected subjects were highly susceptible to HIV. In addition, treatment for helminths reduced HIV plasma viral load in HIV-infected persons (Bentwich et al. 1999). HIV viral load is greater in people from developing countries and is positively correlated with helminth load. Helminths impair immune response, but treating people for worms enables immune response to recover (Borkow et al. 2001). Deworming is cheap, effective, and easily tolerated.

Filaria worm infection is also endemic in countries throughout Asia, Africa, and the Americas, and filariasis is also implicated in greater transmission of HIV. Blood cells of people infected with filaria worms and exposed to HIV show higher levels of HIV proliferation compared to blood cells of healthy persons similarly exposed in vitro. Furthermore, blood cells taken after patients are treated for filarial infection are less susceptible to HIV infection. People infected with worms very likely have increased susceptibility to HIV infection, and "aggressive treatment and control programs for filarial diseases and possibly other helminth infections in areas of Africa, India, and Southeast Asia where the HIV epidemic is rampant" are necessary (Gopinath et al. 2000).

Genital Schistosomiasis

Schistosomiasis is a parasitic disease second only to malaria in its prevalence. It affects more than 200 million people in 74 countries (WHO 1996/2003). Of the five species of waterborne schistosome flatworms, *S. hematobium* is more common in Sub-Saharan Africa than in other regions. Dam construction has caused an increase in schistosomiasis prevalence in a number of African regions, including a threefold increase in some countries (Sharp 2003).

People become infected with schistosomiasis when they are in contact with fresh water in lakes and slow-moving streams infested with snails that harbor the schistosome worms. The worms enter through the skin and locate in the intestines (*S. mansoni* generally) or the urinary tract (*S. hematobium*). The worms leave eggs that further infect those regions. Because people use such streams for bathing, washing clothes, recreation, or collecting aquatic plants for food or thatching houses, schistosome infection is widespread.

With the possible exception of malaria, schistosomiasis, also known as bilharzia, is probably the most significant parasitic cofactor of HIV transmission because some schistosome species colonize the genitourinary tracts. Urinary and intestinal schistosomiasis are generally the more recognized variants, but the importance of genital infection with schistosome worms and eggs has been known for decades. The interaction of female genital schistosomiasis with and contribution to HIV transmission was clearly described as early as 1995 (Feldmeier et al. 1995) and has been demonstrated in numerous studies reported in scientific journals since then, and yet schistosomiasis treatment and eradication are not addressed in HIV-prevention programs. The coincidence of schistosome-endemic areas with zones of high HIV prevalence provides epidemiologic support for a biological mechanism by which the parasite increases vulnerability to HIV transmission (Harms and Feldmeier 2002). Schistosomiasis is so highly endemic that it can be overlooked as a cofactor for other locally endemic conditions.

Prevalence in endemic zones is extremely high. In one endemic area of Tanzania, for example, 63 percent of residents were infected with *S. hematobium,* and 34 percent with *S. mansoni* (Poggensee et al. 2000). Sixty to 75 percent of women with *S. hematobium* (urinary) have genital manifestations, with infestation of worms and ova in the vagina, uterus, vulva, or cervix (Feldmeier, Helling-Giese, and Poggensee 2001; Harms and Feldmeier 2002; Mosunjac et al. 2003).

In spite of numerous references in the medical literature, female genital schistosomiasis (FGS) has been overlooked and has often been mistaken for a sexually transmitted disease (Attili, Hira, and Dube 1983). The presumption by medical professionals and the local population that the symptoms of FGS were in fact symptoms of sexually transmitted diseases has inhibited women from seeking medical care and contributed to stigmatization of women with FGS symptoms (Feldmeier et al. 1995). Even in regions with prevalence of schistosomiasis exceeding 40 percent of the population, such as on the shores of Lake Victoria, people feel that the infection is a shameful condition. Because of its location in the genital organs, they consider it an STD in spite of its transmission in water and the increasing prevalence with proximity to the lake (Mwanga et al. 2004).

Female genital lesions from schistosomiasis bleed spontaneously and from contact. In young girls, lesions are generally located in the vulva and vagina. At sexual maturity, the lesions become more numerous and cluster in the cervix, which is the area most vulnerable to HIV infection in young women (Marble and Key 1995). Genital schistosomiasis promotes the transmission of HIV not only through the general effect of parasite load on nutritional balance and immune activation but also through its direct effect on the immune system barriers (skin and mucosa) and on the cell-mediated response. The numerous lesions produced by the eggs of the schistosome worm on the cervix, the vulva, and the vagina provide direct access to the bloodstream for the HIV virus (Feldmeier et al. 1995). Both viable and dead ova also produce an inflammatory reaction in the tissue and attract $CD4^+$ T cells, which are HIV-susceptible (Poggensee et al. 2000; Mosunjac et al. 2003), to those sites. FGS lesions and inflammation can promote both male-to-female and female-to-male transmission of HIV.

HIV is more prevalent in areas with high schistosome prevalence than in low-prevalence areas (Feldmeier et al. 1995; Marble and Key 1995). Much has been made of the role of commerce in facilitating HIV transmission in Kenya, Uganda, and Tanzania in the regions around Lake Victoria. The emphasis has been on sexual partner change that might accompany the trade in goods across the lake. But the extremely high prevalence of schistosomiasis in the area around the lake has been virtually ignored except by tropical disease specialists.

Genital schistosomiasis in men has been less studied, but there are also indications that it can promote HIV transmission through inflammation of the genital area. In one study in Madagascar, 43 percent of semen samples of a cross-sectional community-based study showed the presence of schistosome eggs. Bleeding associated with male genital schistosome infection is less often noticed than with urinary schistosomiasis, and so the genital form has been overlooked. In HIV-infected men, such bleeding also promotes viral shedding (Feldmeier et al. 1999; Leutscher et al. 2000). In Africa alone, 200 million people, men and women, are afflicted with genitourinary schistosomiasis (Feldmeier et al. 1999), constituting a very large population with increased susceptibility to HIV or more virulent infections of HIV.

In the HIV literature and in global AIDS policy, there is a great deal of attention paid to the notion of risk behaviors. It is clear from the data we have about schistosomiasis and other parasites that one of the riskiest activities in Africa is to be a little girl or boy who gathers water for the family in a slow-moving stream or helps with the family laundry at creekside or bathes or plays in fresh water. When he or she grows up, that child will have a much higher risk of sexual transmission or acquisition of HIV because of a schistosome infection than a healthy person with similar sexual behavior. AIDS policy needs to address the mundane risks of growing up in Sub-Saharan Africa, Asia, and Latin America that burden people with sickness and make them more vulnerable to HIV.

The connection between parasite infection and HIV transmission makes treatment of schistosomiasis and other parasites a very high priority in an HIV-prevention program (Wolday et al. 2002). Effective treatment for schistosomiasis can be delivered for less than 25 U.S. cents per adult and even less for children (WHO 1996/2003). Treatment, however, provides only temporary relief unless there are also parallel improvements in better water, sanitation, and health education. The demonstration that parasite infection interacts with HIV viral load and HIV transmission makes a recalculation of the cost-effectiveness of eradication of *Schistosoma* and other parasites even more urgent. Eradication through water and sanitation investments is also attractive because once high-cost environmental measures are in place, they generate relatively low recurrent cost (Chandiwana and Taylor 1990).

Conclusion

The same conditions that promote high prevalence of other infectious diseases and parasites are responsible for the spread of the AIDS epidemic in poor populations. Programs to prevent HIV transmission will be unsuccessful unless they address the underlying causes of the spread of AIDS. HIV prevention must be based on scientific evidence regarding cofactor conditions, not, as they currently are, on unproven assumptions about the primacy of behavioral factors. Poverty eradication is ultimately the most important means for stopping AIDS epidemics. Investments in food security, sanitary infrastructure, and education are integral parts of a program of poverty eradication. Food security, deworming, schistosomiasis prevention and treatment, and malaria control programs must be incorporated into HIV prevention.

Inexpensive means and organizational support are already available for achieving these goals and can be integrated with AIDS programming.

For 25 years, global AIDS policy has been divorced from the accumulated knowledge and experience in the field of public health. The limited menu of AIDS interventions evidences little understanding of this complex epidemic. Global health policy is trammeled by reliance on tools of epidemiology and health economics that are too rudimentary to understand a complex epidemic. (For a longer analysis of the limitations of methodology, see Stillwaggon 2006.) Randomized controlled trials and cost-effectiveness studies are useful when the relationships to be studied are simple and easily isolated. Public health problems of populations in poverty are interrelated and synergistic. Furthermore, those conditions may be nearly ubiquitous in poor populations. Attempts to isolate the effects of vitamin A or malaria or worms on HIV transmission may be confounded by other endemic conditions. Treatment of only one condition may not produce measurable results because of the persistent impact of other maladies. Global AIDS policy is paralyzed because epidemiologic methods demand a "smoking gun" as evidence of relationships between HIV and the endemic conditions of malnutrition, parasites, and infectious disease. Such a burden of proof is inappropriate because interventions to reduce malnutrition, parasite load, and infectious diseases are beneficial in themselves and because a century of health research has demonstrated that they are necessary to prevent new epidemics, such as HIV/AIDS.

References

Attili, V. R., S. Hira, and M. K. Dube. 1983. Schistosomal genital granulomas: a report of 10 cases. *British Journal of Venereal Disease* 59: 269–272.

Beisel, W. 1996. Nutrition and immune function: Overview. *Journal of Nutrition* 126: 2611S–2615S.

Bentwich, Z., A. Kalinkovich, Z. Weisman, G. Borkow, N. Beyers, and A. Beyers. 1999. Can eradication of helminthic infections change the face of AIDS and tuberculosis? *Immunology Today* 20 (11): 485–487.

Borkow, G., Q. Leng, Z. Weisman, M. Stein, N. Galai, A. Kalinkovich, and Z. Bentwich. 2000. Chronic immune activation associated with intestinal helminth infections results in impaired signal transduction and anergy. *The Journal of Clinical Investigation* 106 (8): 1053–1060.

Borkow, G., Z. Weisman, Q. Leng, M. Stein, A. Kalinkovich, D. Wolday, and Z. Bentwich. 2001. Helminths, human immunodeficiency virus and tuberculosis. *Scandinavian Journal of Infectious Disease* 33: 568–571.

Chandiwana, S., and P. Taylor. 1990. The rational use of antischistosomal drugs in schistosomiasis control. *Social Science and Medicine* 30 (10): 1131–1138.

Chandra, R. K. 1997. Nutrition and the immune system: An introduction. *American Journal of Clinical Nutrition* 66: 460S–463S.

Corbett, E., R. Steketee, F. ter Kuile, A. Latif, A. Kamali, and R. Hayes. 2002. HIV-1/AIDS and the control of other infectious diseases in Africa. *Lancet* 359: 2177–2187.

Cunningham-Rundles, S. 1998. Analytical methods for evaluation of immune response in nutrient intervention. *Nutrition Reviews* 56 (1, Part 2): S27–S37.

Fawzi, W. W., and D. J. Hunter. 1998. Vitamins in HIV disease progression and vertical transmission. *Epidemiology* 9 (4): 457–466.

Fawzi, W. W., G. I. Msamanga, D. Spiegelman, E. Urassa, N. McGrath, D. Mwakagile, G. Antelman, R. Mbise, G. Herrera, S. Kapiga, W. Willett, and D. Hunter. 1998. Randomised trial of effects of vitamin supplements on pregnancy outcomes and T cell counts in HIV-1-infected women in Tanzania. *Lancet* 351: 1477–1482.

Feldmeier, H., G. Helling-Giese, and G. Poggensee. 2001. Unreliability of PAP smears to diagnose female genital schistosomiasis. *Tropical Medicine and International Health* 6 (1): 31–33.

Feldmeier, H., P. Leutscher, G. Poggensee, and G. Harms. 1999. Male genital schistosomiasis and haemospermia. *Tropical Medicine and International Health* 4 (12): 791–793.

Feldmeier, H., G. Poggensee, I. Krantz, and G. Helling-Giese. 1995. Female genital schistosomiasis. *Tropical and Geographical Medicine* 47 (2, Supplement): 2–15.

Friedman, J., J. Kurtis, R. Mtalib, M. Opollo, D. Lanar, and P. Duffy. 2003. Malaria is related to decreased nutritional status among male adolescents and adults in the setting of intense perennial transmission. *The Journal of Infectious Diseases* 188: 449–457.

Friis, H., and K. F. Michaelsen. 1998. Micronutrients and HIV infection: A review. *European Journal of Clinical Nutrition* 52: 157–163.

Gopinath, R., M. Ostrowski, S. Justement, A. Fauci, and T. Nutman. 2000. Filarial infections increase susceptibility to human immunodeficiency virus infection in peripheral blood mononuclear cells in vitro. *Journal of Infectious Diseases* 182 (6): 1804–1808.

Harms, G., and H. Feldmeier. 2002. Review: HIV infection and tropical parasitic diseases—deleterious interactions in both directions? *Tropical Medicine and International Health* 7 (6): 479–488.

Hedberg, K., N. Shaffer, F. Davachi, A. Hightower, B. Lyamba, K. Paluki, P. Nguyen-Dinh, and J. Breman. 1993. *Plasmodium falciparum*-associated anemia in children at a large urban hospital in Zaire. *American Journal of Tropical Medicine and Hygiene* 48 (3): 365–371.

Hoffman, I., C. Jere, T. Taylor, P. Munthali, J. Dyer, J. Wirima, S. Rogerson, N. Kumwenda, J. Eron, S. Fiscus, H. Chakraborty, T. Taha, M. Cohen, and M. Molyneux. 1999. The effect of *Plasmodium falciparum* malaria on HIV-1 RNA blood plasma concentration. *AIDS* 13: 487–494.

John, G., R. Nduati, D. Mbori-Ngacha, J. Overbaugh, M. Welch, B. Richardson, J. Ndinya-Achola, J. Bwayo, J. Krieger, F. Onyango, and J. Kreiss. 1997. Genital shedding of human immunodeficiency virus type 1 DNA during pregnancy: Association with immunosuppression, abnormal cervical or vaginal discharge, and severe vitamin A deficiency. *The Journal of Infectious Diseases* 175: 57–62.

Khandait, D. W., N. D. Vasudeo, S. Zodpey, D. Kumbhalkar, and M. Koram. 1998. Subclinical vitamin A deficiency in undersix children in Nagpur, India. *Southeast Asian Journal of Tropical Medicine and Public Health* 29 (2): 289–292.

Landers, D. 1996. Nutrition and immune function II: Maternal factors influencing transmission. *Journal of Nutrition* 126: 2637S–2640S.

Leutscher, P., C.-E. Ramarokoto, C. Reimert, H. Feldmeier, P. Esterre, and B. Vennervald. 2000. Community-based study of genital schistosomiasis in men from Madagascar. *The Lancet* 3555: 117–118.

Marble, M., and K. Key. 1995. Clinical facets of a disease neglected too long. *AIDS Weekly Plus* August 7: 16–19.

McMurray, D. 1998. Impact of nutritional deficiencies on resistance to experimental pulmonary tuberculosis. *Nutrition Reviews* 56 (1, Part 2): S147—S152.

Mosunjac, M., T. Tadros, R. Beach, and B. Majmudar. 2003. Cervical schistosomiasis, human papilloma virus (HPV), and human immunodeficiency virus (HIV): A dangerous coexistence or coincidence? *Gynecologic Oncolgy* 90 (1): 211–214.

Mwanga, J. R., P. Magnussen, C. Mugashe, R. Gabone, and J. Aagaard-Hansen. 2004. Schistosomiasis-related perceptions, attitudes and treatment-seeking practices in Magu District, Tanazania: Public health implications. *Journal of Biosocial Science* 36: 63–81.

Nimmagadda, A., W. O'Brien, and M. Goetz. 1998. The significance of vitamin A and carotenoid status in persons infected by the human immunodeficiency virus. *Clinical Infectious Diseases* 26: 711–718.

Poggensee, G., I. Kiwelu, V. Weger, D. Göppner, T. Diedrich, I. Krantz, and H. Feldmeier. 2000. Female genital schistosomiasis of the lower genital tract: prevalence and disease-associated morbidity in northern Tanzania. *The Journal of Infectious Diseases* 181: 1210–1213.

PPC (Partnership for Parasite Control). 2002. Rome meeting notes, 2002. http://www.who.int/wormcontrol/about_us/en/mtgnotes/april2002.pdf.

Rowland-Jones, S., and B. Lohman. 2002. Interactions between malaria and HIV infection—an emerging public health problem? *Microbes and Infection* 4: 1265–1270.

Ruel, T., J. A. Rivera, M. Santizo, B. Lönnerdal, and K. Brown. 1997. Impact of zinc supplementation on morbidity from diarrhea and respiratory infections among rural Guatemalan children. *Pediatrics* 99 (6): 808–813.

Scrimshaw, N., and J. P. SanGiovanni. 1997. Synergism of nutrition, infection, and immunity: An overview. *American Journal of Clinical Nutrition* 66: 464S–477S.

Semba, R. 1998. The role of vitamin A and related retinoids in immune function. *Nutrition Reviews* 56 (1, Part 2): S38–S48.

Semba, R., P. Miotti, J. Chiphangwi, A. Saah, J. Canner, G. Dallabetta, and D. Hoover. 1994. Maternal vitamin A deficiency and mother-to-child transmission of HIV-1. *Lancet* 343: 1593–1597.

Shankar, A. H., B. Genton, R. Demba, M. Baisor, J. Paino, S. Tamja, T. Adiguma, L. Wu, L. Rare, J. Tielsch, M. Alpers, and K. West Jr. 1999. Effect of vitamin A supplementation on morbidity due to *Plasmodium falciparum* in young children in Papua New Guinea: A randomised trial. *Lancet* 354: 203–209.

Sharp, D. 2003. Dam medicine. *The Lancet* 362: 184.

Solomons, N. 1998. Plant sources of vitamin A and human nutrition: Red palm oil does the job. *Nutrition Reviews* 56 (10): 309–311.

Sommer, A., K. West, K. West, and A. Ross. 1996. *Vitamin A deficiency: health, survival, and vision.* New York: Oxford University Press.

Stephensen, C. B., J. O. Alvarez, J. Kohatsu, R. Hardmeier, J. Kennedy Jr., and R. Gammon Jr. 1994. Vitamin A is excreted in the urine during acute infection. *American Journal of Clinical Nutrition* 60 (3): 388–392.

Stillwaggon, E. 2006. *AIDS and the ecology of poverty.* New York: Oxford University Press.

Whitworth, J., D. Morgan, M. Quigley, A. Smith, B. Mayanja, H. Eotu, N. Omoding, M. Okongo, S. Malamba, and A. Ojwiya. 2000. Effect of HIV-1 and increasing immunosuppression on malaria parasitaemia and clinical episodes in adults in rural Uganda: A cohort study. *Lancet* 356: 1051–1056.

WHO (World Health Organization). 1996 last updated/2003. *Schistosomiasis.* Fact Sheet No. 115, http://www.who.int/inf-fs/en/fact115.html.

Wolday, D., S. Mayaan, Z. Mariam, N. Berhe, T. Seboxa, S. Britton, N. Galai, A. Landai, and Z. Bentwich. 2002. Treatment of intestinal worms is associated with decreased HIV plasma viral load. *Journal of Acquired Immune Deficiency Syndromes* 31: 56–62.

Woodward, B. 1998. Protein, calories, and immune defenses. *Nutrition Reviews* 56 (1, Part 2): S84–S92.

World Bank. 1997. *Confronting AIDS: Public priorities in a global epidemic.* Oxford: Oxford University Press.

181 - 197

Zambia

I30
I12
015 J16
018

Chapter 10

Stigma When There Is No Other Option: Understanding How Poverty Fuels Discrimination toward People Living with HIV in Zambia

Virginia Bond

Introduction

Based on qualitative fieldwork in urban and rural Zambia (see Bond et al. 2003), this chapter aims to demonstrate that HIV-related stigma and discrimination are fueled by the practicalities of limited resources and narrow options and, in this wider context of poverty and household fatigue, that the poor, women, orphans, and rural dwellers are particularly vulnerable to HIV-related stigma and discrimination. It is apparent that a significant proportion of discriminatory actions are caused by the fact that HIV and AIDS can be so very hard to manage in the context of poverty. Significant differences between the urban and rural sites that emerged in our material, with overall less stigma manifested in the urban site and more pronounced stigma in the rural site, suggest that it is possible to alleviate household stress and reduce this type of stigma and discrimination by providing services and support.

Poverty and stigma have a peculiar relationship: it is easy to "understand" decisions in the context of poverty that result in discriminatory actions, for example, a decision to withdraw orphans from education because the household cannot afford to educate them. The decisions themselves are not always stigma per se, but the actions are experienced as stigmatizing. For example, orphans feel stigmatized by being out of school, and, the consequences of the actions can be damaging. And often the decisions are voiced through a language of attribution and blame.

The Wider Context

The intersections between poverty and stigma related to HIV and AIDS reinforce the fact that stigma cannot be isolated from other social processes and phenomena and that it must be understood in the context of other things happening (Wallman 1988), including, in Zambia, a process of "community unraveling" (Scudder 1983), hunger, deprivation, and limited capacity to cope (Bond 1998). Zambian society is staggering under the weight of economic hardship, the impact of HIV, poor education and health services, and widening inequality. These stresses are reflected in rising incidences of violence, alcohol abuse, accusations of Satanism and witchcraft, and family breakdown. As Whiteside and de Waal (see Barnett and Whiteside 2002) highlight in their "new variant famine" argument, HIV compounded with other problems, such as hunger, is a lethal combination.

These wider stresses lend themselves to the process of stigma. Others have written convincingly about how stigma is "allowed" to unfold within a context of inequitable power relations (Link and Phelan 2001), where stigma plays the role of separating "us" (the morally upright and socially pure) from "them" (the deviant and impure) and reinforces social stereotypes. This chapter aims to demonstrate the synergy between "diverse forms of inequality and stigma" (Parker and Aggleton 2003), as evident in the added vulnerability of the poor, women, and orphans to the dimension of stigma under the lens in this chapter. Castro and Farmer (2005) write, "poverty, already representing an almost universal stigma, will be the primary reason that poor people living with HIV suffer from greater AIDS-related stigma," and "social forces determine not only risk of HIV infection but also risk of AIDS-related stigma." But this chapter aims to make one additional point: that in the context of poverty, people stigmatize people living with HIV and AIDS because they have no other option.

What Is Stigma?

Stigma is a spoiled identity resulting from "an attribute that is deeply discrediting" (Goffman 1963), though, as Goffman further points out, it is a language of relationships, not attributes, that is really needed (Goffman 1963). A person's whole identity can be tainted by an attribute. Disease stigma is "negative social 'baggage' associated with a disease" (Deacon, Stephney, and Prosalendis 2005). In relation to HIV, stigma is the social process of combining the assumed presence of HIV virus in a person or group with "a perceived notion of culpability" (Scrambler 2004). As suggested above, HIV stigma is also often layered on preexisting stigma toward marginal or powerless groups (Herek and Glunt 1988; Parker and Aggleton 2003). The critical elements of HIV-related stigma to consider are causes of stigma, experiences of stigma, consequences of stigma, and strategies to cope with stigma.

The dimension of stigma being examined here is poverty as a cause of stigma. The experiences of stigma catalyzed by poverty revolve around experiences of devaluation, exclusion, and disadvantage (Sartorius 2004), which may be internalized in the forms of self-hatred, self-isolation, and shame (Alonzo and Reynolds 1995). Family members may also find they are "all obliged to share some of the discredit of the stigmatized person to whom they are related" (Goffman 1963).

Background to the Study

The Zambian research "Understanding HIV and AIDS-Related Stigma and Resulting Discrimination" was part of a multicountry study led by the International Centre for Research on Women (ICRW)[1] in collaboration with local partners in Ethiopia, Vietnam, Tanzania, and Zambia, which aimed to disentangle stigma and discrimination in an effort to provide entry points for programmers to reduce stigma; it was carried out from 2001 to 2004 (see Nyblade et al. 2003; Ogden and Nyblade 2005).

It is of significance that in this multicountry study, the relationship between poverty and stigma emerged most strongly in the Zambian material where poverty indices and HIV prevalence combined were the highest out of the four countries, and where household fatigue was the most evident.

Poverty in Zambia

Within the SADC region, by 2002, Zambia had the highest level of income poverty and the fourth largest level of human poverty (following Angola, Mozambique, and Malawi) (World Bank 2002). By 1998, overall national poverty stood at 72.9 percent of the population, with 57.9 percent classified as being in extreme poverty (LCS 1998; World Bank 2002). Poverty levels were highest in the rural area, although this disparity was narrowing by the late 1990s because of a rise in urban poverty; by 1998, 36.2 percent of the urban population were in extreme poverty compared to 70.9 percent of the rural population. Certain groups were more visibly poor than others, including small-scale farmers, large households, female-headed households, and women in general. Lusaka had the second highest concentration of the poor (World Bank 2002).

HIV in Zambia

Prevalence rates in adults aged 15–49 years were estimated to be 21.5 percent in 2002, with variations between urban and rural areas, and around one in four households had experienced an HIV-related death (UNAIDS 2002). Young women aged 15–19 were five times more likely to be infected than young men in the same age group (CBOH 1999), and in 2002, 5 percent of rural and 7 percent of the urban population were estimated to have taken an HIV test (Zambia Sexual Behaviour Survey 2002). As a result of HIV, the numbers of orphans were estimated to be at least 690,000, and at least 40 percent of households were looking after one or more orphans (UNICEF 1999; UNAIDS 2002). The number of orphans was highest in rural areas, in small-scale farming households, and in low-cost areas, where poverty indices were also the highest (World Bank 2002). In 2002, there were many more HIV/AIDS programs in urban areas than rural areas (CBOH 1999).

The Research Sites: Rural and Urban Microcosms of Wider Trends

In Zambia, seven months of qualitative research was carried out in 2002 in two adjacent high-density urban compounds in Lusaka, the capital city, and in a rural constituency in Choma district, Southern Province. Lusaka and Southern Provinces have the highest HIV prevalence in Zambia (CSO 2003), and in Lusaka and Southern Provinces, at least 18 percent and 17 percent, respectively, of the child population are estimated to be orphans (UNICEF 1999).

One of the Lusaka sites (Kamwala) is a planned residential area with a population of 30,000, government primary and secondary schools, a clinic (with voluntary counseling and testing services), piped water, and, with residents who are a mixture of middle-class in formal employment and working class whose income is derived from the informal economy. The other adjacent site is a shanty compound (illegal until 1995) called Misisi, with a population of 23,000, poor-quality housing, no government services, and with residents mostly involved in the informal economy, including clandestine activities. A demographic survey in the shanty compound revealed an extremely high level of adult mortality with HIV largely responsible (Kelly et al. 1998). As one resident barber in the study describes the area, "Very few children go to school, and very few people go for work. . . . People are failing to meet eating needs because they fail to find money."

Community-based organizations (CBOs), nongovernmental organizations (NGOs), and research activities related to HIV and AIDS are quite extensive in both compounds, especially the shanty compound, and include home-based care (HBC), a hospice, an orphanage, and a community school.

The rural site is called Mbabala, lying 30 kilometers to the northeast of Choma town in Southern Province. The population numbers around 15,000 people (mostly one ethnic group, the Tonga), and there are 36 villages, 21 resettlement schemes and commercial farms, seven schools, and one health center (with no VCT services at the time of the study). In Choma town, there is a district hospital and, further to the north, a mission hospital. The 2001/02 farming season was difficult because of late rains, and the harvest was poor. People are mainly farming and trading (in fish, farm products, and charcoal). CBO and NGO activities related to HIV and AIDS were slowly being introduced, but there was no active HBC. At one primary school accessed by four villages in the area, 72 of 350 pupils were orphans (21 double orphans), giving an indication of the orphan burden in the area.

A man living with HIV in the area describes the predicament households face when a household member falls sick as follows: "When someone is sick and the family is poor, there are talks over what to eat, small things that need money. This brings problems in the family. Where will the family get the money?"

Methodology

In each site, a series of participatory and community trust building activities were the starting point for the research. These included a stigma workshop with local representatives, community mapping, a stigma transect walk, free listing of terms used for people living with HIV and AIDS, picture discussions, and timelines of TB and HIV. Following a week of these activities, semistructured key informant interviews, and focus-group discussions were carried out with a representative range of community members (TB patients, people living with HIV/AIDS [PLWHA], youth, children, religious leaders, health professionals, caregivers, educators, farmers, employers, and NGO representatives). In total, 68 key-informant interviews and 53 focus group discussions (FGDs) were held.

In addition, eight one-day participatory workshops were held (four urban, four rural) with 72 children. The children were drawn from out-of-school children; school-going (government and community) children; children living with HIV and AIDS; and street children. And in the urban site, six rounds of interviews with 13 households affected by tuberculosis and HIV and AIDS were carried out.

The data were analyzed thematically and managed using QSR N6 software qualitative data package.

Key Dimensions of the Intersections of Poverty and Stigma

People Living with HIV and AIDS Are a Burden in the Context of Poverty

In a "biting economy" (15-year-old boy, urban), people living with HIV and AIDS are considered a "burden" according to respondents because they are not able to contribute to household income when they are sick and they undermine the income generation and progress of the household. During periods of illness, they soak up money, energy, and time. Both they and relatives who come to visit them take up space.

People living with HIV and AIDS are perceived as a burden for other reasons not related to poverty (for example, an emotional burden), but it was largely the economic burden that respondents in these communities focused on.

In order to meet the needs of people living with HIV and AIDS, households fall back on informal coping strategies (selling assets, borrowing, stealing) and can feel overwhelmed to the breaking point. "Your resources are milked," explained rural men farmers. In order to pay for treatment, food, surf (to wash linen), and water,[2] respondents often reported spending money and selling assets and sometimes reported borrowing money or goods or even telling lies and stealing, as young men in the rural site describe, "A lot of money or wealth will be wasted during that nursing period, and, as a result of the illness, you tend to borrow a lot and tell lies."

Sometimes there is simply "no means" of getting money and/or food; these are households where there is often little (and sometimes nothing) to eat or where people are already eating "unrecommendable food." For such households to repeatedly look after a chronically sick household member is unmanageable; as captured by an urban social worker, "people in this area are living under poverty, I can say. Very few people can manage to look after these people [living with HIV and AIDS] if you look at the current situation. As now, people are just feeding on unrecommendable food *ka pamela* per day, *chiwawa,* and *impwa.*[3] They think that if they start again looking after those people they are actually putting themselves in problems."

Complaints about demands for "special food" from people living with HIV and AIDS included "demands" for "chicken," "meat," "fruits out of season," and "tomatoes." Sometimes the treatment that is considered unaffordable is panadol (a painkiller), as described by gatekeepers in rural Zambia: "If I am poor, for example, I will not even afford to buy a panadol for K100,[4] but the rich go very fast and buy medicine, even if there is no cure." As an urban bus owner pointed out, the needs of people living with HIV and AIDS are often not budgeted for, and "a week's supply becomes days only." There is often a desperate concern that you cannot meet the special needs of the sick and that you are unable, if poor, to "accept them fully" (young women, urban). You can want to take them to the hospital, buy the medicine they are prescribed, and buy them the food they ask for, but you just do not have the money.

Relatives from the village (especially men) who come to visit the sick are an added burden, requiring additional food, space, needs, and transport expenses. Space in the house is very often limited. This is especially true if the visitors are men, said urban pregnant women, "the men will just come for luxury and other stuff. Men are a burden." If it is your spouse who is dying or who dies, there is the burden of being the only breadwinner: "both breadwinner and a widow, the burden is very much there" (health workers, urban).

But, even in the context of absolute poverty, there are certain relationships that withstand the strain, in particular parent–child relationships, because as rural elders proclaim, "you cannot throw away your own." People whom you "belong" to (chiefly close blood relatives) are obliged to care for you, especially in the village.

The quality of the past relationship, reciprocal relationships, individual character, and the household status of the sick person also influence care and stigma. It makes such a difference whether the person with HIV and AIDS is an old friend, family member, neighbor, stranger, or someone you never much liked anyway (Bond 2002). "It depends on how the patient used to relate to you before he or she got sick," explain urban TB patients, "If you were not good, you easily become a burden." An urban headmaster makes the same point even more bluntly: "There are some people even when they were okay they were so useless to the family and when such people are found in a situation, yes they are considered a burden." It was evident that how you get treated depends partly on your household status, with previous breadwinners less likely to be stigmatized, and more junior or marginal members more likely to be stigmatized.

Spiraling Poverty, Needs, and Neglect

Caregivers are not able to work while people living with HIV and AIDS are extremely sick. When illness reaches a "climax," it is "very involving, programs come to a standstill" (young men, rural), "your day-to-day duties are disrupted" (young women, rural), "progress and incomes are disturbed" (hospice worker, urban), and, "they shatter all your plans and activities" (secondary school children, urban). Over time, when spiraling poverty is pitted against spiraling needs, "poverty flows in" (pastor, rural), and this can lead to spiraling neglect. It is an illness that "takes too long" (politician rural), involves "very special care" (bar owner, urban), and "even when they are supposed to die it takes time" (community health workers, rural). Underlying this fatigue is the knowledge that HIV is an incurable disease and that no matter what you do, the patient will eventually die. The fact that the illness takes a long time drags households down, and the more you continue to look after a patient, the more money you lose. An NGO manager comments that even if you thought you could manage to care, you gradually lose patience and can eventually give up. Even urban health workers lament, "it can be an added burden, it is too much and especially when they become more sick and when they carry on to get more and more sick, it can become difficult." Rural secondary school girls relay the burden of treatment costs: "booking taxis taking the person to the clinic if the person is very sick. The hospital costs nowadays are very high, and the food [costs]. When the person dies you find that all the money was spent on the sick person."

The language used by households in relation to caring for people living with HIV and AIDS included: "no, I cannot bear with this kind of problem" (NGO manager, rural); "tiresome" (bar owner, urban); "it is burdensome" (traditional healer, rural).

Over time, as fatigue sets in and poverty worsens, households are likely to develop negative attitudes toward people living with HIV and AIDS, who are then more likely to experience different forms of stigma. They are accused of wasting time and money, and basic needs such as treatment, clean clothes, linen, food, and emotional support are not always met or are even cut out. Some people are sent elsewhere including, for urban dwellers, back to the village. Households say they are "not prepared to handle" (health worker, urban) the people living with HIV and AIDS. Young urban men relay, "If someone has been looking after an HIV-positive person for a long time, he will think 'I am just wasting my time. Why should I care for this person? He is just spending my money for nothing; after all, he will die.' . . . After a long time the care will drastically change."

Respondents reported that sometimes you actually want the patient to die or are advised to let the patient die. Traditional healers and young men in the urban area concur that resources are saved for the funeral over and above treatment and care; "other relatives who are spending on that person would advise you to do it roughly so that he dies; then they spend on the funeral" (traditional healers, urban); "They [the caregivers] will start preparing for the funeral and raising money for the coffin instead of buying food and some stuff" (young men, urban).

Powerlessness of Poor People Living with HIV and AIDS

The powerlessness, marginality, and vulnerability of poor people living with HIV and AIDS who are sick was widely acknowledged and attributed to the fact that they have nothing to offer and are therefore "overlooked" (young men, urban). Similar to street kids, children out of school, and sex workers, they are almost invisible and unaccounted for, as reflected in the following quotes: "you who is dog poor, they [community] just pass by you, not looking at you" (TB patients, men, rural); "(people living with HIV and AIDS) are unwanted and unprotected. . . . If there is no-one to help them, the poor die" (young women, urban); "Because of the hunger situation, it is a problem. You find that when one is poor, there are a few to nurse him" (gatekeepers, rural).

The situation of the poor was a sharp contrast to that of the rich. As urban secondary school children candidly observed, "The poor live 1 year, the rich 10." There is a strong sense that having HIV and AIDS is very different for people with money, that their money buys them more space to hide, allows them to live longer, helps cushion the impact, and allows them to more easily find support and love. People living with HIV and AIDS who are poor (living in either dense, urban conditions or in small, rural communities) have less space to hide from stigma when they are sick, they are sick more often, and they "die faster" or "when they are not supposed to" (headman, rural) and occasionally alone. Respondents commented that poor people's funerals are more likely to be shorter, cheaper, and to involve "less crying" (man living with HIV and AIDS, rural). Poor people are more likely to accept humiliation: "the poor keep quiet and accept any treatment" (secondary school pupils, rural).

In the urban area, primary school children mentioned how the rich could exchange their "contaminated blood" for clean blood,[5] and, a number of other respondents mentioned how the rich could go outside the country for treatment. A few respondents mentioned the rich being able to buy antiretrovirals; for example rural secondary school girls remarked, "Since they introduced these ARVs,[6] the rich man can easily manage to get them while the poor can't because they cost a lot of money."

A businesswoman in town commented that the differential treatment of the rich and poor "starts from hospital up to homes." There was evidence that the rich received preferential treatment in clinics, and the ulterior motive of looking after the rich was often mentioned: "people are after his wealth" (primary school boys, rural). Indeed, the rich were reputed to have no problem in finding bedside caregivers, "but if it's a poor person, this one has just a pair of Tropicals [flip-flops]; what can he leave behind? So they abandon him" (secondary school boys, rural). So for people living with HIV and AIDS, as a rural headman so vividly described, "the disease becomes deeper and deeper." Pregnant urban women bluntly state, "With the rich, you find even if he has soiled linen, many people will be willing to wash them, while for the poor, they will just leave everything, being there is no soap, a lack of water nowadays, and the person will be sleeping on dirty linen, and the disease will be even worse."

Poverty, Orphans, and HIV- and AIDS-Related Stigma

As the children's research in Zambia demonstrated (see Clay, Bond, and Nyblade 2003), orphans often experience differential treatment in the household. One of the main causes of this is being an orphan in a poor society. To take in additional children when "the economy is very bad and mostly families are failing. . . . is really heavy" (women TB patients, rural). Their "needs are always a second priority" (development officer, rural), and poor guardians are forced, or decide, to withdraw education, adequate food, and clothing from orphans. Orphans are regarded to be "wasting money" (secondary school girls, rural). You can "have the heart of looking after the children (orphans), but how?" exclaims an urban nursery school teacher. A woman in an urban household admits, "Small ones who can't do things on their own are especially a burden."

An urban headmaster pits duty against poverty: "In our Zambian society, it is our custom to look after people; if my brother has died, it is my duty to look after his children, but because of these economic changes, we are not able to look after the children, because of the economy." An urban peer educator sees it as a choice between educating your own children or looking after orphans: "Yes, they are seen as a burden because it's not possible for one to spend a lot of money on medicine, transport, food, instead of using it on one's own children for school."

Even your own children can be considered a burden in the context of poverty. An ex-TB patient in the household study explains how when he was sick, "my son was a burden because I was not working," and rural women TB patients explain how "Parents don't have enough to give to their own children."

Women, Poverty, and HIV- and AIDS-Related Stigma

Respondents considered women more vulnerable to deepening poverty and stigma. Women have less income-generating power, so if their husband is sick, the "financial problem in the house will be very big, they finish all the money and will end up selling furniture" (secondary school girls, rural), and the wife "will take all the responsibilities" (traditional healers, rural). Urban TB patients think that women are also more dependent than men on relatives for money, and the relatives "easily get fed up, complain, and later stop [giving help]." A member of a drama group in Misisi pointed out that when husbands are sick, women are sometimes forced into sex work in order to raise money for their husband's medicine.

The burden of caring for the sick falls largely on women, and this takes time away from caring for children and earning their own money because their "duty becomes only taking care of that sick person" (community health workers, rural).

If their husband dies first, women and children will often suffer. A widow in the household study said that she worried after her husband died and his business closed that she would not "have the means to look after the children." In the event, she moved out of the house they lived in and owned and rented it to give her an income. The custom of property grabbing[7] can leave women and children in abject poverty; as explained by urban gatekeepers, "usually what I have seen when the man dies, the woman is mistreated, the relatives of the man would want to grab everything from the woman, even forgetting the children. They will sometimes even call her names, or she will be blamed that she is the causer. But when it is the woman who has died, the family from the woman will not bother the man."

The combination of being a woman breadwinner and a widow[8] is brutal, and it is harder for widows both to raise enough money to get by and to remarry. Women, and more especially aunts and stepmothers, were cited by children as perpetuating abuse against orphans, reflecting the immense stress they are under (Clay, Bond, and Nyblade 2003). Urban traditional healers commented that women "shout" at their husband and children "because of HIV."

If poor women themselves fall sick, they are more vulnerable to "being chased" back to their parents, deserted or neglected by husbands, especially if they fall sick first or if they learn of their HIV-positive status first. A rural traditional healer commented that an HIV-positive woman, "will be isolated like a hoe without a person to use it." Rural community health workers commented how household chores grind to a halt when a woman is sick because "not all that a woman does can be done by a man, so it will be at a standstill."

Within poor communities, there is understanding, even coercion, around sex work until women or girls are thought to have HIV and AIDS, at which stage they are chastised, rejected, and blamed, or the mother is blamed for her daughter's transgressions and assumed status. As urban TB patients in Misisi wryly remarked, "For women, people like pinpointing their mothers that they are the ones who used to send them so that she brings money, especially in Misisi." At that stage, the focus is not on the poverty but how she got infected, and she and the mother are blamed for having transgressed. School children were aware of sex as a survival strategy, and how women are blamed if they fall sick. Looking at a picture of a woman seated surrounded by people with their backs to her, urban primary school children commented, "she was naughty, so everyone is reminding others what she used to do for money, and no-one is willing to help her out." Secondary school boys in the same urban site related how "Nowadays, the biggest problem is poverty. You find in a family no-one works or goes to work, so she (the mother) will decide to go and have a temporal affair so she can raise some money."

If women have no close family to return to, they are deeply vulnerable to neglect; as conveyed by urban traditional healers, "If you don't have a mother, no children, you will have problems. Relatives don't usually help. I say so because I witnessed this myself. A woman was sick, her husband ran away from her, she had no children, and only her relatives were there. If you don't have relatives, some women are buried very dirty, masked with feces."

In poor communities, sex workers are extremely vulnerable to not being cared for when they are sick, as illustrated in the following quote from one urban sex worker: "We have no support or visits from neighbors because they regard us as outcasts or 'not human beings' because of our business. . . . If I then get sick, they wouldn't even give me water if I needed it. . . . They always wish us to die. . . . It's not our wish to be sex workers, but it's due to poverty." The only case respondents in town recalled of a woman who died uncared for was of a sex worker, whose death was noticed by neighbors only once her body started to decompose, attracting flies and rats.

Poverty, Blame, and Stigma

Within explanations of poverty, underlying judgments often creep in to justify the stigmatizing actions. The implication is that poor people living with HIV and AIDS, especially poor women and children, are blamed[9] for their predicament. As a nutritionist in the urban area describes, "People are killing their own children very fast. They leave them to die slowly, painfully because they insult them and say bad names—'You alone went making money' and all sorts of words, which makes the patient have depression. They stop buying medicine . . . saying 'we can't manage. . . . If you want this type of food, you have to eat what we have because we have no money. We never costed but you costed all these, all the problems you have brought into this house!' Others are shunned very much."

Often it seems as though people are also aware of what they are doing, almost as though they are justifying why death has selected one person and not another. And there is recognition that blaming and complaining adversely affect the patient.

Rural Poverty and Stigma

Some urban families do not have rural ties, but for those that do (especially the more recent migrants), there is a trend for people suspected to have HIV and AIDS, and orphans, being sent back to the village.[10] A rural traditional healer commented, "the village is now the dumping ground," and young rural men said that people in town were "throwing" the problem to the village. The motives for doing this include spiritual connections,[11] close family ties in the village, and the tradition of care in the village, what rural gatekeepers called being cared for in "your own circles." But other motives are more discriminatory: wanting to grab property in the town; wanting to get rid of the problem; not having enough money to cope; and that funerals are cheaper in the village, where people often die at home and can be buried just in a blanket or a homemade coffin, saving hospital, mortuary, transport, and coffin costs.

The irony of this trend is that, in the face of limited food and services and support, people living with HIV and AIDS will die quicker in the village. There are stories of children resisting attempts to send a surviving parent to the village and comments about how people who are sick in town and return to the village will not have the friends in the village to support them (recognizing that it is especially hard to forge friendships when sick). Returning sick and in need of help to the village is not as life should be: people in the village look to urban kin to support them; as a pastor in the rural area explains, "In the village, we look forward to these people who are in town to help us, but if they come sick, it's an added load, it's a burden." And it is clear that those relatives who had supported rural kin while in town are much more likely to be cared for than those who did not and were "eating their money alone" (transporter, rural). Village kin also worry that they are not able to give their town relatives the lifestyle and food that they are used to.

Seasonal food scarcity and farming activities make it hard to care adequately when people living with HIV and AIDS are sick during the farming season:[12] farming activities cannot be postponed easily, and rural respondents complained bitterly about not being able to farm properly because of the care demanded by people living with HIV and AIDS.[13] Economic options are much more limited in the village, and it is harder to both generate and borrow cash in crisis. This is clear in the following quote from rural women farmers: "This patient at home has disturbed them. They don't finish the work at the fields properly. The patient also complains to them, saying that they take a long time to give him food. They will also say that, 'At the field that is where your food comes from.' They will blame the patient all the time."

Urban Poverty and Stigma

People in the village realize that it is better to be in town if you are HIV-positive and sick. They pinpointed institutional care in hospices, HIV and AIDS activities (clubs, NGOs, HBC), and more HIV and AIDS information as the advantages of being in town and said that people living with HIV and AIDS would live longer in town. There is also more cash in circulation in urban areas, and it is easier to borrow money or raise cash.

In the context of the extreme urban poverty of Misisi, if people are unable to cope with people living with HIV and AIDS, they can and do turn to the hospice, HBC, churches, a training center for girls, and the orphanage. Urban elders state, "If you cannot afford to look after an HIV patient nowadays, we have home-based care centers where they give support. These people will give assistance." There are simply more places to turn to when people can no longer cope at home. For example, urban respondents often mentioned taking patients to the hospice when they could not cope, as reflected in the following comment by urban gatekeepers: "financially, they would rather not keep them at home and will take them to the hospice if they are very sick."

In the urban sites, in comparison to the rural site, there was also more awareness of what people living with HIV and AIDS need, for example, their need for nutritious foods. People living with HIV and AIDS were more visible, and there were fewer cases in the data of extreme discrimination, more openness (including more discussion about disclosure), more awareness of the impact and hurt of stigma and discrimination, and fewer fears around casual transmission. Because these data are qualitative, evidence of reduced stigma in the urban sites emerges from the data but cannot be quantified.

However, looking after people living with HIV and AIDS does deepen poverty in town as well as in the village. It can stop people going to work or force them to take leave. Households may even employ someone to care for the sick person, or, if people are involved in the informal economy (stone crushing, trading), it can result in reduced business. It can be an excuse for relatives to come from the village, and these relatives, unless they are women caregivers, are regarded as an added burden.

Conclusion

This material demonstrates how the poor, orphans, and women are more susceptible to multiple stigmas and HIV-related stigma in Zambia. How HIV-related stigma deepens existing inequalities and exclusions has been expounded by other research and academics (Goffman 1963; Gilmore and Somerville 1994; Bharat 1999; Parker and Aggleton 2003) and is one of the core dimensions of HIV stigma worldwide (Ogden and Nyblade 2005). However, this chapter is making another simple but original point about the relationship between poverty and stigma, namely that the practicalities of poverty fuel stigmatizing actions and stigmatizing experiences. And the stigmatizers, poor and vulnerable themselves, and perhaps in an effort to distance themselves from the consequences of their actions, often adopt a language of blame when they make painful decisions about the allocation of resources. This blaming and shaming serves to deepen the stigma experiences by people living with HIV and AIDS in the context of poverty, and when (as often is the case) the stigmatizers are close relatives, the pain of the stigma experiences is even greater. Urban health workers, discussing how a family with no income and no other support cannot care for people with HIV and AIDS, comment, "you start complaining deep down in your heart, so even the patient won't get well because you are complaining."

However, indications of reduced levels of stigma in the urban site underline how it is possible to tackle this particular cause of stigma through a broader approach: through poverty reduction, women's empowerment, orphans' empowerment, and, through an increase in access to special HIV services (particularly in the rural areas) and to interventions that improve the practical and medical management of HIV. Our material strongly suggests that by giving poor people more pragmatic support to manage household members living with HIV and AIDS, both stigmatizing actions and experiences are likely to decrease.

Acknowledgments

We acknowledge the assistance of the three communities Kamwala, Mbabala, and Misisi; other researchers and research assistants, Annie Chanda, Urban Chileshe, Levy Chilikwela, Martha Chirwa, Janet Chisaila, Sue Clay, Patience Hakamwaya, Titus Kafuma, Neater Malambo, Bertha Milimo, Florence Moyo, Edwin Mwanza, Danny Njovu, Laura Nyblade, Flavia Saili, and Gita Sheth; all support staff at KCTT, ZAMBART, and ICRW; and the funders, USAID, the CORE initiative, GlaxoSmithKline's Positive Action programme, DFID, and SIDA.

Notes

1. The research was funded by USAID, with additional support from the CORE initiative, GlaxoSmithKline's Positive Action programme, DFID, and SIDA.

2. In both urban sites and Mbabala township, people had to pay for water, and water was in short supply.

3. *Ka Pamela,* a small bag of maize meal (usually half a kilogram); *chiwawa,* pumpkin leaves; and *impwa,* small wild yellow eggplants.

4. K 100 is equivalent to 5 cents.

5. This refers to a reported practice at the time of rich people living with HIV and AIDS going to South Africa for blood transfusions.

6. In Zambia, ARVs were not subsidized and available in the government health services until 2004.

7. Property grabbing is a customary practice of a husband's family taking goods from his widow. It was made illegal in Zambia in the late 1980s.

8. Stephen Lewis calls the combination of hunger and HIV the "the most ferocious assault on women ever" (Lewis 2003).

9. See "Experiences of Stigma" for a more detailed discussion of blame.

10. As mentioned in the description of the study sites, the rural fieldwork was conducted during a period of food scarcity, which exacerbated household stress.

11. People may want to die or be buried in the village, close to their ancestors.

12. The farming season starts in October, with clearing the fields, and runs through May, when the fields are harvested. Vegetable gardens and gathering and selling wild fruits are often dry season farming activities, but not so labor intensive.

13. Cliggett (2005) and Moore and Vaughan (1994) write about how old people and young children are often neglected during the farming months and left without adequate food and water in the house while people work in the fields.

References

Alonzo, A. A., and N. R. Reynolds. 1995. Stigma, HIV and AIDS: An exploration and elaboration of a stigma trajectory, *Social Science and Medicine* 41 (3): 303–315.

Barnett, T., and A. Whiteside. 2002. *AIDS in the 21st century: Disease and globalisation.* New York: Palgrave, Macmillan.

Bharat, S. 1999. *HIV/AIDS related discrimination, stigmatisation and denial in India—a study in Mumbai and Bangalore.* Mumbai, India: Unit for Family Studies, Tat Institute of Social Sciences.

Bond, V. 1998. *Household capacity and "coping up" in rural Zambia: Dealing with AIDS, other illness and adversity in Chiawa.* Doctorate thesis, University of Hull.

———. 2002. The dimensions and wider context of HIV/AIDS stigma and resulting discrimination in southern Africa. In *One step further—Responses to HIV/AIDS,* ed. A. Sisask. *Sidastudies* 7: 29–53.

Bond, V., L. Chilikwela, S. Clay, T. Kafuma, L. Nyblade, and N. Bettega. 2003. "*Kanyaka*": "The Lights is On": Understanding HIV and AIDS related stigma in urban and rural Zambia. Report, Lusaka, KCTT and ZAMBART Project, www.icrw.org.

Castro, A., and P. Farmer. 2005. Understanding and addressing AIDS-related stigma: From anthropological theory to clinical practice in Haiti. *American Journal of Public Health* 95: 53–59.

CBOH, 1999, HIV/AIDS in Zambia, background projections, impacts and interventions, Ministry of Health, September.

Clay, S., V. Bond, and L. Nyblade. 2003. *We can tell them: AIDS doesn't come through being together.* Children's experience of HIV and AIDS related stigma in Zambia 2002–2003, Report, KCTT, ICRW, and ZAMBART.

Cliggett, L. 2005. *Grains from grass, aging, gender and famine in rural Africa.* Ithaca, N.Y.: Cornell University.

CSO (Central Statistics Office Zambia). 2003. Demographic and Health Survey 2001–2002. Lusaka: CSO.

Deacon, H., I. Stephney, and S. Prosalendis. 2005. *Understanding HIV/AIDS stigma: A theoretical and methodological analysis.* Human Sciences Research Council Research Monograph. Cape Town: HSRC Press.

Gilmore, N., and M. A. Somerville. 1994. Stigmatization, scapegoating and discrimination in sexually transmitted diseases: overcoming "them" and "us." *Social Science and Medicine* 39 (9): 1339–1358.

Goffman, E. 1963. *Stigma: Notes on the management of a spoiled identity.* New York: Simon & Schuster.

Herek, G., and Glunt, E. 1988. An epidemic of stigma: Public reaction to AIDS. *American Psychologist* 43 (11): 886–891.

Kelly, P., R. A. Feldman, P. Ndubani, K. S. Baboo, I. Timaeus, M. J. G. Farthing, and S. Wallman. 1998. High adult mortality in Lusaka [research letter]. *Lancet* 351: 883.

Lewis, S. 2003. *Keynote Lecture, UN Special Envoy for HIV in Africa, WHO 3 by 5 Initiative.* www.whoint/3by5/partners/Slewis/en/index3.html.

Link, B., and J. Phelan. 2001. *On stigma and its public health implications, stigma and global health: Developing a research agenda.* Washington, D.C.: National Institutes of Health.

LCS (Living Conditions Survey). 1998. *Living Conditions Survey.* Central Statistics Office, Zambia.

Moore, H., and M. Vaughan. 1994. *Cutting down trees: Gender, nutrition, and agricultural change in northern province of Zambia, 1890–1990.* Portsmouth, N.H.: Heineman.

Nyblade, L., R. Pande, S. Mathur, K. MacQuarrie, R. Kidd, H. Banteyerga, A. Kidanu, G. Kilonzo, J. Mbwambo, and V. Bond. 2003. *Disentangling HIV and AIDS stigma in Ethiopia, Tanzania and Zambia.* Washington, D.C.: ICRW Publication with CHANGE-AED, MHRC, MUCHS, ZAMBART, and KCTT.

Ogden, J., and L. Nyblade. 2005. *Common at its core: HIV-related stigma across contexts.* Washington, D.C.: ICRW and CHANGE.

Parker, R., and P. Aggleton. 2003. HIV and AIDS-related stigma and discrimination: A conceptual framework and implications for action. *Social Science Medicine* 57: 13–24.

Sartorius, N. 2004. *Report of the Workshop on Health Related Stigma and Discrimination.* The Royal Tropical Institute, 29 Nov–2 Dec 2004, http://www.dgroups.org/groups/Stigmaconsortium.

Scrambler, G., 2004. *Report of the Workshop on Health Related Stigma and Discrimination.* The Royal Tropical Institute, 29 Nov–2 Dec 2004, http://www.dgroups.org/groups/Stigmaconsortium.

Scudder, T. 1983. Economic downturn and community unravelling: The Gwembe Tonga revisted. *Culture and Agriculture* 18 (Winter): 16–19.

UNAIDS. 2002. *Report on the global HIV/AIDS epidemic July.* Geneva: UNAIDS.

UNICEF. 1999. *Joint USAID/UNICEF/SIDA study fund project, orphans and vulnerable children: A situational analysis, Zambia 1999.* Lusaka: GRZ.

Wallman, S. 1988. Sex and death: The AIDS crisis in social and cultural context. *Journal of AIDS* 1: 571–578.

World Bank. 2002. *Poverty reduction strategy paper (PRSP) and joint assessment.* Zambia, Vol. 1, Report No. 24035.

Zambia Sexual Behaviour Survey. 2000. *Zambia Sexual Behaviour Survey.* CSO, USAID, MEASURE Evaluation, Zambia.

Chapter 11

Scaling up Multisectoral Approaches to Combating HIV and AIDS

Hans P. Binswanger, Stuart Gillespie, and Suneetha Kadiyala

Introduction

The AIDS pandemic is a global crisis with impacts that will be felt for decades to come, demanding massive responses at many levels. Such responses need to continue to be grounded in the three core pillars of prevention, care and treatment, and mitigation. But these responses need to be much larger in scale, far more broadly based, and better connected so as to better match the scale, breadth, and interconnectedness of the pandemic's causes and impacts.

Alarmingly, programs aimed at preventing the spread of HIV reach fewer than one in five people who need them (UNAIDS 2004a). Fewer than 12 percent of the 6 million people estimated to be in immediate need for treatment are receiving it (WHO 2005). Only a tiny fraction of households that are affected by the pandemic are receiving any kind of support. Programs aimed at combating the epidemic generally tend to be concentrated in urban areas.

This deplorable situation is not caused by lack of knowledge of what needs to be done in prevention, care and treatment, and mitigation. On many of these issues there are well-codified scientific and operational guidelines. A few such examples include guidelines on combating the epidemic among men having sex with men (Anyamele et al. 2005; UNAIDS 1998) and HIV/AIDS care and treatment guidelines for resource-limited settings (WHO 2004). Several small- and medium-scale programs are successfully addressing many other issues, such as home-based care for people living with HIV (PLWHAs) or support to street children.

The first part of this chapter focuses on challenges to scaling up. The second part discusses World Bank's experience with scaling up its multisectoral HIV/AIDS initiative. The final part of the chapter illustrates models for scaling up multisectoral prevention and social protection programs to combat HIV and AIDS with a focus on the role of community-driven development.

If It Is So Urgent, and So Much Is Known, Why Is So Little Happening?

Is It the Excessive Cost of Scaling Up?

The annual global costs of scaling up such programs has been estimated by UNAIDS to be around US$12 billion in 2005, and perhaps doubling over the next 20 years in real terms (UNAIDS 2004b, 2005).[1] This compares to annual global military expenditures of $852 billion in 1999, of which developing countries spent $245 million. The annual total cost of agricultural subsidies of OECD countries, including the cost of OECD agricultural policies to their consumers, amounts to an additional $300 billion (OECD 2003). The issue of financing the expenditures to combat HIV/AIDS is not, therefore, a question of affordability but a question of willingness of the national governments of affected countries, and of public and private donors, to pay for the costs of fighting HIV/AIDS. Or to say it differently, there is a lack of political will.

HIV/AIDS: A Slow-Onset Disaster

Amartya Sen has long demonstrated that catastrophes that develop gradually do not elicit the same response as sudden catastrophic events (Sen 1981). Willingness to pay for dealing with the former is much more limited than for the latter, as the public and private responses to the 9/11 attacks and the tsunami in the Indian Ocean amply demonstrate. Other slow-onset catastrophes where action has been slow include hunger and malnutrition, global warming, loss of tropical forests, and depletion of a number of marine fisheries. On global warming, for example, the Kyoto protocol proposes only very modest action in developed countries, does not bind developing countries to any action, and has been rejected by the current U.S. administration.

Stigma

To understand the lack of political will in responding to the spread and impacts of HIV/AIDS, one must also look to the stigma associated with HIV/AIDS and to the religious controversies over sex education and the use of condoms to account for the lack of truly scaled-up action. Stigma systematically impedes scale up of effective HIV/AIDS response strategies. Stigma is internalized by stigmatized people, preventing them from taking action when they could help themselves to deal with the epidemic (Aggleton 2000). More specifically, external and internal stigma:

- contribute to the spread of fear and false information

- prevent many people from seeking the knowledge they need

- impose untold psychological stress and suffering on people who are potentially or actually infected by the virus, on their families, and on their surviving orphans

- reduce the willingness of people to assist people living with HIV/AIDS (PLWHA) and may even lead them to inflict additional harm

- prevent many people from accessing the support, care, and treatment programs that already exist and therefore contribute to additional unnecessary deaths[2]

Stigma thus exercises its influence at the global, national, community, and individual levels and in the hearts of those infected and affected. Even after 25 years of the epidemic, stigma is still rampant, hindering implementation and scaling up of systematic harm reduction approaches. This has and will clearly lead to easily preventable infection with a deadly disease and therefore has and will continue to lead to a large number of clearly preventable deaths from AIDS.

The Challenges Posed by the Program Complexity and the Multisectoral Nature of the Fight against HIV/AIDS

The multisector nature of the HIV/AIDS response,[3] including provision of antiretroviral treatment (ART), poses a challenge to scaling up. As emphasized in the AIDS treatment guidelines of the World Health Organization (WHO), implementing even a treatment program involves many actors and organizations beyond the health professionals and clinics and hospitals for a comprehensive treatment strategy with the following components (WHO 2004):

- Voluntary counseling and testing (VCT) for HIV and regular monitoring of all who are infected

- Healthy living and survival skills, psychosocial support, nutrition, and so on.

- Prevention and treatment of opportunistic infections

- ART and the associated adherence support to the patients

- Prevention of mother-to-child transmission (PMTCT), including treatment of the mothers and infected family members (MTCT-Plus)

Even where ample financial resources for scaling up treatment have been provided, as in the case of Botswana, health sectors find it very difficult to do so on their own (WHO 2003). The most successful treatment programs, such as the one in Brazil, have mobilized capacities both inside and outside the public sector, in the private sector, and NGOs. And they have decentralized the financial resources all the way to the municipal level (Bacon et al. 2004).

The complexities of multisectoral development initiatives are widely recognized and well understood. The lessons from the integrated rural development approach have now paved the way to decentralized and participatory mechanisms of planning and execution, including a much broader range of actors from national to local levels (Box 11.1).

At the 2004 World Bank conference on local development, a consensus emerged that stresses that local development is a coproduction among communities, local governments, the sector institutions, and the private sector (World Bank 2004). Central governments and donors need to find ways to energize and help finance the local arena, so that these various actors can collaborate and be effectively coordinated. A step-by-step approach to scaling up such programs can be found in Binswanger and Nguyen (2006) (also see Box 11.2).

Such local and community-driven development programs have successfully been scaled up to national levels in Mexico, to the entire Northeast of Brazil, and to about half of Indonesia and are growing rapidly in many parts of Africa. And the approach has been integrated into the Multicountry AIDS Program (MAP) for Africa, in which more than half of the resources go to so-called community funds (World Bank 2004).

Scaling Up under the World Bank HIV/AIDS Programs in Africa

Funding and Disbursement

The Multicountry AIDS Program (MAP) of the World Bank for Africa was initiated in early 1999, with the first US$500 million tranche of the program approved by the Board of the World Bank in September 2000.[4] At the end of 2004 the MAP

Box 11.1 Lessons from Multisectoral Integrated Development Projects

Under the leadership of the World Bank in the 1960s, "Integrated Rural Development Projects" became a popular attempt to deal with multiple institutions and sectors involved in rural development until about the mid-1980s. The integrated rural development projects tried to create synergy between the different components of rural development. They relied on central sectoral agencies (such as agriculture, infrastructure, education, health) for the execution of the multiple components of the programs, which were designed in an integrated fashion by design teams rather than by the sectors. The approach failed all over the world and has been abandoned (World Bank 1988).

The first serious weakness of this centralized model was that it failed to mobilize the significant latent capacities at the local and community level and in the private sector. Subsequent decentralized and community-driven programs all over the world have demonstrated that latent capacities available at these levels are indeed very large (World Bank 2002).

Each of the sectors already faces formidable challenges in ensuring that its services reach the widely dispersed populations of their countries. They also have priorities of their own. When they were asked to implement additional projects for which they themselves did not develop priorities, they tended to use the additional resources to help implement their sectoral activities.

To coordinate integrated rural development projects, and to ensure that the sectors would implement the priorities agreed on at project preparation, central project units were set up and given strong powers to manage the financial resources to be used by the involved sectors. But coordinating complex programs in thousands of localities from the center posed nearly insurmountable information problems. It created additional bureaucratic layers, which slowed the disbursement of project resources and implementation to a crawl. The lesson from integrated rural development, therefore, is that it is difficult to scale up multisectoral programs by coordinating central sector agencies for implementation.[a]

In rural development, such centralized approaches have now been replaced with decentralized and participatory mechanisms of planning and execution, including a much broader range of actors. At the community and local levels, there are no insurmountable information problems. What needs to be done and how to do it are often readily apparent, and the cross-sectoral coordination problems are reduced to manageable proportions. Moreover, accountability of service providers and contractors to local populations is easier to achieve than with distant agencies. Responsibility for setting priorities, planning, and execution is transferred to local development committees, which are usually associated with local governments and communities. Local governments and communities plan and execute their own projects using locally available implementation capacities, labor and materials, and matching grants from donors or their own governments. Communities and/or local governments are provided with block grants and/or conditional grants, which they have to match with their own resources in cash and in kind. They obtain training and technical services from government agencies, the private sector, and NGOs. The need for strong central support from the various sectors does not disappear, but the role shifts to the setting of policies and program parameters, standard setting and controls, cofinancing of the programs, facilitation and training, monitoring, and evaluation (World Bank 1997).

[a] At the same time that "integrated rural development programs" were in the ascendant, the multisectoral nutrition-planning paradigm was also dominant. Though advances were made in recognizing the multiple causality of malnutrition, the prescription of a single nutrition-planning unit with a mandate to somehow orchestrate the sectors in top-down, highly planned, multisectoral action plans that required complex coordination also failed.

supported national HIV/AIDS programs in 34 African countries. Total approved funding was US$1,088 million as subsidized International Development Association (IDA) grants and subsidized credits, of which about US$300 million had been disbursed by 2005. MAP has adopted the following principles:

- Empower stakeholders with funding and decisionmaking authority

- Involve actors at all levels, from individuals and villages to regions and central authorities

- Provide support in the public and private sectors and in civil society

- Encompass all sectors and the full range of HIV/AIDS prevention, care and support, and mitigation activities (World Bank 2004)

Box 11.2 Scaling Up Community-Driven Development (CDD): Key Lessons

- Overall, keep in mind and build on country context, institutional arrangements, capacity, and the triggers and different processes of scaling up. Build a library of well-documented context-specific experiences through good monitoring, evaluation, and operational research. Use these to advocate for improvements in the contextual environment.

- To sustain CDD, anchor it within existing contextual systems (government), frameworks (e.g., PRSP), and processes (decentralization), even where these may be imperfect. Ultimate aim is to weave and embed sustainable CDD in the national social, political, cultural, and institutional fabric. Donors and governments need to focus more on the institutions and processes to manage CDD programs (not the project per se) and on transformation or transition (not exit strategies). Community-driven is citizen-driven, not client-driven.

- Capacity is pivotal and is more than simply resources; it includes institutional arrangements, motivation, and commitment, which necessitate appropriate incentives at all levels. Capacity development takes time and resources but is an essential investment. The capacity and commitment of local governments, facilitators, and local leaders is particularly important.

- Learn by doing and by communicating, monitoring, evaluating, and changing. Learn from failure, but learn faster from success. Start with the positive (what is working) not the problem (what is not) and build on that. Be adaptive, flexible, and open to change. Anticipate and address trade-offs. Apply realistic time horizons (10- to 15-year, not 5-year, cycles).

Source: Gillespie (2004).

In each country, the IDA resources support the implementation of the national HIV/AIDS strategy and program. Financing can be used for any of the national program components and virtually all categories of expenditures including community grants, salaries, vehicles, condoms, and HIV/AIDS drugs. IDA resources can therefore be used by national HIV/AIDS programs to fund unfunded or underfunded components; that is, IDA acts as a funder of last resort.

The program finances both HIV/AIDS programs of central ministries and decentralized expenditures of NGOs, faith-based organizations, the private sector, local governments, and communities. Most programs have two separate funds, a "sector fund" and a "community fund," with the community funds typically accounting for more than 50 percent of the planned expenditures.

From the beginning it was recognized that one of the main objectives of the program had to be to develop the funding and implementation mechanisms that would allow the transfer of resources to thousands or tens of thousands of implementing organizations while maintaining financial accountability and ensuring quality programs. Fully developing the disbursement and procurement mechanisms that would be able to do this has been the major objective as well as a major challenge during the first years of program implementation. Based on the experience so far, a comprehensive generic operational manual has been produced that summarizes the best practices for designing and implementing a scaled-up response (World Bank 2004).

The community funds have typically been designed using the following principles:

- Build on available culturally adapted models. In most countries, and on virtually all components of the fight against HIV/AIDS, existing small projects and programs have had many years to develop culturally adapted best practices. Their staffs and volunteers can provide their insights during the design phase and training during the scale-up phase of programs.

- Identify all existing and latent capacities, design the programs so that they can participate, and obtain the necessary financial resources. These include local or district governments, government agencies and services, private firms, persons living with HIV/AIDS, community-based organizations such as PLWHAs associations, churches, producer associations, local chambers of commerce, and NGOs.

- Facilitate learning by doing rather than insist on fully developed capacities before granting funding.

- Rely on community participation and decentralized coordination. Within broad guidelines and priorities defined by national AIDS councils, local and district stakeholder AIDS committees plan and coordinate local programs. The committees assign responsibilities and resources for different program components as well as to local implementers such as communities, organizations, and services.

- Provide the HIV/AIDS funds to local coordinating committees as fungible block grants or envelopes that can be used for all components of the fight against HIV/AIDS.

- Once their proposals have been approved, directly transfer funds into bank accounts of all implementing organizations.

- Use simplified procurement mechanisms.

- Promote accountability. Transparent budgeting, disbursement, and accounting procedures need to ensure accountability to end users of the services and to the government.

- Encourage additional resource mobilization by providing resources as matching grants to implementing organizations and communities.

A recent interim review of the MAP finds that in less than four years, just over US$1 billion has been committed to 28 countries in Sub-Saharan Africa: one subregional project and eight additional country projects are in the final stages of approval (World Bank et al. 2004).

Implementation Experience

The review finds that in its concept and design, MAP has been a major achievement: It is the largest single commitment to HIV/AIDS ever undertaken by the World Bank. Disbursement levels under the program approach those of other health and social sector projects financed by the World Bank, but they are not nearly as fast as would have been necessary in the case of the HIV/AIDS crisis or as anticipated at the inception of the program.

Implementation experience has been mixed. The decentralized community components and the NGO components have been the most successful part of the program. "Community-based and targeted interventions managed by civil society organizations and visited by the review team were often inspiring" (World Bank et al. 2004, p. 16).

Over 50,000 communities in Africa have now been reached with financial resources. Significant capacity exists in civil society and the private sector to implement the program. Echoing the disappointment in integrated rural development, the sectoral components have been disappointing with almost identical action plans by the ministries focusing on the initial stages of workplace programs rather than on beneficiaries.

Other principal findings of the review were as follows:

The objectives, approach, and design of the MAP Program have generally been appropriate. The original objectives are in the process of being realized. Experience with implementation of individual projects and subprojects has been mixed and often disappointing. However, most projects are new and need time to mature. The context for dealing with the HIV/AIDS epidemic in Africa has changed significantly since the Program was launched in 2000. Consequently, the future MAP program will need to become more strategic, collaborative and evidence-based. (World Bank et al. 2004)

The interim review stresses that most MAP projects are new. The six projects visited have an average age of 12.5 months. Perhaps the most important objective in the coming period will be to allow the new institutions and mechanisms created by the governments with Bank support to mature, ensuring that the fundamental mechanisms and systems are in place as noted above. In other words, the first priority is to stay the course (World Bank et al. 2004, p. 12).

The report notes that since MAP started four years ago the context has significantly changed, with other funders having committed significant resources.

Under these changing circumstances, the future approach of the MAP Program will need to be more strategic. While retaining the very positive aspects of the current approach—flexible, client-driven, community-based and delivered through the civil society—the future Program should be an instrument to reinforce the national approach advocated by UNAIDS, referred to as "The Three Ones"—one national authority, one strategic framework, and one monitoring and evaluation system to manage the HIV/AIDS response. The MAP program is operating within this framework, and should encourage others such as the Global Fund and PEPFAR to adopt this approach. Working with other development partners, it can assist national authorities to build a more effective, accountable authority, revise the strategic framework and introduce a simple, manageable and useful M&E system for HIV/AIDS. (World Bank et al. 2004, p. 7)

Scaling Up Prevention

The desired outcomes of prevention programs include changes in sexual practices toward fewer partners, a single partner, delayed initiation of sex by youth, or abstinence and adoption of safer sex techniques, in particular condoms.[5] They also may include changes in community norms of male dominance and tolerance, violence, and abuse.

Parents and communities must accept that their children be provided with thorough sex and prevention education enabling them to protect themselves as and when they start to have sex. For women it involves giving them the self-confidence to demand condom use by their regular partners or husbands. Global experience suggests that AIDS education and awareness programs, although clearly necessary, rarely bring about behavior change without intensive participation by those whose behavior is to be changed (UNAIDS 2004a, Chapter 4). In rural areas of Africa, the most successful interventions required not only interpersonal communication but participatory involvement of whole communities, such as the model of TANESA, which was scaled up to all villages in an entire district.[6] As the following list of 10 elements of a comprehensive prevention program illustrates (UNAIDS 2004a), prevention programs not only need to approach behavior change from many different angles, but also include a number of additional elements:

- AIDS education and awareness

- Behavior change programs, especially for the young, those at higher risk of HIV exposure, and people living with HIV

- Promoting male and female condoms

- Voluntary counseling and testing

- Preventing and treating sexually transmitted infections

- Prevention of mother and child transmission

- Harm reductions programs for injecting drug users

- Measures to protect blood supply safety

- Infection control in health care settings

- Community education and changes in laws and policies to counter stigma and discrimination, and vulnerability reduction through social, legal, and economic change

Although it includes highly targeted interventions, MAP financed by the World Bank has taken a whole-population approach to prevention interventions. For this it has recently come under criticism, both by internal evaluations and outside publications (World Bank et al 2004; Mallaby 2004). The internal evaluators in particular stress that there are enormous variations in the nature and extent of the AIDS epidemic, that the qualities of the subprojects it supports are very mixed, and that the program could be improved by better taking these variations into account and focusing more on interventions that have the highest payoffs. Now that many countries are coming closer to having the implementation and financial mechanisms in place for scaling up the HIV/AIDS response, MAP has to deal with these criticisms. Without abandoning prevention efforts for the population at large, the third tranche of MAP became more adaptive and evidence-based in the choice of interventions to be favored.

There are a number of examples of prevention effort under MAP that have gone beyond mass communication and achieved coverage of other prevention methods to a significant scale, including in Ethiopia, Kenya, Ghana, and Burkina Faso. Within the broad MAP principles discussed above, they use somewhat different implementation mechanisms.

Design of a Community-Driven Multisectoral Prevention Initiative:
Scaling Up in Burkina Faso

Burkina Faso has developed an approach for covering all villages and urban neighborhoods within each province with intensive prevention efforts including interpersonal communication and community participation. Under the Burkina Faso approach, provincial authorities have set up HIV/AIDS committees at the provincial level (as a subcommittee of the general provincial development committee), district level, and community levels (i.e., village or urban neighborhood level). Membership in these committees involves all stakeholder groups from government, the private sector, and civil society. At all levels membership in the committees is based on demonstrated interest of individuals to serve on them and on selection of the committees by actors at that level (CCISD 2002). After a successful initial pilot project in the particularly poor province of Poni in 1990, the program has been expanded to the 13 provinces with the highest populations. Eight thousand communities have received training and funds and used them primarily for prevention efforts.

Training the community committees in submission of proposals, setting up a bank account, financial management, monitoring, and the ABCs of HIV/AIDS and its prevention took a training course of two weeks. The volume of training required is huge. From each community two men and two women have been trained, and among them one adult and one youth. For the 8,000 communities already trained, this meant training 32,000 community members. In addition, NGOs that want to support the program, local staff in the public and private sector, and all members of the district and provincial committees have to be trained, perhaps 300 people per province, or another nearly 4,000 people so far. Scaling up to the 44 provinces of Burkina Faso will therefore imply a total training effort of between 80,000 and 100,000. In the provinces covered so far, the resulting logistics problem was solved by cascade training, with a team of trainers of trainers at the provincial level, and training teams in each district. The provincial and the district committees put in place these training teams and supervise their work. The training teams usually consist of retired teachers and other government officials, educated spouses, and educated youth. In order to minimize travel and transport costs, they are all recruited in the district in which they work. It is a testimony to the significant latent capacities at this highly decentralized level that it has not been difficult to find good people to do this work on a part-time basis. All committee and training team members are volunteers and are paid a unified and low per diem for their training or workdays. They can be mobilized again for subsequent training efforts.

Once trained, community HIV/AIDS committees were given a budget envelope of US$1.00 per capita. They submitted a simple project proposal for funding to the district committee for a preliminary approval. The district committee then sent the set of approved community proposals to the province level for inspection and final approval. The same process was used for proposals from NGOs, the private sector, and local offices of government agencies such as education and health. Once approved, the provincial authorities gave their bank a disbursement order to transfer the approved budgets to the communities and other implementing entities.

The process evaluation of the pilot program in the province of Poni (CCISD 2002) has concluded that this novel approach has functioned well and indeed has been able to cover practically all communities in the pilot province. The cost of reaching one person with face-to-face HIV/AIDS and prevention education via this approach was about US$0.60 and that between 60 and 100 percent of the population was reached. There is as yet no evaluation available for the Burkina Faso approach of its impact on behavior and HIV transmission.

Scaling Up Social Protection

Many impacts of HIV and AIDS are revealed through the responses that individuals, households, and communities adopt. Some of these responses are examples of resilience, but many derive from distress. The first line of defense has been communities, many of which have responded in very innovative ways. Documented responses include labor sharing, orphan support, community-based childcare, community food banks, credit schemes for funeral benefits, and new ways of reducing the time and energy of domestic tasks, such as fuel and water collection and food preparation (Mutangadura, Mukurazita, and Jackson 1999; Donovan et al. 2003; Drimie 2003; NAADS 2003; Gillespie and Kadiyala 2005).

Social protection interventions to combat HIV/AIDS can be targeted at vulnerable communities, families, or individuals. They include interventions to make them less susceptible to HIV infection as well as interventions to deal with the consequences of the disease itself. Examples include support to the production and income generation of vulnerable individuals and households so that they are less likely to have to engage in sex work or are able to recover from the loss of working-age adults, food and nutrition interventions, home-based care, assistance with schooling and health needs of orphans and other survivors, and outright cash transfers.

To maximize food and nutrition security in the context of HIV/AIDS the overriding dual principle should be to (1) augment community and household resistance and resilience as far as possible and (2) ensure there are safety nets in place for those who are unable to "cope" otherwise. The emphasis in mitigation strategy needs to be on strengthening resilience, the ability of households and communities to adapt livelihood strategies so as to bounce back from the shock of HIV/AIDS. Policy needs to draw on what is working already in communities where proactive responses are under way. Where households' and communities' capacity to "cope" has been exceeded, a broad-based social security system offering minimal benefits or specifically targeted welfare programs may in the short and medium term be important for mitigation. There is a need to move from an "individual-infected" model to a "community-affected" one and to focus on strengthening community capacity.

Thus, understanding community responses and capacities is a crucial first step in developing a long-term, comprehensive, and expanded strategy for social protection. Although there are several studies of community-driven responses to HIV/AIDS (Mutangadura, Mukurazita, and Jackson 1999; Foster 2002; Hamazakaza and Kauseni 2002; Hsu, Du Guerny, and Marco 2002; Silomba 2002; White 2002), there are only limited analyses of experiences in scaling up such initiatives (Phiri, Foster, and Nzima 2001; Hunter 2002; International HIV/AIDS Alliance 2002; Kadiyala 2004).

Although most social protection programs have been narrowly focused and adopt a service delivery model, the paradigm is slowly shifting. Kadiyala (2004) discusses how the Scaling Up HIV/AIDS Interventions through Expanded Partnerships (STEPs) initiative, supported by Save the Children U.S.A. (SC), in Malawi has evolved from a service delivery model to provide material support to orphans into a scaled-up community-driven multisectoral initiative (Box 11.3).

Box 11.3 Scaling Up HIV/AIDS Interventions through Expanded Partnership (STEPs)

Supported by USAID and Save the Children U.S. (SC), STEPs started in 1995 (then called COPE, Community-based Options for Protection and Empowerment) as a service-delivery program in one district in Malawi to assist children affected by HIV/AIDS. Through evaluations, SC realized such an approach was not sustainable, cost-effective, or scalable.

On the basis of recommendations from the evaluations and the field experience, the program revitalized the dormant decentralized AIDS committees (at the district, community, and village levels) and their technical subcommittees under the National AIDS Commission (NAC), in the Namwera community in Mangochi to mobilize collective action to combat the epidemic. Based in turn on the positive experience in Namwera, the program changed its initial strategy to that of an external agent for change, assisting communities with community mobilization and capacity building so that communities become empowered to act collectively to address their own problems.

Village AIDS Committees (VACs) identify the vulnerable and plan responses on the basis of the nature and magnitude of vulnerability within the villages, the needs of the vulnerable, and the capacity within the villages to respond. They also monitor the program's activities and mobilize resources. Because the needs of the most affected communities are multiple, the program has evolved into a truly multisectoral program, offering prevention, care, support, and mitigation activities. Through its experience with STEPs, SC has also influenced national policies related to HIV/AIDS and children. For example, it played a critical role in drafting National Orphan Care Guidelines and coordinated Malawi's first national child abuse study in partnership with the National Task Force on Child Abuse. Save the Children was also instrumental in formation of the Wills and Inheritance National Task Force. It actively monitors the orphans, widows, and widowers component of the National Strategic Framework. Through partnerships and training, other NGOs and CBOs (community-based organizations) in the program approach of community mobilization and facilitating collective action, STEPs, and similar models aim to cover 75 percent of Malawi's population.

Source: Kadiyala (2004).

Contextual factors that are critical for scaling up this community-driven model include an enabling policy environment with a strong commitment of the current government, especially NAC, to a multisectoral approach to combating HIV/AIDS. Organizational factors enabling scaling up include a well-trained and motivated staff; adoption of a community mobilization model through capacity building of district, community, and village AIDS committees; commitment to documenting and disseminating lessons learned; and reaching more affected populations through partnerships. Factors specific to communities include leadership within the community, whether the communities are urban or rural (rural communities are easier to mobilize), the nature of livelihoods, and the history and culture of the communities with respect to collective action. Planning along with the communities for a phasing down of SC's presence and scaling up of the role and responsibilities of the AIDS committees and funding mechanisms have also been identified as critical in enabling and sustainably scaling up collective action (Kadiyala 2004).

Important factors that threaten or limit the scaling up of STEPs include the magnitude of the epidemic, which is eroding community resources; recurrent food crises, which divert resources to sheer survival; the gap between the resources that communities need and what they have, which undermines the spirit of volunteerism; weak commitment of donors to a truly community-driven multisectoral response; and the overall context of poverty and underdevelopment, which makes it more difficult to mobilize communities and build their capacities to respond to the multiple challenges of the AIDS epidemic (Kadiyala 2004). The STEPs experience shows that scaling up multisectoral, community-driven responses to HIV/AIDS is possible but highly challenging. Building such responses in high-HIV/resource-poor settings is both resource- and time-intensive. But promoting community ownership and building local capacity is essential for action to be sustained. Using similar principles as the STEP program discussed above, Burkina Faso is currently preparing a social protection pilot for a truly scaled-up community-driven approach (Box 11.4).

Conclusions

There is significant consensus on how to prevent, mitigate, and treat HIV and AIDS, well summarized in recent guidelines and best practice papers of UNAIDS, WHO, UNICEF, and other organizations. Nevertheless, scaling up of actions recommended in these documents has been slow. In this chapter we conclude that the slow speed cannot be explained by absence of the required knowledge or by the prohibitively high costs of scaling up; scientific consensus exists in many areas, and the world could well afford the funding needed. Instead, explanations must be sought in the slow-onset nature of the catastrophe, the enormous stigma surrounding

Box 11.4 A Burkina Faso Proposal for Scaling Up Social Protection

When the Burkina Faso community-driven prevention program was first set up, communities were allowed to put in place social protection components. Few ever did, and it became clear that communities would not be able to do so on their own. Several barriers to community management of the social protection efforts need to be resolved. A learning-by-doing program to cover the entire province of Sanmatenga is currently in the design phase and trying to overcome these barriers.

1. Communities and individual families are already part of an informal, if inadequate, social protection system. But they do need additional resources and support to expand these informal mechanisms into a more systematic effort. These resources should be provided as matching grants to the communities, with the latter providing the matching resources in cash or in kind. Rural communities that are provided with cash to assist with health and education expenses will be asked to provide the food needed for their most vulnerable members, either in kind or in cash.

2. Although communities all over Africa are able to identify vulnerable families and classify them by degree of need, they are not able to carry out proper needs assessment for these families, a task that normally is done by a social worker. In Sanmatenga there are nearly 300 villages and urban neighborhoods but only three trained social workers, and there is no way the Ministry of Social Welfare can hire enough social workers to assist communities to do this job. The learning-by-doing program will therefore ask communities to select one or several members to be trained in basic family needs assessment and supervision skills, and they will then be remunerated via daily allowances for their work out of the community grants. The ministry is currently developing a curriculum and training program for them.

3. Assisting the chronically ill, orphans, and the families that take care of them will require significant additional training of enough community members to manage the tasks. These community members cannot work as volunteers for a long period of time and need to be provided with modest remunerations, such as per diems for every day they work or home visit they make.

4. The community members will encounter situations that they and the community as a whole cannot handle, such as medical emergencies or child abuse. To deal with these cases requires the putting in place of proper referral systems so that difficult cases can be handled by health professionals, social workers, or educators with the required skills. These same specialists need to be involved in designing and delivering the training and to be available for facilitation and training on demand.

5. The same committee structures that were used for prevention at the provincial, district, and community level, the same training teams, and the same financing mechanisms can be reinforced and used to coordinate, manage, and monitor the social protection program. In particular, the committees can coordinate and provide financial resources to the NGOs and local offices of the respective government services so that they can become the facilitators, trainers, and referral system.

Source: Hans Binswanger, personal observations.

HIV/AIDS, and the multiplicity and complexity of the actions required in the areas of prevention, care and treatment, and social protection.

Regarding the latter, we show that implementation of parallel vertical intervention by different central sector agencies is not a practical way of scaling up. Integrated rural development is the classic example of the failure of such a strategy. It floundered on the lack of real participation and buy in from the beneficiaries, the impossibility of centrally coordinating local actions of different sectors, the inability or unwillingness of sector agencies to deliver services locally according to an agreed and coordinated program, and the prohibitive cost of parallel service delivery mechanisms and personnel. The approach has been supplanted by local and community-driven development approaches in which implementation and coordination of many actions are delegated to communities and development committees associated with local governments, with the assistance of sector agencies and the private sector. Information at the local level is much more readily available, and therefore coordination at that level becomes feasible. The deep involvement of communities and existing local implementers sharply reduces cost, increases willingness to cofinance the interventions, and improves commitment and understanding of the programs.

The community funds of the Multicountry AIDS Program financed by the World Bank in around 30 countries of Africa have been designed along the lines of this model. Early implementation experience, although not yet conclusive, shows that such implementation mechanisms can mobilize significant local capacities in communities and at local levels and can be scaled up at more affordable costs. Impact evaluation, however, lags behind. The WHO treatment guidelines for HIV/AIDS also incorporate principles of decentralization and strong community participation. A social protection program in Malawi and a scaled-up prevention program in Burkina Faso provide additional examples of affordable and feasible community-driven implementation strategies.

It is urgent that such strategies for scaling up be subject to further evaluation, of the scaling up mechanisms involved, how to further improve them, as well of the impact on slowing down the epidemic and dealing with its health and socioeconomic consequences. Research along these lines will require that researchers participate early on in the design of the monitoring and evaluation systems, the required baselines, sampling and data collection strategies for impact evaluation, and the continuous feedback of research results back into the programming environment.

Notes

1. These figures include the cost of comprehensive prevention effort and care and support of people living with HIV, including ART for about half of those in need of treatment, it being assumed that all those in need cannot be reached.

2. ACT-UP, the coalition of AIDS activists that over the past 20 years has put enormous pressure on governments to fight AIDS, has often used the slogan "Stigma=Death," and rightfully so. The most dramatic illustration of internalized stigma is well known by treatment practitioners in the field: A significant number of AIDS patients refuse to acknowledge their status and, as a consequence, fail to seek treatment for AIDS. Hans Binswanger has personally witnessed the death of seven people, three of whom were employees of the World Bank, who knew perfectly well that they could be treated but failed to seek it or even refused it.

3. This section draws on Binswanger (2000).

4. For extensive documentation on the program, see http://www.worldbank.org/afr/aids/map.htm.

5. In addition, prevention includes blood and injection safety and prevention of mother-to-child transmission (MTCT). Because the standard for MTCT programs has come to include antiretroviral treatment of the mother and her infected family members, the latter is discussed as part of the treatment section.

6. For information on the TANESA program, see http://www.kit.nl/projects/pr_sheets/pr_sheet17.asp and www.kit.nl/projects/resource/pub/87.mht.

References

Aggleton, P. 2000. *HIV and AIDS-related stigmatization, discrimination and denial.* UNAIDS. Available at www.unaids.org.

Anyamele, A., R. Lwabaayi, T. Nguyen, and H. Binswanger. 2005. *Sexual minorities, violence and AIDS in Africa.* World Bank, Africa Region Working Paper.

Bacon, O., M. L. Becoraro, J. Galvao, and K. Page-Shafer. 2004. *HIV/AIDS in Brazil.* San Francisco: University of California San Francisco, AIDS Policy Research Center.

Binswanger, H. P. 2000. Scaling up HIV/AIDS programs to national coverage. *Science* 288: 2173–2176.

Binswanger, H. P., and T. Nguyen. 2006. *Scaling up community-driven development: A step-by-step approach.* Washington, D.C.: World Bank.

CCISD (Centre de Coopération Internationale en Santé et Développement). 2002. *Mission d'appui à la documentation et l'évaluation de la phase pilote du Programme Multisectoriel de lutte contre le VIH/SIDA et les IST dans la Province du Poni, Saint Foi, Quebec.* ccisd@ccisd.org.

Donovan, D., L. Bailey, E. Mpyisi, and M. Weber. 2003. *Prime-age adult morbidity and mortality in rural Rwanda: Effects on household income, agricultural production, and food security strategies. Research report.* http://www.aec.msu.edu/agecon/fs2/rwanda/index.htm.

Drimie, S. 2003. HIV/AIDS and land: Case studies from Kenya, Lesotho and South Africa. *Development Southern Africa* 20 (5): 647–658.

Foster, G. 2002. Understanding community responses to the situation of children affected by HIV/AIDS. In *One step further. Responses to HIV/AIDS,* ed. A. Sisask. SIDA Studies. Stockholm and Geneva: Swedish International Development Cooperation Agency (SIDA) and UN Research Institute for Social Development (UNRISD).

Gillespie. S. 2004. *Scaling up community driven development: A synthesis of experience.* Food Consumption and Nutrition Division Discussion Paper 181. Washington, D.C.: International Food Policy Research Institute.

Gillespie, S., and S. Kadiyala. 2005. *HIV/AIDS and food and nutrition security: From evidence to action.* Food Policy Review 7. Washington, D.C.: International Food Policy Research Institute.

Hamazakaza, P., and R. Kauseni. 2002. *Annotated bibliography of study of reports and past activities on the impact of HIV/AIDS on poverty, agriculture and food security in Zambia.* Rome: Farming Systems Association of Zambia and FAO.

Hsu, L. N., J. Du Guerny, and M. Marco. 2002. *Communities facing the HIV/AIDS challenge: From crisis to opportunity, from community vulnerability to community resilience.* Bangkok, Thailand: UNDP South East Asia HIV and Development Programme.

Hunter, S. 2002. *Supporting and expanding community-based HIV/AIDS preventions and care responses: A report on Save the Children U.S. Malawi COPE project.* Washington, D.C.: Save the Children Federation/U.S.

International HIV/AIDS Alliance and Family AIDS Care Trust. 2002. *Expanding community-based support for orphans and vulnerable children.* Brighton, U.K.: University of Sussex.

Kadiyala, S. 2004. *Scaling up HIV/AIDS interventions through expanded partnerships (STEPs) in Malawi.* Food Consumption and Nutrition Division Discussion Paper 179. Washington, D.C.: International Food Policy Research Institute.

Mallaby, S. 2004. *The world's banker: A story of failed states, financial crises, and the wealth and poverty of nations.* Washington, D.C.: Council on Foreign Relations and Penguin Press.

Mutangadura, G., D. Mukurazita, and H. Jackson. 1999. *A review of household and community responses to HIV/AIDS epidemic in rural areas of Sub-Saharan Africa.* UNAIDS Best Practice Collection. Geneva: UNAIDS.

NAADS (National Agricultural Advisory Services). 2003. *The impact of HIV/AIDS on the agricultural sector and rural livelihoods in Uganda.* Rome: Integrated Support to Sustainable Development and Food Security Programme (IP), FAO.

OECD. 2003. *Agricultural policies in OECD countries: A positive reform agenda.* OECD Policy Brief, Paris.

Phiri, S. N., G. Foster, and M. Nzima. 2001. *Expanding and strengthening community action: A study of ways to scale-up community mobilization interventions to mitigate the effect of HIV/AIDS on children and families.* Washington, D.C.: U.S. Agency for International Development.

Sen, A. 1981. *Poverty and famines: An essay on entitlement and deprivation.* Oxford: Clarendon Press.

Silomba, W. 2002. HIV/AIDS and development. In *One step further. Responses to HIV/AIDS,* ed. A. Sisask. SIDA Studies. Stockholm and Geneva: Swedish International Development Cooperation Agency (SIDA) and UN Research Institute for Social Development (UNRISD).

UNAIDS. 1998. *AIDS and men who have sex with men.* Geneva: UNAIDS Point of View.

———. 2004a. Bringing comprehensive HIV prevention to scale. Chapter four in *2004 Report on the global AIDS Epidemic.* Geneva: UNAIDS.

———. 2004b. *Report on the global AIDS epidemic.* Geneva: UNAIDS.

———. 2005. *AIDS in Africa: Three scenarios to 2020.* Geneva: UNAIDS.

White, J. 2002. *Facing the challenge: Experiences of mitigating the impacts of HIV/AIDS in Sub-Saharan Africa.* Kent, U.K.: Natural Resources Institute, University of Greenwich.

———. 2003. *Treating three million people by 2005: Making it happen, the WHO strategy.* Geneva: WHO.

———. 2004. *Scaling up antiretroviral therapy in resource-limited settings: Treatment guidelines for a public health approach.* Geneva: WHO.

———. 2005. *"3 by 5" Progress Report.* Geneva: WHO.

World Bank. 1988. *Integrated rural development: The World Bank experience 1965–86.* Washington, D.C.: World Bank, Operations Evaluation Department.

———. 1997. *Rural development: From vision to action.* Washington, D.C.: World Bank.

———. 2002. *Community-driven development: From vision to practice. A technical sourcebook.* Washington D.C.: World Bank.

———. 2004. *Turning bureaucrats into warriors: Preparing and implementing national HIV/AIDS programs in Africa, a generic operations manual.* Washington, D.C.: World Bank.

World Bank, DFID, UNAIDS, and MAP International. 2004. *Interim review of the multi-country AIDS program for Africa.* Washington, D.C., available on www.worldbank.org/aids.

Chapter 12

Multisectoral HIV/AIDS Approaches in Africa: How Are They Evolving?

Sarah Gavian, David Galaty, and Gilbert Kombe

Introduction

The response to HIV/AIDS in Africa has evolved considerably since the first cases were reported on the continent in the early 1980s. After the initial medical and public health responses through the mid-1990s, there was an enormous expansion in the scope of the strategic approaches and level of political and financial commitment to fight the disease. In the absence of a vaccine or cure, the global response expanded far beyond the traditional confines of the health sector. Perceiving strong links between AIDS and the greater development processes, national and international organs reached out to a wide array of stakeholders to implement a broad multi-sectoral agenda. This expansion in vision was accompanied by a corresponding development of institutional structures and coordination mechanisms. Efforts to extend, harmonize, and improve the management of the multisectoral response are very much continuing today.

Early in the new millennium, a very powerful new intervention was introduced into the arsenal against global HIV/AIDS. Already available in the developed countries, antiretroviral treatment (ART) was shown to effectively delay the progression of the disease in low-resource developing country conditions. A combination of medical advances, research, advocacy, and a very substantial upswing in donor funding allowed the global community to commit to universal access to these life-saving medications by 2010. The myriad of challenges to such a huge campaign, once seen as entirely insurmountable, is now seen as merely daunting.

These major trends have resulted in an HIV/AIDS landscape characterized by high-level international commitment to combating HIV/AIDS in a coordinated, multisectoral, participatory, large-scale, evidence-based manner. In this chapter we describe the evolution of multisectoral HIV/AIDS (MSHA) in the context of the rapid scale-up of the international response to HIV/AIDS and the introduction of ART. We identify the challenges and opportunities for the next phase of HIV/AIDS in the context of this mounting response.

We find that the multisectoral approach has moved beyond rhetoric into national and donor strategies but that it needs a more substantial conceptual framework as well as mechanisms for tracking, evaluating, and prioritizing multi-sectoral interventions. This is especially true as increased resources are flowing into the costly campaign to provide universal access to AIDS treatments. Examining this evolution from the broader development perspective, we also argue for the need to reevaluate the conceptual separation of HIV/AIDS and public health and consider resituating it in the domain of public health with strong conceptual and organiza-tional links to other important national development efforts toward the Millennium Development Goals.

The Health Response

The first cases of AIDS in Africa were reported in the early 1980s (WHO 2001). HIV sentinel surveillance systems began to be established at that early stage, pri-marily drawing data from pregnant women at antenatal clinics. Financed and led primarily by National Ministries of Health and treated as emergency measures, initial control efforts focused primarily on blood safety protocols. For example, in 1987, a short-term emergency plan was invoked in Zambia to ensure safe blood and blood product supplies.

In the mid- to late 1980s, preliminary scientific evidence began to appear sug-gesting that HIV in Africa primarily affected unmarried young and middle-aged people, most severely along specific transmission routes. Simultaneously, this period saw a steady trend of global mobilization against AIDS characterized by increas-ingly widespread attempts to measure seroprevalence and prevention campaigns emphasizing education, information, and human rights. In Africa, the World Health Organization's Global Program for AIDS had by 1990 provided technical assis-tance to 123 countries to develop short-term plans and had mobilized funds for 65 countries primarily for national public education campaigns and HIV surveillance, with some focus on blood screening, guidance care and counseling, and manage-ment strengthening (Slutkin 2000, pp. S26–S27). Progress was limited, however, and resources were scarce.

The early 1990s, however, saw dramatic increases in the number of people living with HIV/AIDS in Africa. In 1992, the South African National Health Department reported that the number of recorded HIV infections had increased 60 percent in the previous two years, and the number was expected to double in 1993 (London School of Hygiene and Tropical Medicine 1993). This explosion caught the world by surprise. According to WHO, the infections that had occurred by the year 2000 were three times greater than 1991 expectations (WHO 2001). The rapid spread of the virus during the 1990s was then followed by waves of rising death rates and growing numbers of orphans.

As a result, HIV/AIDS began to be recognized as a long-term issue requiring a more comprehensive public health approach. At the same time, research was providing new understandings about the virus. Several studies indicated that HIV was disproportionately affecting young women in their reproductive ages. Antenatal surveillance in several countries indicated high HIV prevalence among pregnant women. And, in 1994, medical research established ways to prevent mother-to-child transmission of HIV/AIDS through cesarean sections (Dunn et al. 1994), AZT (Connor et al. 1994), and Nevirapine (HIVNET012 trials). By the middle of the 1990s, broader public health interventions came to the fore: interventions to change sexual behavior; the prevention and treatment of sexually transmitted infections; programs to reduce risk and harm among injecting drug users; and initiatives to reduce the risk of mother-to-child transmission.

Rethinking the Fight Using Multisectoral Approaches

At the beginning of the 1990s, the battle against HIV/AIDS was being waged primarily by ministries of health through clinics and hospitals. As the prevalence continued to soar and the multiple waves of impacts devastated communities of Southern and Eastern Africa, responses restricted purely to the health sector seemed inadequate. The mounting pressure led to a great expansion of the battle conceptually, organizationally, and financially, with a focus on multisectoral approaches.

Multisectoral Stakeholders and Activities

Although the AIDS literature never rigorously defines the term, multisectoral approaches to HIV/AIDS are those seeking to reduce HIV prevalence, provide care and treatment to persons living with HIV/AIDS (PLWHA), and mitigate the impacts of the epidemic on affected populations by employing an appropriate mix of health- and non-health-based interventions and involving a broad array of stakeholders in their design and implementation.

By the mid-1990s, governments in the hardest hit countries in Africa started extending AIDS-focused public health interventions throughout government agencies and, eventually, beyond. They set up workplace AIDS policies and programs to promote prevention in other line ministries (agriculture, justice, etc.), usually through an AIDS focal point. Interventions included HIV/AIDS awareness and education campaigns carried out in ministries, offices, schools, and farmer field schools. Likewise, condoms started being distributed to high-risk populations at sites such as truck stops, border crossings, and places of work. Testing, counseling, and treatment services were extended in nontraditional workplace settings (Nathan 2002). As nongovernmental actors emerged as key players in global HIV/AIDS, thinking around HIV/AIDS evolved and resulted in widening recognition of the important role of NGOs, FBOs, CSOs, and the private sector in the HIV/AIDS response. At the same time, administrative reforms under full swing in many African countries led to the creation of AIDS task forces at district level or lower. Thus, public health interventions began to be mainstreamed through all levels of government and throughout the economy.

Simultaneously, as studies were released on the impact of AIDS on various sectors of the economy, the nature of HIV/AIDS responses was modified in a subtle way. Recognizing these impacts, government ministries, NGOs, and private sector firms alike developed responses motivated by the need to protect their own operations rather than simply serving as venues for ministry of health efforts to reduce HIV prevalence. Some of these actions focused on prevention, such as the addition of an HIV/AIDS awareness component to the 1999/2000 Zambian postharvest survey for survey field staff to be passed on to survey respondents to reduce losses in agricultural productivity (USAID 2003). Others combined prevention and mitigation, such as toolkits for small businesses to use in developing workplace AIDS programs designed to assess and lessen the economic impact of the disease on their operations.

Over time, multisectoral programming became more sophisticated. NGOs in particular piloted programs to support PLWHA and their families through a continuum of care, treatment, and mitigation efforts related to home-based care, psychosocial support to address emotional needs, home gardens and food aid to improve nutrition and incomes, vouchers for legal services to protect assets, and lighter plows and subsidized fertilizers to support incomes (USAID 2003).

As the portfolio of HIV/AIDS interventions expanded, there was increasing recognition of the need to link interventions by providing a comprehensive package of HIV and non-HIV services to target populations. The best examples come from the domain of support for orphans and vulnerable children. The 2004 *Framework for the Protection, Care and Support of Orphans and Vulnerable Children Living in a World with HIV/AIDS* brings together five strategic pillars: strengthening family capacity, mobilizing community-based responses, providing essential services, improving policy and legislation, and advocating for a supportive environment (UNAIDS 2004e).

National and International Multisectoral Organizations

As the concept of multisectoral HIV/AIDS (MSHA) evolved, so too did the national and international institutional architecture governing the HIV/AIDS response. In keeping with the underlying public health approach, the early HIV/AIDS efforts were coordinated nationally by ministries of health and internationally by organizations such as the World Health Organization. Over time, and reflecting what would become known as the "exceptional nature of HIV/AIDS" (UNAIDS 2005b), an entirely new set of institutional arrangements has sprung up.

As the HIV/AIDS crisis gained momentum, African governments in heavily afflicted countries set up national AIDS councils (NACs), largely under the supervision of ministries of health. Towards the late 1990s, however, fueled by the need to mobilize the entire public sector, NACs came under the direct supervision of the executive (either the president or prime minister) and represented at the ministerial level by all line ministries. With the increasing profile of nongovernmental actors, most NACs formed technical committees composed of the broader array of stakeholders.

In general, NACs are responsible for (1) guiding the elaboration, approval, and revision of national HIV/AIDS strategy and action plan, (2) defining policies, (3) approving large projects with a national scope, (4) reviewing and approving annual workplans and global budgets, (5) reviewing progress in the implementation of the program, and (6) serving as the lead advocate for attention to the HIV/AIDS epidemic (Brown, Ayvalikli, and Mohammad 2004, p. 21). Multisectoral from their inception, NACs oversee all aspects of strategic planning, decisionmaking, and resource allocation around HIV/AIDS in their respective countries. By 2004, 21 of 27 UNAIDS country offices reporting from SSA had a NAC (UNAIDS 2004c).

The creation of multisectoral structures at the national level was accompanied by a parallel set of changes at the international level. Set up in 1986, WHO's Special Program on AIDS, using resources from the Global Program on AIDS trust fund, focused primarily on the public health measures described above. From 1987 to 1990, the program contributed to developing the first national strategies, promulgating widespread public information campaigns, and promoting human rights as well as emphasizing the need for a rapid, massive, and multisectoral response. In mid-1993, six United Nations organizations, including WHO, began to seek agreement on forming a novel joint and cosponsored UN program on HIV/AIDS

(WHO 1995). In July 1994, the Economic and Social Council of the United Nations resolved to form a coordinating group to spearhead the global response to the epidemic, reinforce national capacities to develop comprehensive strategies, implement effective HIV/AIDS activities across a wide range of sectors and institutions, and raise funds and commitments for the response (UN 1994). The resulting body, UNAIDS was made operational in 1996 and at the time of this writing, in 2005, describes itself as having driven "a unique, multistakeholder response" (UNAIDS 2005b, p. 4). The UNAIDS multisectoral response includes supporting the effectiveness of the UN system, working closely with AIDS-related civil society and people living with HIV, and engaging nontraditional partners in fighting AIDS, such as the media, faith-based organizations, business, sports organizations, uniformed services, and the labor movement (UNAIDS 2005b, p. 12).

Although not strictly speaking an institution, the World Bank's Multicountry AIDS Program (MAP) for Africa has been specifically designed to support implementation of national multisectoral HIV/AIDS strategies and action plans (World Bank 2002, 2004). In fact, the existence of a NAC became a prerequisite for participation in the program. MAP's purpose is to avert millions of HIV infections, alleviate suffering for tens of millions, and help preserve the development prospects of a large number of African countries. The first phase, MAP1 was approved in 2000, funded at US$500 million, and put into operation in 2001. In Fiscal Year 2001, the World Bank's contribution to HIV/AIDS in Africa was greater than in all previous years combined. Particularly supporting the decentralized aspects of multisectoral approaches, a large share of MAP resources are directed to local communities for designing and implementing HIV activities tailored to their specific conditions. In the second phase of its estimated 12- to 15-year commitment, the World Bank has committed another US$500 million under MAP2 to expand efforts to new countries, to pilot test ARTs, and to support cross-border initiatives (World Bank 2002).

As follow-up to the 2001 UN General Assembly Special Session on AIDS, the Global Fund to Fight AIDS, Tuberculosis, and Malaria (GFATM) was established at the beginning of 2002 (GFATM 2004). By the end of 2004, the Global Fund had disbursed US$402 million for HIV-related grants (UNAIDS 2005a), representing 56 percent of total Global Fund disbursements (31 percent and 13 percent going to malaria and tuberculosis, respectively). Sixty-one percent of the HIV/AIDS funds went to Sub-Saharan Africa; 49 percent of HIV/AIDS funds disbursed through the Global Fund during this period were earmarked for drugs and supplies (e.g., ARV drugs). Finally, in many cases, many NACs also serve as the Country Coordinating Mechanisms for GFATM activities.

Greater Political and Financial Commitments

Globally, there has been a growing recognition and formal commitment to the idea that effective responses to the HIV/AIDS epidemic include multisectoral approaches to preventing the disease, caring for and treating its victims, and mitigating its effects. The Abidjan Declaration of 1997 committed African mayors and municipal leaders to promoting and co-coordinating local multisectoral approaches for HIV prevention and the care of infected and affected people. The Abuja Declaration of April 2001 signed by African heads of state acknowledged the role played by poverty, poor nutritional conditions, and underdevelopment in increasing vulnerability to HIV/AIDS. In June 2001, 189 countries of the United Nations General Assembly Special Session (UNGASS) signed the Declaration of Commitment on HIV/AIDS to ensure the development and implementation of multisectoral national strategies and financing plans for combating HIV/AIDS by 2003. This commitment has continued to accelerate (Fig. 12.1). Global spending on AIDS programs in low- and middle-income countries has increased nearly 15-fold since 1996, when UNAIDS was founded to coordinate all AIDS-related activities of the UN system. Although not shown in the figure, annual institutional spending on HIV/AIDS rose even further in 2004 to US$6.1 billion.

This amount represented contributions in 2003 from domestic sources (national governments and households, 42 percent), bilateral donors (23 percent), international nongovernmental organizations (NGOs), and the multilateral (Global Fund, UN, and the World Bank, 26 percent). A large portion of these funds comes from just a few donors. The most recent data (2004) indicate that the United States contributes nearly 50 percent of all bilateral contributions to global HIV/AIDS in developing countries (excluding funds for GFATM and research), and the United Kingdom 21 percent; the European Union as a whole, Canada, Germany, and Japan contribute shares of about 3 to 4 percent each (UNAIDS 2004a,b,f, 2005a).

Although funding continues to surge, it falls well behind the ever-increasing costs of combating the epidemic. UNAIDS estimates there will be a funding gap of at least US$18 billion from 2005 to 2007 (UNAIDS 2005a). Addressing this gap raises several key issues. First is the ongoing need to greatly improve financial tracking and costing. Great strides are being made by UNAIDS, World Bank/MAP, donors, and in-country NACs, but there is a long way to go. At present, it is very difficult to track the true costs and available funding for the full multisectoral response to HIV/AIDS. Some of the problems arise from the sheer difficulty of gathering reliable information on key components of spending. Others are more bureaucratic, such as developing codes for dual-purpose interventions (OECD/DAC and UNAIDS 2004), which many multisectoral activities are, or putting in place

Figure 12.1 Institutional HIV/AIDS spending, 1996–2002

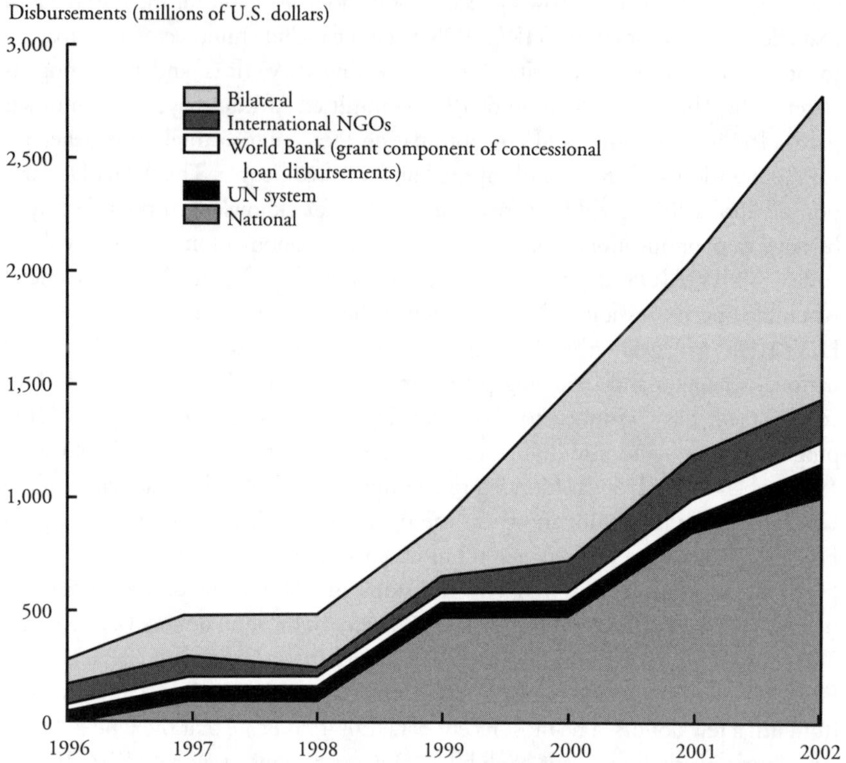

Disbursements (millions of U.S. dollars)

Source: UNAIDS (2004b, p. 15).

the data collection and analysis processes needed to budget and monitor the implementation of national strategic plans. Finally, there are strategic issues. Most donor strategies reflect a strong multisectoral orientation either explicitly or by endorsing a wide array of multisectoral interventions (CIDA 2002; GTZ 2003; DFID 2004a,b; GTZ 2005). The rules governing the disbursement of funds under the U.S. government's PEPFAR program make it difficult to use these funds for multisectoral interventions (United States Department of State 2004, 2005a,b; USAID 2004).

The Era of ARVs

Recent results presented at the 11th World AIDS Conference in 1996 in Vancouver established the efficacy of antiretroviral therapy (ART), and in the course of the next few years, antiretroviral (ARV) drugs became a major tool in the arsenal for combating HIV/AIDS in developed countries (Katzenstein, Laga, and Moatti 2003, p. S1). To the great frustration of many in Sub-Saharan Africa, the high cost of the drugs and the considerable logistic challenges of rolling out drugs to such a large, impoverished community seemed insurmountably daunting.

In May 2000, the Accelerating Access Initiative (AAI) was launched as a cooperative endeavor of UNAIDS, the WHO, UNICEF, UNFPA, the World Bank, and five (later six) pharmaceutical companies. The purpose was to find ways to expand safe access to affordable HIV medicines in developing countries. The drug companies rapidly lowered prices as countries negotiated batch orders; the companies also gave large price reductions to NGOs, private sector employers, and health care providers. At the same time, all of the 19 national governments that entered into supply agreements under the AAI lifted taxes and trade barriers to the medications. Some also brought in highly price-competitive generic drugs from the Indian drug manufacturer Cipla (WHO 2002).

The effect of these initiatives on ARV prices in Africa was dramatic (see Fig. 12.2), falling from about $12,000 in 1999 to $300 per person per year in 2004. Falling ARV prices provided treatment advocates with the momentum for building political and financial commitment to widespread drug access in the developing world. So too did evidence from initial trials in Cote d'Ivoire, Senegal, and Uganda that drug resistance in Africa could be kept to levels at or below levels in Western countries (Katzenstein, Laga, and Moatti 2003, p. S1), and the argument, drawn in part from the experience of cities such as San Francisco, is that the availability of treatments motivated people to prevent and test for HIV. ARVs continue to be seen as a critical tool for mitigating the impacts of HIV on affected communities by extending lives and livelihoods.

International commitment to treatment grew rapidly. As early as 1997, the World Bank published a groundbreaking report (*Confronting AIDS: Public Priorities in a Global Epidemic*) proclaiming that treatment needed to be an integral part of AIDS strategies. In addition to its express commitment to multisectoral approaches, the Declaration of Commitment to HIV/AIDS signed unanimously by all 189 UN members in 2001 recognized the right of all people living with HIV in low-income countries to care and treatment. Widespread commitment emerged at the International AIDS Conference in Barcelona in July 2002 to the goal of extending ARV treatment to millions of people in developing countries. This consensus was rapidly consolidated by the end of the year in the World Health Organization/UNAIDS "3 by 5" Initiative (WHO 2005) to ensure that 3 million people living with HIV/AIDS in developing countries have access to antiretroviral treatment by the end of 2005 (UNAIDS 2004a). In July 2003, at their special summit on

Figure 12.2 Prices (US$/year) of a first-line antiretroviral regimen in Uganda, 1998–2003

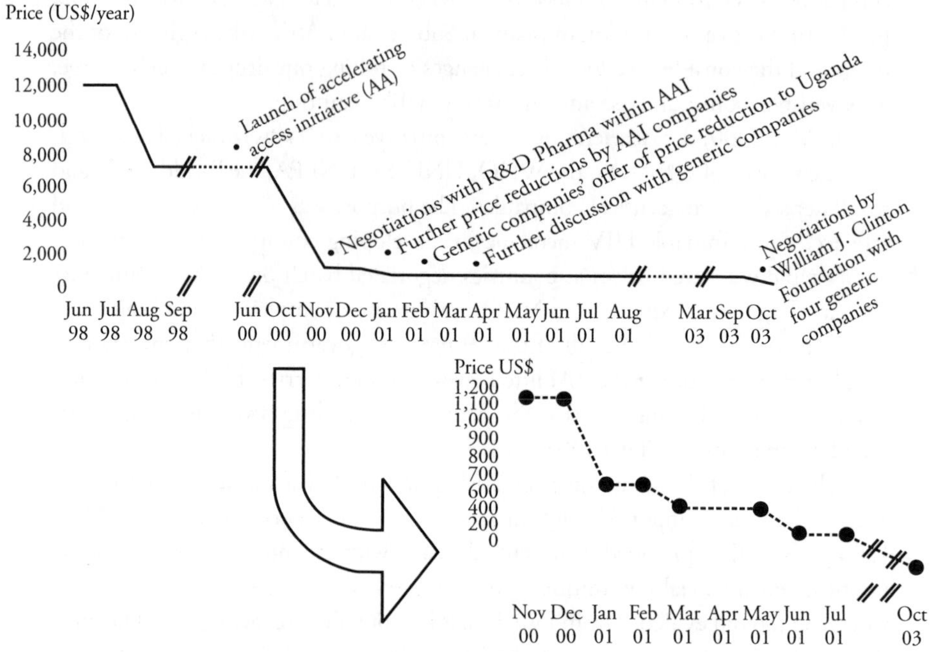

Source: http://www.unaids.org/html/pub/topics/epidemiology/slides12/bkk04slide034_en_ppt.ppt#256,1, Slide 1.

HIV/AIDS, the Southern African Development Community (SADC) countries issued the "Maseru Declaration," which combined an explicit multisectoral approach to combating HIV/AIDS with a strong priority on scaling up care, treatment, and access to antiretroviral drugs (SADC 2003).

Donors responded by funding treatment programs. In early 2001, Uganda was one of the first countries to start using World Bank/MAP money for providing ART. Since its inception, the Global Fund has disbursed US$272 million for HIV/ AIDS in Africa (49 percent of total Global Fund disbursements go toward drugs and supplies). Initiated in January 2003, the U.S. President's Emergency Plan for HIV/AIDS Relief (PEPFAR) represents one of the largest sources of ARVs in the developing world. One of the main PEPFAR goals is to use 55 percent of its resources to provide treatment for 2 million HIV-infected people in the first five years of the program.

As a result of this tremendous organizational focus, WHO estimates that the number of Africans receiving ARV therapy approximately doubled from 150,000 to 325,000 between June and December 2004. Coverage, however, remains very low. Only 8 percent of those currently requiring medications are receiving them (WHO 2005).

Challenges and Opportunities Going Forward

The urgent need to stop the rapid spread of the incurable, deadly, and devastating HIV virus has prompted great activity and experimentation on the part of the national and international communities. An initial health-based response was followed, in the absence of vaccines, cures, or even effective treatments, by broad-based multisectoral efforts involving to varying degrees all levels of government and stakeholders. After a slow start, life-extending ARVs are becoming available to the vast number of HIV-infected persons in developing countries, including the 66 percent who live in Sub-Saharan Africa.

This complex and rapidly evolving situation requires immediate efforts to harmonize concepts, priorities and strategies, implementation plans, measures for monitoring and evaluation, and resource tracking. Responding to the cacophony of actors and approaches, UNAIDS and its partners are promoting the "Three Ones" principles, which call for one agreed-on national framework of action against AIDS in each country that unifies all partners; one national AIDS coordinating authority, with a broad-based multisectoral mandate; and one agreed-on country-level monitoring and evaluation system. The growing commitment to the "Three Ones" poses significant challenges and opportunities going forward.

Aligning Strategic Frameworks

If the many players in the AIDS arena in each country are to operate under a unified national framework, that framework must be up-to-date, robust, and clearly prioritized, with meaningful objectives, monitoring plans, and resource allocation processes. Aligning strategic frameworks requires efforts on many levels.

First is to integrate the modalities of extending universal access to ARV therapies. By the late 1990s, most of the high-prevalence African countries had drafted comprehensive, multisectoral national AIDS strategies and policies. Because only 43 percent of these have been updated in the last two years (UNAIDS 2004c), many of the older national strategies do not yet reflect plans for extending ARVs. Countries need strategies to deal with the many moving pieces: procurement and supply management, strengthening health systems, training health workers, assuring quality and accreditation, monitoring treatment and drug resistance, supporting home-based care, developing appropriate nutritional components, and ensuring equitable treatments for women and children (WHO 2005).

Second, NACs also need to work with their stakeholders to put a more solid foundation under the multisectoral components of their strategies. Multisectoral responses have been formally introduced in a large number of ministries, typically 20 or more in each country, but the quality and implementation of those plans has been uneven. Some sectors have had more success mainstreaming an HIV/AIDS response than others. Predictably, health ministries have been most active in designing and implementing programs to address HIV issues faced by their staff and their constituencies (World Bank 2004; Futures Group, Research Triangle Institute, and the Centre for Development and Population Activities 2002). A review of SADC HIV/AIDS policies conducted in 2002 found that the education ministries were also widely engaged to the extent of having detailed implementation strategies. Other ministries tended to have policies but no action plans (Futures Group, Research Triangle Institute, and the Centre for Development and Population Activities 2002). A 2003 UNAIDS survey in 63 countries (worldwide) found only 13 percent had actually made progress in implementing sectoral plans (UNAIDS 2004a). In 2004, World Bank evaluations found these sectoral efforts to be "somewhat half-hearted . . . cookie cutter" plans that do not reflect local situations (Brown, Ayvalikli, and Mohammad 2004; World Bank 2004). Further, although ministries often have workplace action plans and programs, many have not taken the next steps to address the HIV/AIDS issues related to their interactions with their constituencies (e.g., farmers, students, trade associations).

Third, revised multisectoral strategies must find a way to motivate genuine private sector involvement. Although studies show that private households bear a tremendous share of the costs associated with HIV/AIDS (see Box 12.1), involvement by the business community appears to be fairly modest (Fig. 12.3). The figures shown do not capture the contribution African businesses may make to HIV/AIDS prevention, care and treatment, and mitigation in their own work settings. However, a recent study by the World Economic Forum suggests that such investments are also fairly limited, especially in relation to the high level of concern about HIV impacts expressed by the business managers surveyed (World Economic Forum 2005).

There are many reasons for what B.A. Brink, senior vice-president for health at Anglo-American, calls the "disappointing global business response to HIV/AIDS" (World Economic Forum 2005, p. 4). At present, there are few incentives. To address the problems of poverty and inequity, donors are directing huge sums of public funding through governments and NGOs to subsidize AIDS-related drugs

Box 12.1 Out-of-Pocket Spending on HIV/AIDS by African Households

- In Burkina Faso in 2003, household spending was 14.3 percent of the total expenditure on AIDS; this constituted 98 percent of total private expenditures on HIV/AIDS and almost double the government's share.

- In Kenya in 2002, households were 45 percent of the total.

- In Rwanda in 1998, households bore 93 percent of all HIV/AIDS spending; by 2002, a large influx of donor funding reduced the burden on households to 13 percent. But even at that level, households still far outspent government, which accounted for only 8 percent of total HIV spending.

- In Zambia as in Burkina Faso, the household share was nearly twice the government's share (29 versus 17 percent for Zambia; 20 versus 10 percent for Burkina Faso).

  These patterns are repeated around the world.

Source: Data are from UNAIDS (2004d).

and health services, undercutting the potential for the private sector to compete in these domains. In addition, not all companies have the wherewithal to undertake their own programs. Finally, the private sector often faces high "transaction costs" of dealing with bureaucratic NACs (Brown, Ayvalikli, and Mohammad 2004).

Carrying through on a multisectoral response to the AIDS epidemic that sustainably involves the private sector requires radical thinking on how to improve incentives for partnership and even handover. WHO, UNAIDS, and USAID are experimenting with approaches to expand the private sector's role in delivering AIDS services to the general public. World Bank reports recommend a combination of subsidies and contracts to private businesses to increase their involvement while addressing critical public sector constraints. Brown et al. note that smaller enterprises that are willing but unable to provide HIV/AIDS services outside to their staff "should be treated as any civil society NGO and receive full grant financing" (Brown, Ayvalikli, and Mohammad 2004, p. 52). Noting the key role of the private sector in supply chains for health services and drugs the World Bank has

Figure 12.3 Contributors to HIV/AIDS spending in 2003

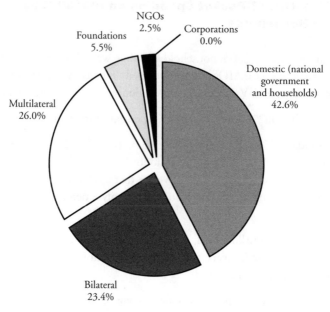

Source: UNAIDS (2004f).

experimented with in MAP projects with contracting financial management services (Senegal), AIDS-related accounting and other traditional project management services (Cape Verde and Zambia), and disbursement services for civil society grants (Kenya) (Brown, Ayvalikli, and Mohammad 2004, p. 78). In addition to evaluating and extending these pilot efforts, there is an ongoing need for substantial studies and debate on how to motivate the private sector to play a sustained, profitable, and equitable role in the rollout of ARVs.

Ongoing efforts to improve national coordination provide an important opportunity for donors and other stakeholders to improve the national and sectoral strategies themselves.

Governing a Multisectoral Response

The "Three Ones" calls for one national AIDS-coordinating authority with a broad multisectoral mandate. As implemented, NACs tend to be exceptional government structures, outside the usual chain of ministerial command. Although such interagency bodies have precedent in Africa and indeed elsewhere, some analysts voice concern that they may circumvent, rather than strengthen, normal government functions. In its ongoing reviews of its MAP program, the World Bank has repeatedly signaled the problem that "the placing of the NAC Secs outside the Ministry of Health has caused resentment and confusion among health officials" (World Bank 2001, p. 12). In his assessment of AIDS governance issues, Putzel writes that

> [t]he organizational template being imposed by UNAIDS, the World Bank, and the Global Fund is not necessarily conducive to developing an effective battle against the epidemic. . . . The national commissions called for by the Bank and the Global Fund have tended to weaken government and overly marginalize the health sector and medical profession. (Putzel 2003, p. iv)

The large-scale rollout of ARVs again underscores the key role of the health sector in contributing to the HIV/AIDS response. As with any complicated health problem, AIDS demands the involvement of actors and interventions outside the strict confines of the health sector. But the ongoing need for a broadly participative, multisectoral approach does not obviate the basic principles of public sector management and responsibility. The World Bank recommends that NACs and NAC secretariats stick to facilitation rather than control and avoid competing with or duplicating the key role of the health sector in responding to the epidemic (World Bank 2001). Over time, there is an opportunity to learn from the success of multisectoral NACs and consider whether better linkages among all ministries on a broad range of interrelated development issues may not be a better approach focusing coordination on one "exceptional" disease.

Developing Robust Multisectoral Monitoring and Evaluation

Consistent with the final stipulation of the Three Ones principles, there is consensus that monitoring and evaluation (M&E) is critical to producing the scientific data and strategic information needed to guide the response. M&E forms integral components of World Bank, Global Fund, and PEPFAR HIV/AIDS activities. Perhaps the greatest strides have been made in Uganda, which has well-defined M&E activities, a budget, an implementation plan, indicators, and benchmarks as part of its HIV/AIDS strategic framework (Government of Uganda 2000). However, this is not the case elsewhere. The World Bank argues that "In the future, arguably the single most important role for a NAS will be to develop an integrated, fully costed, annual project implementation plan . . . with clear definition of responsibilities, outputs and budgets" (Brown, Ayvalikli, and Mohammad 2004, p. 25).

Huge sums of money are now being invested in multisectoral approaches with weak statements of how those funds are truly going to address the AIDS problem in a sustained manner. There have been extensive efforts to assess the effectiveness of the traditional public health interventions (such as condoms, VCT, STI, abstinence, PMTCT, blood safety, etc.) in terms of prevalence rates, numbers of infections averted, or cost per infection averted.[1] At present, the goals for most care and treatment interventions are tracked in terms of their outputs, not their impacts: thus, number of employees reached with workplace AIDS programs, number of patients receiving treatment, or number of home-based care visits. M&E for mitigation is at a very rudimentary stage. The major M&E systems and resource tracking models used by UNAIDS include few mitigation activities beyond orphans and vulnerable children. M&E plans typically lack indicators related to household or community food security and nutrition (beyond orphans and vulnerable children), incomes, economic productivity, livelihood and assets protection, the coverage and equity of social service provision, stigma and discrimination, and gender-based violence. Furthermore, when included, mitigation indicators typically do not capture impacts but rather only inputs and outputs such as number of orphans schooled or number of PLWHA associations formed.

There are two major reasons for this poor tracking. First, there is no clear, agreed-on, definition of multisectoralism in HIV/AIDS and how it leads to prevention, treatment and care, and mitigation. Most proclamations and donor and national strategies fail to provide a clear definition or conceptual framework for their multisectoral approach. They tend to focus on "who": government line ministries and their decentralized organs, nongovernment groups, and others. Most statements are mute on the specific objectives (expected outcomes) of their multisectoral approach and on who needs to do what to accomplish those objectives.

Thus, if AIDS funds are to be effectively directed to preventing the epidemic and lessening its impacts, the full basket of interventions must be evaluated in similar terms against well-defined goals. Efforts to refine M&E plans, now further motivated by the Three Ones, offer an opportunity to address these difficult issues. The first step must be to clarify the goals of HIV prevention, care and treatment, and mitigation. Such efforts must start with laying out a basic conceptual framework for each of these concepts that shows the distinct roles for a broad range of health and nonhealth approaches.

- For prevention, once the linkages among various multisectoral determinants of infection are explicitly formalized, they must be tested against the same standards used for other public health interventions (e.g., infections averted, prevalence). At present, there are few studies of multisectoral interventions that express outcomes in terms of these standard HIV measures, in part because of the great complications in linking socioeconomic conditions to infections in a rigorous manner across a highly diverse range of environments and attenuating circumstances.

- For care and treatment, measures of mortality, morbidity, and disability-adjusted life years (DALYs) are likely to become more important with broader use of ARVs.

- For mitigation, some of the newer OVC indicators, which include nutritional status and other measures of welfare, may provide an opening for expanding the monitoring and evaluation of mitigation efforts beyond this one group of affected people.

The second reason for the difficulties tracking MSHA interventions is that such interventions usually have multiple objectives. The full value of their benefits cannot be captured solely in terms of their impacts on HIV/AIDS because they were designed to allow other sectors to attain their objectives in spite of HIV/AIDS. Evaluating the effectiveness of a workplace program solely in terms of number of infections prevented will miss other important impacts it may have on motivation, productivity, recruitment, and, ultimately, the bottom line for all businesses, profitability.

More profoundly, there are many development interventions that fall well outside the traditional set of HIV/AIDS activities that are likely to have a very significant impact on decreasing prevalence, improving care and treatment, and mitigation impacts. Although evidence on the direct effects of poverty on HIV is mixed, it is clear that the impoverishment of African countries has eroded their ability to put in place the health systems needed to prevent and treat the disease. Nor have these countries succeeded at creating the social and economic opportunities needed to mitigate the impacts of HIV/AIDS and potentially contribute to prevention in the first place. As terrible as the HIV/AIDS epidemic truly is, it is not the only terrible problem plaguing Africa. In spite of a plethora of studies on HIV/AIDS, there are few assessments of its impacts relative to other health problems and other nonhealth challenges to people's well-being, such as drought, food crises, corruption, wars, and slow economic growth. It may be that the next best way to improve the human condition in Africa is to invest in the roads, schools, and farms needed to eradicate poverty, hunger, and poor health conditions. At present, we simply do not have the evidence to say. Even in the face of international cries and commitments to increase development assistance across the broad array of Millennium Development Goals, there have been few strategic or analytic efforts by either donors or national government to lay out consistent, costed, sequenced, and monitored multipronged development strategies.

Thus, one of the greatest challenges going forward is the need to develop a more robust set of M&E indicators that reflect the multiple impacts of a broad-based HIV/AIDS program that can be used to better allocate scarce funds among competing objectives. It is therefore imperative to develop the analytic framework and tools to situate HIV/AIDS in the greater development context. A truly multisectoral approach requires rigorous assessments of the returns to varying types of interventions not only in terms of HIV outcomes but also in terms of other development outcomes as described in the Millennium Development Goals, such as poverty reduction, incomes, and hunger. Such analyses should be carried out in a framework that (1) sums up joint returns of multisectoral investments in terms of their health and nonhealth impacts and (2) provides meaningful comparisons of the returns from different HIV and non-HIV interventions against a broad range of development goals.

Only with such information can scarce resources be sensibly invested among the sectors, within the health sector itself, and among the wide span of activities designed for prevention, care and treatment, and mitigation. There is great demand for this kind of information at all levels. Political discussions at the highest international levels (such as July 2005 G-8 discussions on development in Africa) as well as the ongoing technical revisions to M&E plans currently being undertaken by PEPFAR and the UNAIDS Monitoring and Evaluation Resource Group provide important opportunities to tighten the effectiveness of multisectoral HIV/AIDS investments going forward.

Summary

There have been rapid and impressive advances in the science, organizational approach, and funding to HIV/AIDS in the last two decades. National governments, with their UN and other partners, have exhibited strong multisectoral commitment and momentum, engaging a broad range of stakeholders through participatory and decentralized processes. The focus on locally driven multisectoral approaches has been supported by the creation of flexible institutional structures, such as UNAIDS, World Bank MAP, and GFATM. Donor funding has soared. In addition to donor commitments to multisectoral interventions, there have sprung up innovative management and funding arrangements, such as contracted services, pooled funding, and community funding channels designed to strengthen the multisectoral response.

However, there are still some major challenges. HIV prevalence continues to rise worldwide and, despite some important successes, in Africa. Although broadly espoused, the MSHA approach lacks a tested conceptual framework linked to defined outcomes with clear linkages to effective interventions. As a result, there is a "cookie-cutter" approach to sectoral strategies and fairly rudimentary (but improving) MSHA M&E. The rapid advance of the epidemic, the corresponding inflow of massive resources into many health and nonhealth intervention approaches, and the recent commitment to universal extension of costly treatment programs requires a careful balancing act. Although useful, broad stakeholder representation at the national level is not enough to ensure results-oriented, evidence-driven decisionmaking or effective implementation. Within the AIDS community, there is already lively discussion of the issues involved in balancing investments within the broad range of HIV activities aimed at prevention, treatment and mitigation, and research. Multisectoral approaches provide a solid foundation for designing ARV outreach programs as well as maintaining the political pressure needed to ensure equitable distribution of treatment services. However, the gaping weaknesses in the health infrastructure required to meet the 3×5 targets have refocused attention on the need to invest beyond HIV in strengthening the health sector more generally (WHO 2005). There is a need for better M&E information in order to make optimal choices. Unless interventions can be shown to have direct and measurable impacts on HIV/AIDS, the single largest donor, the United States, will remain cautious about using AIDS money for multisectoral interventions. Increasing commitment to the Three Ones provides a critical impetus to efforts to harmonize strategic plans, priority setting, implementation, terms, methods, and monitoring and evaluation.

There are many opportunities for both health and nonhealth specialists to work together to improve the effectiveness of multisectoral approaches to combating HIV/AIDS in this rapidly changing landscape. Possible forums include the technical committees of NACs and the Global Fund CCMs, where nonhealth specialists can provide input into strategic dialog, priority setting, implementation, and results tracking for HIV/AIDS. Mounting awareness of the links between HIV/AIDS and nutritional status creates an opportunity for nutrition and food security experts to develop these conceptual links lacking in current MSHA frameworks, provide an empirical basis for assessing impacts and costs, propose indicator and monitoring systems, and design appropriate targeted food interventions. Likewise, the food and nutrition security community is well suited to offer a broader operational definition of mitigation beyond orphans and vulnerable children.

Further, with the world focused on the calls to greatly increase the quantity and quality of assistance to Africa, the broader development community also has an important role to play in the working with the health community to ensure the best allocation of public funds across a wide range of development goals.

Notes

The authors thank Cosmas Musamali and Patricia Banda of the USAID/Zambia Health Systems Strengthening Project, Alex Simwanza of the Zambian National AIDS Council, Charles Hakoma and Michael Chanda of the USAID/Zambia SHARe project, and Robert Kauka of the Ugandan Ministry of Agriculture, Animal Industries and Fisheries for sharing their ideas and assistance. We, of course, take full responsibility for the research and perspectives expressed in this chapter.

    1. Libraries of such studies as well as links to AIDS costing models based on the results of such studies can be found at the web pages of the International AIDS Economics Network (www.iaen.org).

References

Brown, J. C., B. Ayvalikli, and N. Mohammad. 2004. *Turning bureaucrats into warriors: Preparing and implementing multi-sectoral HIV-AIDS programs in Africa. A generic operations manual.* Washington, D.C.: The International Bank for Reconstruction and Development (World Bank). http://www.worldbank.org/afr/aids/gom/manual/World%20Bank%20GOM%20Final%20June.pdf. Accessed June 24, 2005.

CIDA (The Canadian International Development Agency). 2002. *CIDA takes action against HIV/AIDS around the world.* Quebec.

Connor, E., R. S. Sperling, R. Gelber, P. Kiselev, G. Scott, M. J. O'Sullivan, R. VanDyke, M. Bey, W. Shearer, and R. L. Jacobson. 1994. Reduction of maternal–infant transmission of Human Immunodeficiency Virus type 1 with zidovudine treatment. *New England Journal of Medicine* 331: 1173–1180.

DFID (Department for International Development). 2004a. *Taking action: The UK's strategy for tackling HIV and AIDS in the developing world.* http://www.dfid.gov.uk/Pubs/files/HIVAID-Stakingactionsummary.pdf.

———. 2004b. *Responding to HIV/AIDS. Report by the Comptroller and Auditor General. Executive Summary.* HC 664 Session 2003–2004: 18 June 2004. London: Stationery Office. http://www.dfid.gov.uk/news/files/st-responsetonaoreport.asp.

Dunn, D. T., M. L. Newell, and M. J. Mayaux. 1994. Perinatal AIDS collaborative transmission studies: Mode of delivery and vertical transmission of HIV-1: A review of prospective studies. *Journal of Acquired Immune Deficiency Syndrome* 7: 1064–1066.

Futures Group, Research Triangle Institute, and the Centre for Development and Population Activities. 2002. *National and sector HIV/AIDS policies in the member states of the Southern Africa Development Community.* Prepared for the SADC/HSU by the POLICY Project.

GFATM (The Global Fund to Fight AIDS, Tuberculosis and Malaria). 2004. *A force for change: The Global Fund at 30 months.* http://www.theglobalfund.org/en/files/publications/forceforchange/bangkok_2004_overview.pdf. Accessed April 7, 2005.

Government of Uganda. 2000. *The National Strategic Framework for HIV/AIDS Activities in Uganda: 2000/1–2005/6. Uganda.* Prepared in partnership with the Uganda AIDS Commission and the Joint United Nations Programme on AIDS. http://www.aidsuganda.org/pdf/Annex_2_TWG_2_Report.pdf.

GTZ (Deutsche Gesellschaft für Technische Zusammenarbeit). Undated. *Mainstreaming anti-HIV/AIDS measures within agriculture and rural development in Africa.* http://www.gtz.de/de/dokumente/en-hiv-aids-agriculture-and-rural-development.pdf. Accessed March 7, 2005.

————. 2003. *The fight against HIV/AIDS: the GTZ contribution.* Division 4300. Eschborn. http://www.gtz.de/de/dokumente/en-gtz-contribution-to-fight-hiv-aids.pdf. Accessed June 21, 2005.

Katzenstein, D., M. Laga, and J.-P. Moatti. 2003. The evaluation of the HIV/AIDS drug access initiatives in Côte D' Ivoire, Senegal and Uganda: How access to antiretroviral treatment can become feasible in Africa. *AIDS* 17 (Suppl 3): S1–S4. http://www.aidsonline.com/pt/re/aids/fulltext.00002030-200317003-00001.htm;jsessionid=CFrZF5133L0OSdDRW6HNOwN MkqpJ5vu2Mb111QBZTFHNOIJ1ipmC!512964740!-949856031!9001!-1?&fullimage=true. Accessed July 1, 2005.

London School of Hygiene and Tropical Medicine. 1993. *AIDS newsletter.* Bureau of Hygiene & Tropical Diseases. Vol. 8 (7/8): May 31.

Nathan Associates Inc. 2002. *Economics of HIV/AIDS: Multisectoral impacts and programmatic implications.* USAID Bureau of Economic Growth, Agriculture and Trade (EGAT) briefing paper prepared under the Trade Capacity Building (TCB) Project., contract No. PCE-I-00-98-00016, Task Order 13. June 18, 2002.

OECD/DAC and UNAIDS. 2004. *Analysis of aid in support of HIV/AIDS control: 2000–2002.* http://www.oecd.org/dataoecd/57/60/32159448.pdf.

Putzel, J. 2003. *Institutionalising an emergency response: HIV/AIDS and governance in Uganda and Senegal.* A report submitted to the Department for International Development. May. http://www.crisisstates.com/download/HIV/Putzel.pdf. Accessed April 5, 2005.

Slutkin, G. 2000. Global AIDS 1981–1999: the response [The Pittsfield Lecture] *The International Journal of Tuberculosis and Lung Disease* 4 (2 s1): S24–S33.

SADC (Southern Africa Development Community). 2003. *Final communiqué 2003 SADC heads of states and government summit on HIV/AIDS.* Maseru, Lesotho.

UNAIDS. 2004a. *Report on the global AIDS epidemic.* Geneva. http://www.unaids.org/bangkok2004/GAR2004_pdf/UNAIDSGlobalReport2004_en.pdf. Accessed March 6, 2006.

————. 2004b. *A joint response to AIDS.* Geneva. http://www.sahims.net/doclibrary/2004/05_May/14/Regional/A%20joint%20response%20to%20AIDS.pdf. Accessed March 6, 2006.

————. 2004c. *UNAIDS at country level: Progress report.* UNAIDS Country and Regional Support Department, Geneva. http://www.youandaids.org/unfiles/countrylevelProgressReport.pdf. Accessed March 6, 2006.

————. 2004d. *National spending for HIV/AIDS 2004.* Geneva. http://data.unaids.org/Publications/IRC-pub06/JC1023-NationalSpending2004_en.pdf?preview=true. Accessed March 6, 2006.

———— 2004e. *Children on the brink 2004.* With UNICEF and USAID. Produced by the Population, Health and Nutrition Information Project of USAID, under contract no. HRN-C-00-00-0004-00. http://www.unicef.org/publications/files/cob_layout6-013.pdf. Accessed March 6, 2006.

———— 2004f. Financing the expanded response to AIDS. http://data.unaids.org/publications/IRC-pub06/JC1022-FinancingResponse2004_en.pdf. Accessed March 6, 2006.

————. 2005a. *Resource needs for an expanded response to AIDS in low and middle income countries.* Presented at the Programme Coordinating Board Seventeenth Meeting, Geneva, 27–29 June 2005. http://data.unaids.org/publications/irc-pub06/resourceneedsreport_en.pdf. Accessed March 6, 2006.

————. 2005b. An exceptional response to AIDS. Geneva. http://www.unaids.org/html/pub/publications/irc-pub05/jc1117-exceptionalresponse_en_pdf.pdf. Accessed March 6, 2006. http://www.unchina.org/unaids/exceptionalresponse_en_pdf.pdf.

United Nations. 1994. Resolution 1994/24 of the Economic and Social Council: Joint and co-sponsored United Nations programme on human immunodeficiency virus/acquired immunodeficiency syndrome (HIV/AIDS). July 26.

United States Department of State. 2004. The President's emergency plan for AIDS relief: U.S. five-year global HIVAIDS strategy. Office of the United States Global AIDS Coordinator. Washington, D.C. http://www.state.gov/documents/organization/29831.pdf. Accessed March 21, 2005.

————. 2005a. Engendering bold leadership: The President's emergency plan for AIDS relief first annual report to Congress. Washington, D.C.: Office of the United States Global AIDS Coordinator. http://www.state.gov/documents/organization/43885.pdf. Accessed April 5, 2005.

————. 2005b. *U.S. AIDS campaign reports success in first year.* The United States Diplomatic Mission to Nigeria. Press release, March 24.

USAID (United States Agency for International Development). 2003. Multisectoral responses to HIV/AIDS: A compendium of promising practices from Africa USAID-PVO steering committee on multisectoral approaches to HIV/AIDS. Produced by the Academy for Educational Development (AED) for the USAID-PVO Steering Committee on Multisectoral Approaches to HIV/AIDS. Washington, D.C.

———. 2004. *Guidance on the definition and use of the child survival and health programs fund and the global HIV/AIDS initiative account. FY 2004 Update.* http://www.usaid.gov/policy/ads/200/200mab.pdf.

World Bank. 2001. The US$500 million multi-country HIV/AIDS program (MAP) for Africa progress review mission, FY01. http://www.worldbank.org/afr/aids/map/prog_rpt_01.pdf. Accessed April 5, 2005.

———. 2002. Second multi-country HIV/AIDS program (MAP2) for Africa. AIDS Campaign Team for Africa, Africa Regional Office. Draft. http://www.worldbank.org/afr/aids/map/mapII_abstract.pdf on April 5, 2005.

———. 2004. Interim review of the multi-country HIV/AIDS program for Africa. October. http://www.worldbank.org/afr/aids/map/MAP_Interim_Review-04.pdf. Accessed April 5, 2005.

World Economic Forum. 2005. Business and HIV/AIDS: Commitment and action? A global review of the business response to HIV/AIDS 2004–2005. Global Health Initiative. In collaboration with UNAIDS and Harvard School of Public Health. http://www.unaids.org/html/pub/topics/partnership-menus/wef-ghi_businesshiv-aids_05_en_pdf.pdf.

World Health Organization. 1995. *Global Programme on AIDS, progress report 1992–1993,* p. viii. Geneva: WHO.

———. 2001. *HIV surveillance report for Africa 2000.* Regional Office for Africa, Harare, Zimbabwe. November. http://www.who.int/hiv/strategic/surveillance/en/hivsurvafr2000.pdf. Accessed June 29, 2005.

———. 2002. *Global health-sector strategy for HIV/AIDS 2003–2007: Providing a framework for partnership and action.* http://www.who.int/hiv/pub/advocacy/GHSS_E.pdf.

———. 2005. *"3 by 5" progress report.* Jointly published with UNAIDS. Geneva. http://www.unaids.org/html/pub/cosponsors/who/who_3by5-progressreport_dec04_en_pdf.pdf. Accessed June 22, 2005.

Chapter 13

The Rural HIV/AIDS Epidemic in Ethiopia and Its Implications for Market-Led Agricultural Development

Clare Bishop-Sambrook, Nigatu Alemayehu, Yirgalem Assegid, Gebremedhin Woldewahid, and Berhanu Gebremedhin

The seriousness of the HIV/AIDS epidemic in Ethiopia is widely acknowledged. Since the first HIV case was recorded in 1986, prevalence rates rose rapidly during the 1990s. By the end of 2003, it was estimated that 1.7 million people in the country (with a total population of over 70 million) had already died from AIDS and a further 1–2.3 million were living with the disease (UNAIDS, UNICEF, and WHO 2004). In addition, it is estimated that there are around 700,000 children under the age of 17 who have lost either one or both parents to AIDS. Ethiopia is classified (along with Nigeria, China, India, and Russia) as belonging to the "next wave countries" with large populations at risk from HIV infection, which will eclipse the current focal point of the epidemic in central and southern Africa (NIC 2002).

The disease is taking its toll on life expectancy and is undermining the country's efforts to reduce poverty. There have been substantial efforts recently by the government of Ethiopia to address the disease through a multisectoral approach, with increasing attention being paid to reaching the rural areas. However, addressing the epidemic is particularly challenging in such a poor country, where per capita expenditure on health is in the order of US$6, including out-of-pocket contributions (CCM 2004). It is estimated that over 50 percent of government hospital beds are occupied by AIDS patients (GoE 2004). The problem of caring for and supporting people living with AIDS and orphans has surpassed the capacity of traditional coping mechanisms. Since the turn of the new millennium, the government recognizes that "investing adequately in HIV/AIDS prevention is now a precondition for virtually all other development investments to succeed" (GoE 2001).

Little work has been done on the nature of the disease in rural areas, despite the fact that 85 percent of the population lives in rural areas. This essential gap in information has been noted by many (Ministry of Health 2002; Mitike et al. 2002; Garbus 2003; Bishop-Sambrook 2004a; Pankhurst 2004). The agricultural sector plays a central role in the Ethiopian economy and lies at the heart of government initiatives to accelerate nationwide economic growth. Even though rural prevalence rates are lower than urban rates (2.6 percent and 12.6 percent, respectively, Ministry of Health 2004), they are rising, and the potential scale of the rural epidemic requires an urgent response. At the household level, the impact of the disease diverts attention and resources from productive activities to caring for the sick and surviving the aftermath of the death of key household members. If left unchecked, the disease reduces the availability and quality of household labor, changes the composition of rural communities, and alters the priorities of farming households, thereby making many of the traditional production-oriented extension messages irrelevant. One significant aspect of the rural epidemic is the extent to which it may undermine efforts to improve agricultural productivity and achieve market-led development.

This chapter discusses the rural epidemic in the context of the Improving Productivity and Market Success (IPMS) of Ethiopian Farmers Project, a five-year CIDA-funded project focusing on technology transfer, improved extension, input supply, rural finance, farmer organizations, and marketing arrangements in support of a market-led integrated agricultural development strategy. The principal sources of risk of HIV infection for rural communities and impacts of the disease are identified in three project *woredas* (administrative districts), with particular attention paid to any increased risk of infection or vulnerability to impacts arising from agricultural marketing. The chapter concludes by considering measures to contain the spread of the disease in the context of the IPMS project.

Stages of the Epidemic

There are three principal stages of the epidemic that a community may pass through: AIDS-initiating, with very low HIV prevalence rates and no AIDS impacts; AIDS-impending, where HIV prevalence rates are rising but the majority of infected people are still in the asymptomatic phase before becoming ill; and AIDS-impacted, when households and communities feel the impact of AIDS as infected people succumb to AIDS-related illnesses and eventual death (Barnett and Topouzis 2003). One of the greatest challenges of working in many rural communities is that HIV/AIDS data are relatively scarce. Identification of the stage of the epidemic is more difficult when some of the classic indicators of heavily impacted communities are not relevant because of the characteristics of the local farming and livelihood systems. The picture may be further confused by the community's response to the epidemic if they do not know the symptoms of the disease or are in a state of denial about its presence.

This chapter sets out to examine three questions:

- What are the sources of risk of HIV infection for people in the project communities?

- To what extent are these communities and their livelihood systems already AIDS-impacted?

- What may a production- and market-oriented project, such as the IPMS, offer to address the epidemic?

The findings are based on qualitative studies undertaken in three to four communities in each of three *woredas* participating in the project: Atsbi-Wemberta in the highlands in northern Tigray; Fogera adjacent to Lake Tana in western Amhara; and Ada'a Liben in the cereal-livestock systems of Oromia in the central highlands to the east of Addis Ababa. Information was gathered from interviews with key informants, such as government and NGO staff, and from group discussions with farmers, traders, and the rural youth. Groups typically comprised 10–25 people, of whom between one-third and one-half were women. The fieldwork was conducted between late 2004 and early 2005, using a range of participatory methods, including mapping, timelines, matrices, and semistructured interviews (Bishop-Sambrook 2004b). The data focused on reviewing potential sources of risk of HIV infection and examining the extent to which the *woredas* are already impacted by AIDS or their vulnerability to possible future impacts. It should be noted that the findings presented below are based on the interpretation of qualitative data, and attempts have been made to strengthen their validity by conducting the survey in a total of 10 communities.

Sources of Risk of HIV Infection

In order to understand the nature of the rural epidemic, a careful analysis of who is most at risk of becoming infected and how they could become infected is required

(Pisani et al. 2003). The dominant mode of transmission is through heterosexual contact (estimated to account for 87 percent of infections) and mother-to-child transmission (MTCT) (10 percent of infections) (GoE 2004). Blood transfusion, harmful traditional practices, and unsafe injections are all recognized to be a small risk at present but require attention (GoE 1998).

Prevalence rates indicate there are significantly lower levels of HIV infection in rural communities than are found in urban areas. However, the disease may be concentrated in subpopulations within the rural community but not well established within the general population. In this case, the source of risk for the majority of rural residents is through bridging populations, people who are at higher risk and provide substantial links with other subpopulations who have lower-risk behavior. These linkages may provide a conduit for the virus to move into the general population (UNAIDS and WHO 2000). Thus, there are three steps in identifying the extent to which rural communities are at risk from HIV infection: the status of the epidemic in the urban hinterland, the presence of bridging populations, and norms and practices within a community that place people at risk. Risks specifically associated with agricultural marketing are considered separately.

Urban Hinterland and *Woreda* Hotspots

In order to examine the dynamics of HIV/AIDS in rural areas, it is essential to place rural communities in the context of their urban hinterland. The disease is well established in many of the principal regional towns throughout the country, where prevalence rates typically range from 10 percent to 20 percent (Ministry of Health 2004). The extent to which the farming community interacts with this high-risk environment (and engages in unprotected sex with infected people) will have a major bearing on the development of the rural epidemic. This would appear to be borne out by the evidence from the three project *woredas*. The high urban HIV prevalence rate in Amhara is mirrored in the high rural prevalence rate of over 5 percent; whereas the more moderate urban rates of 12.4 percent in Tigray and 10.3 percent in Oromia are reflected in lower rural rates of 2.8 percent and 1.8 percent, respectively (Ministry of Health 2004). HIV-risky environments are not only urban phenomena but also exist within *woredas,* such as administrative and trading centers, military camps, and major transport routes.

Bridging Populations

There are three types of bridging population, who may link low-prevalence rural areas with higher-prevalence communities. The first are adults and the youth who link their rural communities to higher-risk urban hinterlands for employment, education, or social reasons. Because these activities take place away from home and the confines of community norms, the lack of social cohesion and anonymity may be a contributory factor that encourages them to engage in activities outside their social norm. The group includes seasonal migrants who seek alternative employment during the quiet months in farming, for example, working as casual laborers in the construction industry in Bahir Dar, on major road construction in Amhara, in the industrial zone on the outskirts of Addis Ababa, or on large commercial sesame farms in western Tigray. In Atsbi some men have dual livelihoods, farming for part of the year and working in town as skilled carpenters or masons during the summer months. Long-term migrants include students attending further education, the youth in Atsbi migrating to Saudi Arabia (but this is less common today), and women working as housemaids. Weekly migrants include adolescents attending senior secondary schools usually located in the *woreda* town. Ad hoc movements include visits to relatives; school dropouts and military returnees moving between small towns and their rural community; administrators and government employees attending meetings or training outside the *woreda;* and farmers staying in town if there are bottlenecks in registration, screening, and disbursement of seeds and credit by the Bureau of Agriculture. People usually stay with relatives or friends, in rented accommodations, or in the home of the employer. Many men leave their wives in the villages and take on a new "wife" in their new residence. They may also stay in local drinking houses.

The second bridging population are those who may carry the virus from outside into rural communities. This includes professionals working in rural communities such as agricultural development agents, teachers, and health workers, who are often unaccompanied by their families; politicians visiting rural areas for sensitization and mobilization purposes for extended periods; the military posted to rural camps; commercial sex workers who follow the seasonal migration of people, seasonal income flows, and the military; long-distance truck drivers and their assistants on overnight stops; seasonal migrants assisting with crop harvests; long-distance salt traders stopping for one or two nights in Atsbi en route while selling salt in local markets; visiting relatives; and distributors of food relief.

The third group relates to those moving within and between neighboring rural communities. Such movement is associated with daily living (such as fetching wood, water, milling, public meetings, and community development works), attending to administrative matters (for example, rural administrators visiting the main *woreda* town or elders mediating in conflicts), and social affairs (visiting relatives, attending wedding and burial ceremonies, special church meetings or holidays). With the exception of social events and overnight stays in administrative centers, the risk of sex associated with daily aspects of rural living is considered to be very small.

Cultural Norms and Practices within Communities

Once the virus is present within a rural community, cultural and social practices may contribute to its spread between people. Such practices that potentially place people at risk for HIV infection differ widely between communities and between regions. Many are now reported to be on the decline, partly as a result of efforts spurred by the epidemic.

- *Marriage:* Various forms exist, such as early marriage (girls may be as young as 10 to 12 years old, particularly in Amhara), marriage by abduction, polygamy, and widow inheritance. Many of these arrangements disadvantage women and place them at risk of infection through their husbands. The Demographic and Health Survey (DHS) of 2000 found that although it was quite common for young rural men to have premarital sex, it was rare for young rural women to do so (13 percent compared to 1 percent) (CSO 2000).

- *Multiple sex partners:* The practice of multiple sexual partnerships varies between regions, sex, and marital status. Fieldwork discussions suggest that extramarital affairs have been relatively common in the project *woredas,* but many are now reported to be on the decline. However, it has been found that communities tend not to associate their customary sexual practices with the risk of HIV infection because they are conducted within community norms, including inherent elements of trust (Miz-Hasab Research Centre 2004).

- *Use of condoms:* The DHS found urban residents were much more likely to use a condom during potentially high-risk sex than rural residents. This would appear mainly to be related to a general reluctance to use them (because of a lack of familiarity or cultural taboos of adultery associated with their use) rather than their availability (they are sold in shops in rural market centers or available for free in administrative offices, health centers, and some restaurants and bars).

- *Alcohol consumption:* Drinking alcohol, especially in bars and drinking houses, is often closely related to casual sex. Men do not usually pay for sex in the village but rather pay in kind by establishing friendships with young women working in drinking houses (who are often recent divorcees from early marriages) and supporting their business. Excess alcohol consumption is often more acute among the landless and unemployed young people.

- *Wedding parties, religious occasions, and holidays:* These events are celebrated by young men and women dancing and singing during the night and possibly having a sexual relationship with a new partner. The holiday of Epiphany is traditionally taken as an opportunity to be introduced to someone and start a relationship.

- *Harmful traditional practices:* Several harmful traditional practices (HTPs) are very common in the project regions, including uvulectomy and milk tooth extraction (Jeppsson, Tesfu, and Persson 2003). Although on the decline, female genital cutting is still widespread, with 80 percent of women aged 15–49 years being circumcised (CSO and ORC Macro 2001). Almost all male Ethiopians are circumcised. Other practices are regionally specific, such as incision of the eyelid in Tigray, vein punctures in Tigray and Amhara, and tattooing of women in Tigray. Ethiopian health officials fear that the use of unsterilized instruments to perform these practices aggravate the HIV/AIDS epidemic (GoE 1998); however, the few data available have not found an association between HTP and HIV infection (Garbus 2003). There is increasing action to deter people from practicing HTPs, for example, through the work of the National Committee on Traditional Practices in Ethiopia, and there have been some successes.

- *Suckling young babies:* Sometimes women suckle another's young baby if the mother is out of the village for a day or more, possibly leading to the risk of HIV infection through breast milk.

- *Gender imbalances:* Women and girls are more vulnerable to HIV infection not only biologically but also socially because of discriminatory social and cultural practices (INRI 2004). They generally have low rates of literacy, leave school earlier than boys, and have little opportunity to participate in decisionmaking. They are also disadvantaged with regard to using and controlling economic resources in the household. As a result of their weak social position and the dominance of men, women are either unaware or unable to insist on condom use or to negotiate for safe sex. Gender inequalities also affects women's ability to use treatment and care services, to disclose their HIV status, to discuss issues of sexuality and safe reproductive behavior with their families, and to receive support for adherence of ARV therapy in the family and community (CCM 2004).

- *Awareness and understanding about HIV/AIDS:* The Behavioural Surveillance Survey of 2002 found farmers to be the least well informed about preventative methods, to have the highest levels of misconceptions about how it could be transmitted, and nearly all farmers had at least one stigmatizing attitude toward people living with HIV/AIDS (PLWHA) (Mitike et al. 2002). Rural women were found to be the least well informed about preventative methods, which places them at risk both during sex and as caregivers of PLWHA. There has been a change in the level of intensity of awareness-raising activities during the last five years in rural communities. Whenever people gather together, government officials, religious leaders, and village leaders spend some time talking about HIV/AIDS. Development agents, health workers, teachers, peer educators, and serial radio dramas are also important sources of information. Village HIV/AIDS clubs and students perform drama on market days and at school events. Some *woredas* have found that the first-hand experiences by local PLWHA are proving very effective in stimulating behavior change. In contrast, when messages about HIV/AIDS are closely intertwined with religious beliefs, it can sometimes result in confusion regarding appropriate preventative action and effective care.

• *Infrastructure:* Although the number of voluntary counseling and testing centers based in rural areas has increased significantly in the last year, services are still relatively limited. Even when they are available, the fear of stigma and the potential breach of confidentiality encourage some people to travel to major towns for HIV tests rather than use the local center.

Marketing-Related Risks

Certain aspects of agricultural marketing may play a major role in driving the rural epidemic. Marketing involves much movement of sellers and buyers both into and from rural areas, on journeys that may be completed within a day or over several days. Weekly rural markets in the *woreda* are a major social gathering, drawing people together, typically from a 10- to 15-kilometer radius. Market days are often a source of recreation, even if there is no business to conduct, and are acknowledged as an opportunity to meet secret lovers. Drinking on market days is a common and long-established practice and may lead to casual unprotected sex. Activities are heightened during the harvesting season, when money is available and commercial sex workers move into market centers. Indeed, in Ada'a it was reported that many male teenagers have their sexual debut during the months after selling the *teff* harvest, when money is readily available. Larger markets attract people from further afield and may result in overnight stays. Livestock traders from Ada'a are reported to have women in some towns they visit who are known *kimite* ("a woman waiting for a particular man") and share their household expenses. Occasionally, if buyers are busy, they pay farmers a nominal sum on delivery of their produce and settle the balance in the evening, requiring farmers to spend the whole day waiting around the market.

Engagement with the market, and hence market-related risk of infection, is strongly influenced by gender roles because women and men usually occupy distinct niches in the marketing chain. Women sell small volumes (of the main cash crops, vegetables from their home gardens, small livestock and their products, and honey) according to household needs, usually in the local market on a regular basis. Men tend to sell the majority of the cash crops, fattened cattle, and other livestock; when selling in bulk, they often travel further afield to major markets to get better prices. Women and girls are potentially at risk from unwanted sexual advances while they travel to and from markets, and many travel in groups to improve their security. They may also encounter pressure to have sex when they stay away from home while trading, and, culturally, they are in a weak position to refuse.

Summary of Risks by Person

From the above analysis of bridging populations and cultural norms, it is evident that the source of HIV infection differs between household members and is strongly influenced by age and sex. Those at highest risk are married men and the youth, at moderate risk married women and women heading households, and at relatively low risk, the elderly, children, and babies.

- *Babies and children* under the age of 5 are most at risk of infection from their mothers during pregnancy, birth, and breastfeeding (occasionally other women) and possible infection through contact with infected blood and other body fluids (through circumcision or HTPs such as tonsillectomy).

- *Children* from 5 to the age at which they become sexually active are at risk from infected blood and other body fluids (for example, through HTPs including milk tooth extraction).

- *Adolescents,* once sexually active, are at risk through unprotected sex (at dances, weddings, casual laboring, urban migration, and secondary school) and from infected blood and other body fluids (through HTPs). Young men are particularly at risk from visiting town for work, trade, recreation, and drink. Young women face additional risks through abduction, rape, early marriage, and female genital cutting.

- *Married men* are the highest-risk group: they have more opportunities for casual sexual relationships because of their greater mobility, propensity to migrate seasonally, and access to cash; and if they have extramarital affairs they are likely to have several different partners.

- *Married women* are generally a much lower-risk group than men in terms of their behavior, although they are at risk of infection through their husbands: they migrate less, tend not to travel unaccompanied, and tend not to stay away from home overnight; however, in some cultures it has been common for them to have extramarital affairs within the community; they may also be at risk through caring for PLWHA.

- *Female heads of household* are at moderate risk of infection: they may form relationships with men in order to gain assistance with farm work; and if they migrate to town, they may end up working in bars and having sex with customers.

- *Elderly men* are a low-risk group: they do not usually stay away from home overnight, but if they do have extramarital affairs when they go to town to market or attend court cases, they are most likely to have a stable relationship. In Fogera, there has been a tradition for elderly men to form relationships with widows, but this is on the decline.

- *Elderly women* are at minimal risk of HIV from sexual encounters, but as caregivers of people living with AIDS, they are at risk if they do not understand how the disease is transmitted.

Impacts of AIDS on Communities and Livelihood Systems

The section above clearly demonstrates that all rural communities are at risk from HIV infection because of both their close linkage with the external world and practices within the community. However, it is often difficult to identify the stage of the disease in the community, largely because of denial and stigma. Although levels of awareness about the disease are high, there is a reluctance to admit that people from their community are infected or dying from AIDS, although it may be something that is affecting neighboring *woredas*. In addition, as a result of high levels of stigmatization and misconceptions about the modes of transmission, PLWHA who are displaying symptoms of AIDS are often not seen in the community because of self-exclusion or marginalization by others.

Despite the propensity to deny the presence of HIV/AIDS, recent changes in behavior suggest that many people recognize the threat the disease poses. The most common change has been toward multiple sex partners by reducing the number of extramarital affairs, the use of prostitutes, and polygamous marriages. However, it was noted that this change is also taking place for economic reasons and not just as a result of HIV/AIDS awareness. People are also taking steps to reduce their risk of exposure by decreasing the remarriage of divorcees, widows, and spouses and avoiding unnecessary overnight stays away from home. The youth would appear to be among the more committed to change, expressing an interest in establishing one-to-one partnerships, taking premarriage HIV/AIDS tests, and having less extramarital sex. Nevertheless, the use of condoms continues to be extremely low despite their availability.

Another indication of the reality of the rural epidemic is reflected in the changing composition of communities. In all three *woredas,* it was noted that during the last 5 to 10 years there have been fewer polygamous marriages (now accounting for 5–15 percent of total households in the study communities), a growth in monogamous households (40–60 percent), and fewer remarriages among widows and widowers. Female-headed households (15–25 percent) have experienced the highest rate of growth, and households headed by single men, orphans, and grandparents have also increased (each typically accounts for 5–10 percent). Not all these changes can be attributed to the impact of AIDS because there are other reasons that account for the growth in single-adult-headed households, such as the migration of husbands in search of work, an increase in divorce, war (in Atsbi), and a land shortage (Fogera).

Changes in livelihood systems may also indicate the impacts of AIDS. Livelihoods appear to be reasonably buoyant in Ada'a, which may mask, possibly only temporarily, the impact of AIDS. Ada'a benefits from proximity to centers of economic activity, including the industrial zone of Addis Ababa, offering nonfarm employment opportunities and access to major agricultural markets. Poorer households with very small holdings or no land are increasing their nonfarm activities (brewing, distilling, pottery, weaving, silversmithing, and grain trading) or migrating to town. More children are attending school, and, as a result, parents are taking over their farming and household activities. However, it is likely that Ada'a is AIDS-impending because the community is potentially at high risk as a result of its location (with the major urban center of Debre Zeit and the Addis Ababa–Djibouti highway) coupled with a strong tradition of extramarital affairs and high alcohol consumption. An indication of possible times to come is reflected in one busy market center where it was noted that less time is now spent on funerals because of the high number of deaths.

During the last five years in Atsbi, the agricultural sector has been characterized by leading farmers increasing their land under small-scale irrigation, growing an increased range of crops (including vegetables, fruits, spices, and pulses) and adopting improved crop and livestock breeds (such as poultry and dairy cows). The area under fallow has been reduced because of population pressure, and there has been a shift from cattle to smaller livestock because of pressure on grazing land. The practices of reciprocal labor and sharecropping are decreasing because farmers find it more productive to work their own land. All households are increasing their nonfarm activities (such as trading, brewing, selling food, and construction works) except those headed by women and grandparents. The highest level of denial about AIDS was expressed by men and youth in Atsbi. The *woreda* is likely to be at the stage of AIDS-initiating or AIDS-impending.

In contrast, Fogera is already AIDS-impacted with the disease taking its toll on rural livelihoods. Poor and female-headed households are struggling to survive the loss of key adults and asset depletion (particularly the sale of livestock) during illness. They are resorting to sharecropping, hiring out their children for farm work, brewing local drinks, collecting and selling fuelwood, or migrating to town and receiving alms. In some communities, relatives, close friends, and neighbors assist with farming activities; they may also lend money or contribute to supplement food shortages. Some widows weed other people's land in exchange for assistance with plowing, but reciprocal labor groups are becoming less popular because of the labor shortage. Today, there are indications that only relatives and close friends attend funeral ceremonies.

Within communities the impact of AIDS differs between occupational and wealth groups. Those who depend on their physical well-being or appearances for their livelihood are particularly vulnerable. Farmers and transporters of produce lack the physical energy to do their work. Customers shy away from buying from retailers or sellers who look ill because of stigma and misunderstanding regarding the transmission of the disease. Once the signs of the disease become evident, infected individuals often withdraw from public space, including visits to the market. The disease makes many poor livelihoods untenable, whereas the opportunities for recovery are much stronger in resource-rich households with the options of remarrying, hiring home help, and hiring labor to work on the farm.

Opportunities for Addressing HIV/AIDS through Market-Led Growth Strategies

The recommendations below specifically focus on opportunities available to address HIV/AIDS through improving agricultural productivity and marketing. They are relevant to the IPMS project and may be implemented with the support of local resources such as the *woreda* HIV/AIDS prevention and control offices. The review in the preceding section highlights the need to tune interventions first to the needs of different communities, depending on the stage of the epidemic, and second to different groups within the community, depending on their specific sources of risk.

Raising Awareness and Understanding about HIV/AIDS

The focus varies between AIDS-initiating and AIDS-impending communities (modes of transmission, local sources of risk, and methods of prevention) and AIDS-impacted communities (safe care and nutrition needs of PLWHA).

- Train agricultural staff; members of farmer organizations, cooperatives, and marketing groups; and members of trade associations about HIV/AIDS and its implications for agriculture.

- Work with groups associated with agricultural production and marketing initiatives who are traditionally overlooked by HIV/AIDS awareness and outreach activities because they do not usually belong to formal associations, such as petty traders and retailers, ambulant traders, transporters, and owners of hotels and drinking houses.

- Use occasions when people are gathered together (for example, market days, seasonal migrants working on farms, or commercial sex workers moving into an area during harvesting season) to educate them about HIV/AIDS and its prevention.

- Hold intensive awareness campaigns during seasons of high risk, such as harvesting and holidays.

- Distribute HIV/AIDS leaflets to members of cooperatives and farmer groups.

Reducing Risk of Exposure to HIV Infection

This is relevant for all communities regardless of the stage of the epidemic; the main emphasis is to reduce the risk of activities leading to unprotected sex with infected people.

- Reduce the need to migrate through improving food and nutrition security by increasing output, improving the quality of produce, widening the range of products, and making more efficient use of inputs (including labor).

- Reduce the wish to migrate by increasing livelihood options in and around the community and extending the growing season through developing small-scale irrigation, product diversification, agroprocessing, strengthening existing and creating new market linkages, and developing the farm input supply chain.

- Reduce the need to travel to markets by bringing the marketing chain closer to the producer (market information readily available in rural community and new modes of market engagement such as forward contracts).

- Reduce the behaviors of high alcohol consumption and extramarital affairs by training farmers how to manage their market earnings through savings and investment, and broaden their horizons to improve the well-being of their whole family.

- Reduce women's weak bargaining position regarding unwanted sexual encounters by empowering them economically through income-generating activities and gender training. Make the marketing chain more women-friendly and secure.

- Encourage rural youth to participate fully in the opportunities of market-led agricultural development.

- Introduce methods of payment for products that reduce the time spent at market.

Reducing Vulnerability to AIDS Impacts

This is relevant for AIDS-impacted communities.

- Overcome barriers to participating in agricultural production and marketing by infected and affected households, such as their depleted resource base, the need to be close to home to tend to the sick, loss of key skills, and their inability to undertake risk.

- Develop market opportunities for crops and livestock that are suited to the resource base of infected and affected households.

- Provide assistance to infected and affected households to overcome constraints imposed by HIV/AIDS on their market-related activities (for example, transporting produce to market, processing, and forming retailing groups among petty retailers in the market).

- Promote crops and livestock that contribute to balanced diets for PLWHA and prolong their lives through the provision of antiretrovirals.

- Use cooperatives and farmer organizations as an entry point for mitigation, care, and support activities in communities, for example, by developing income-generating activities, savings, health insurance, or establishing a social fund to provide care for orphans.

Conclusion

Initiatives to strengthen the market orientation of agricultural production present both an opportunity and a threat to the rural HIV/AIDS epidemic. Although any contributions toward reducing poverty and the need to migrate may reduce susceptibility to HIV/AIDS, there are very real risks that the additional cash and the stimulus to travel further afield to market produce could result in increasing the risk of exposure to HIV. Hence, activities associated with promoting the marketing of agricultural products need to be designed with care to ensure they play a role in arresting, rather than hastening, the spread of the disease in rural communities.

References

Barnett, T., and D. Topouzis. 2003. *FAO and HIV/AIDS, towards a food and livelihoods security based strategic response.* Rome: FAO.

Bishop-Sambrook, C. 2004a. *The challenge of the HIV/AIDS epidemic in rural Ethiopia: Averting the crisis in low AIDS-impacted communities, findings from fieldwork in Kersa woreda, Eastern Hararghe Zone, Oromiya Region.* Rome: FAO.

———. 2004b. *Addressing HIV/AIDS through agriculture and natural resource sectors: a guide for extension workers.* Rome: FAO Socio-economic and Gender Analysis Programme (SEAGA).

CCM. 2004. *Application for global fund, fourth call for proposals.* Addis Ababa: Country Coordinating Mechanism.

CSO. 2000. *Ethiopia demographic and health survey.* Addis Ababa: Central Statistical Office.

CSO and ORC Macro. 2001. *Ethiopia and demographic health survey 2000.* Addis Ababa: Central Statistical Office and U.S.A.: ORC.

Garbus, L. 2003. *HIV/AIDS in Ethiopia.* Country AIDS Policy Analysis Project. San Francisco: AIDS Policy Research Center, University of California.

GoE (Government of Ethiopia). 1998. *Policy on HIV/AIDS.* Addis Ababa: GoE.

———. 2001. *National strategic framework 2001–2005.* Addis Ababa: GoE.

————. 2004. *A comprehensive strategic plan to combat HIV/AIDS epidemic in Ethiopia (2004–2007),* Final Report. Addis Ababa: GoE.

INRI. 2004. Ethiopia: Efforts underway to achieve gender parity, in *INRInews,* UN Office for the Coordination of Humanitarian Affairs.

Jeppsson, A., M. Tesfu, and L. A. Persson. 2003. Health care providers' perceptions on harmful traditional health practices in Ethiopia. *Ethiopian Journal of Health Development* 17 (1): 35–44.

Ministry of Health. 2002. *AIDS in Ethiopia,* 4th ed. Addis Ababa: Disease Prevention and Control Department, MOH.

————. 2004. *AIDS in Ethiopia,* 5th ed. Addis Ababa: Disease Prevention and Control Department, MOH.

Mitike, G., W. Lemma, F. Berhane, R. Ayele, T. Assefa, T. Michael, F. Enqusellase, A. Alem, Y. Abebe, and D. Kebede. 2002. *HIV/AIDS behavioural surveillance survey,* Ethiopia Round One. Ethiopia: Department of Community Health, Addis Ababa University, and Ethiopian Public Health Administration.

Miz-Hasab Research Centre. 2004. *HIV/AIDS and gender in Ethiopia: The case of 10* wereda *in Oromia and SNNPR.* Addis Ababa: Miz-Hasab Research Centre.

NIC (National Intelligence Council). 2002. *The next wave of HIV/AIDS: Nigeria, Ethiopia, Russia, India and China.* Washington, D.C.: NIC.

Pankhurst, A. 2004. *Conceptions of and responses to HIV/AIDS: Views from twenty Ethiopian rural villages,* Paper presented at Second International Conference on the Ethiopian Economy organised by Ethiopian Economic Association at United Nations Conference Centre, June 3–5, 2004, Addis Ababa.

Pisani, E., G. P. Garnett, N. C. Grassly, T. Brown, C. Hankins, N. Walker, and P. D. Ghys. 2003. Back to basics in HIV prevention: Focus on exposure. *British Medical Journal* 326: 1384–1387.

UNAIDS, UNICEF, and WHO. 2004. *Ethiopia, epidemiological fact sheets on HIV/AIDS and sexually transmitted infections.* Geneva: WHO.

UNAIDS and WHO. 2000. *Guidelines for second generation HIV surveillance, second generation surveillance for HIV: The next decade.* Geneva: UNAIDS.

Chapter 14

AIDS and Watersheds:
Understanding and Assessing
Biostructural Interventions

Michael E. Loevinsohn

Introduction

Over the past 15 years, evidence has accumulated of how HIV/AIDS impacts rural people who depend for their food and livelihood on agriculture and the management of natural resources. Evidence is also available, though less extensive, of how changes in the rural environment influence the dynamics of HIV/AIDS. It is striking, however, how little this understanding has yet to contribute to the methods used in the struggle with HIV/AIDS. The "expanded response" that UNAIDS is spearheading to meet the targets set by the UN General Assembly Session on HIV/AIDS in 2001 includes no reference to agricultural or natural resource–based measures for prevention, treatment, and care (Stover et al. 2002). This is hardly surprising because there is as yet little documented evidence of their effectiveness in HIV/AIDS control terms or feasibility on a wide scale. Much less is it clear how such efforts might be financed. Across the sectoral divide, agricultural and natural resource management policies and programs are aimed at enhancing food security, improving nutrition, and expanding livelihood opportunities. However, the decisionmakers responsible for the most part have a very limited understanding of how these may be affecting HIV/AIDS risks, positively or negatively, and how these inadvertent effects can be optimized. Few have a clear understanding of how HIV/AIDS is affecting or will in the future affect attainment of the objectives they now pursue and what adjustments will be necessary to keep these in sight.

The base of evidence and experience is gradually deepening as some of the presentations at this conference demonstrate; however, the profile of this body of work remains very low. A new term, biostructural intervention, may help to clarify the nature and potential of what is at stake. In public health, a structural intervention is one that addresses the determinants of health problems situated in the social, political, or economic environments. With respect to HIV/AIDS, structural interventions have most frequently been considered in relation to factors that impede or facilitate an individual's efforts to avoid HIV infection (Parker, Easton, and Klein 2000; Sumartojo et al. 2000) but can also address treatment and care of PLWHA and mitigation of AIDS' impacts. A biostructural intervention (BSI) can be defined as a structural intervention that draws on efforts to enhance the benefits people derive from living natural resources such as through agriculture, fishing, or forestry / and that seeks to ensure that a part of these benefits supports public health objectives, in the present context those of HIV/AIDS control.

The contribution that BSIs can make is growing as HIV epidemics are becoming increasingly rural in character in Sub-Saharan Africa and other regions (NAC 2003; PFI/PRB 2003). They offer a number of potential advantages in comparison to individually focused medical and public health interventions or structural interventions that do not draw on renewable natural resources but can also complement them. They also present certain difficulties and challenges. The balance needs to be assessed in each situation, drawing on the best information available, making decisions, and refining them in the light of improved understanding: applying what Loevinsohn and Gillespie (2003) term an "HIV/AIDS lens."

An example can help clarify the kinds of advantages and drawbacks a BSI may offer. In Lesotho, CARE and the Ministry of Agriculture are in the early stages of a program to support households and schools in taking up intensive homestead gardening and water harvesting (Abbot et al. 2005). Focusing on households affected by AIDS and providing home-based care to people living with HIV/AIDS, the initiative promotes local foods that enhance nutrition and bolster immune function. If these households indeed manage to take up and adapt the approaches to their particular conditions, sustainable improvements in nutrition and increased longevity for those living with HIV/AIDS are possible, at a cost probably lower than achievable through nutrition supplements. The fit to local and individual conditions can be hastened to the extent that households draw on their agricultural knowledge, experiment, and exchange their experiences, features less readily available to other interventions. Local institutions, formal and informal, can support such experimentation and exchange and also mobilize collective action to enable the weakest to benefit. Importantly, a successful homestead garden increases the resources available to affected households which they can use for other purposes—related or not to HIV/AIDS. Again, such flexibility is generally not a feature of other interventions.

On the other hand, a program such as home garden promotion can take longer to roll out and to get food into people's mouths than one based on supplements. People under considerable stress and with little time are less likely to be able to experiment (Loevinsohn, Meijerink, and Salasya 2001). Local institutions may themselves be under great strain in high-prevalence situations such as Lesotho, and their ability to support the weakest may be undermined. Power relations and divisions within communities can further marginalize the weakest, as can the stigma attaching to AIDS, though this may be less an issue where prevalence is high and no family is untouched.

A supplement program in support of home-based care can be implemented by a health ministry, possibly in collaboration with health-oriented NGOs. A program that includes home gardens needs the support of the ministry of agriculture and of NGOs with agricultural skills, inevitably increasing the difficulties of coordination. The agricultural organizations will also need to acquire new skills and perspectives. They will need to work with some of the poorest of households, often headed by women, to foster their participation and facilitate experimentation. These skills prove to be among the most difficult for large organizations to acquire and to practice effectively, particularly as pilot programs are taken to scale. The erosion of experience within organizations as a result of AIDS makes the challenge all the greater.

Finally, the agricultural organizations need to ensure that they maintain a reasonable balance within and among their various objectives. HIV/AIDS is not the only impoverishing force affecting rural areas, and a proper concern with equity requires that people also be addressed who are poor as a result of causes other than HIV/AIDS and who may be differently situated. This will be particularly important where the prevalence of HIV and AIDS is still low but increasing. It will also be important for the organizations to ascertain to what extent responding to the needs of people at risk of HIV and AIDS entails compromise with objectives such as supporting agricultural productivity and environmental integrity. These issues are likely to play out differently in different contexts.

This chapter examines these issues in greater depth in relation to one potential BSI, watershed development (WSD) in India. WSD is an evolving approach that seeks to conserve and harmonize the use of soil, water, pasture, and forest resources while increasing agricultural productivity within an area, typically of a few hundred to several thousand hectares, that is drained by a common outlet. Over the past several decades, increasing attention has been paid to ensuring local participation and to concerns such as employment creation and equity for women, the landless, and other vulnerable groups. More than US$500 million is invested annually in WSD programs across the country by the central and state governments and donors (Singh 1994; Turton 2000; Kerr 2002).

The assessment focuses on two main questions:

- What is the contribution, potential and actual, of WSD and related efforts to HIV/AIDS control?

- How might taking on HIV/AIDS control support or undermine achievement of the objectives that WSD programs are currently pursuing?

The analysis is intended to be strategic and to provoke reflection by the stakeholders of both WSD and similar programs and of HIV/AIDS control. It makes use of an epidemiologic model and recent data on the epidemiologic context of HIV in South India and on the social impact of WSD to create and compare realistic scenarios, buttressed by qualitative analysis. Scenario modeling adds to the HIV/AIDS lens concept a new degree of both rigor and flexibility. WSD is highlighted because it is an approach widely practiced in South Asia and other regions and because there is a substantial literature available on its social impacts. However, the same analysis could, in principle, be carried out on other approaches that have sought to buttress food and livelihood security, indeed whether or not explicitly linked with improved natural resource management. The primary focus is on the contribution of food and livelihood security to HIV prevention, a dimension that has been relatively neglected by research (Loevinsohn and Gillespie 2003) and one that is of critical importance in India where prevalence nationally is still low, less than 1 percent, but increasing and now reaching significant levels in some areas, especially in the four large southern states of Maharashtra, Andhra Pradesh, Karnataka, and Tamil Nadu (UNAIDS 2004). However, it is no less relevant to Africa, where prevalence is higher and many of the same situations of risk can be identified.

Watershed Development and Its Social Impacts

A variety of WSD programs have been designed over the past several decades by states and the central government, some with the assistance of foreign donors. The approaches have differed, depending on conditions in the regions targeted and the orientation of the leading organizations. All have been concerned with improving water availability to people, crops, and livestock and with conserving soils. The preoccupation in the early years with production and productivity and the emphasis on implementation of physical structures have, with time, been balanced by social objectives: relieving distress in areas of chronic water scarcity and soil degradation and achieving greater equity among farmers cultivating different parts of the watershed, the landless, and those dependent on pasture and forest resources, often women and *adivasis* (Hanumantha Rao 2000; Shah 2001a,b; Kerr 2002).

The visual impact of WSD is often striking. Within a few seasons, once dry, bare hillsides are covered in grass, shrubs, and young trees; wells that ran dry not long after the rains now provide drinking water all or most of the year, and fields whose crops withered when the rains faltered now yield one and often two harvests a year under irrigation. Among the first steps in WSD typically is to restrict access to pastures and forests in the upper parts of the watershed to permit the vegetation to recover and water to infiltrate and recharge wells and reservoirs. Those who benefit first and in greatest measure are generally farmers with fields in the lower reaches. People who depend on the fodder and forest products from the upper parts— women, the landless, and *adivasis*—will be hurt by the restrictions. These groups typically are also not well represented in village councils. Some of the pioneering WSD projects such as Sukhomajri and the *Pani Panchayats* and efforts elsewhere, particularly NGO-led, have sought innovative ways to avoid this structural inequality. These have included granting water rights to the landless, which they can trade to farmers or use on rented land, and expanding employment opportunities based on natural resources. Fostering the emergence of institutions that can give voice to the interests of these groups has also been key. These ideas have spread and influenced practice widely, but equity and broad-based participation remain major challenges in WSD programs (Fernandez 1994; Shah 2001a,b; Kerr 2002; Fernandez 2003).

For some rural households, particularly those relatively well placed in terms of land and connections in urban areas, seasonal migration can be part of a deliberate strategy to diversify livelihoods. However, for many of the rural poor, seasonal migration is a key dimension of distress. Reliable estimates of its prevalence are available for only a few rural areas; for example, 65 percent of households in 42 villages in Madhya Pradesh, Gujarat, and Rajasthan (Mosse et al. 2002) and 35 percent of households in one village in West Bengal (Rafique and Rogaly 2003) had at least one member involved in migration. Similar or higher levels have been reported elsewhere (Srivastava, Sasikumar, and Giri 2003; Washington et al. 2004a). Men, married or single, typically form the bulk of migrants, though in some cases women in significant numbers and even whole families are involved. Distress migration often has significant social and environmental costs in the source areas, for example, reducing the labor available for land improvement and increasing the burden on family members who remain behind. In the destination areas, migrants often face low wages and poor housing and sanitation. Women are exposed to sexual abuse

(Shah 2001b; Mosse et al. 2002; Srivavstava, Sasikumar, and Giri 2003). Migrants are typically found to have higher rates of HIV (Decosas et al. 1995) or to engage more frequently in risky sexual behavior than nonmigrants, as recent work in Rajasthan has shown (Washington et al. 2004a).

The extent to which seasonal migration, or at least its most pernicious and dangerous forms, has been curtailed is one of the social criteria that is often used to assess WSD's impact. In some of the early projects such as Sukhomajri, complete elimination is claimed, at least in years of reasonable rainfall.[1] One of the few wide-scale assessments is from Andhra Pradesh, where, in some 2,000 watersheds in a year of below-average rainfall (1988–89), migration was found to have been reduced by 10 to 40 percent (Hanumantha Rao 2000). Several observers are skeptical about the extent to which these benefits are shared by the landless and marginal farmers. Significant increases in employment, beyond the initial construction phase, have, in general, proven more difficult to achieve than has improved water availability and extended irrigation in the lower reaches of watersheds (Shah 2001a,b; Joy and Paranjape 2004). In his survey of watersheds in Andhra Pradesh and Maharashtra, Kerr (2002) found that as many as one-third of the landless claimed that they had been harmed by WSD in some of the large government programs. Whether this additional distress translates into a net increase in migration from the watershed is not clear. Projects implemented by NGOs or by NGOs and government jointly were more likely to have been judged beneficial by the landless.

The Epidemiologic Context

With more than 1 percent of their adult populations estimated to be infected with HIV, the four southern states of Maharashtra, Andhra Pradesh, Karnataka, and Tamil Nadu are deemed to harbor generalized HIV epidemics. A striking feature of these epidemics is that prevalence in rural areas, as measured at antenatal surveillance sites, is similar to or higher than that in urban areas (PFI/PRB 2003; Washington et al. 2004b).[2] In Africa, infection rates are typically substantially higher in urban areas (UNAIDS 2004). Among attendees at STD clinics in Karnataka, HIV prevalence in those working in the agricultural sector was more than 70 percent above the median (18.6 percent vs. 10.8 percent) and greater than that in people working in the transport sector (15.9 percent), a high-risk group in many parts of the world. Migrant workers were found to be particularly affected (Washington et al. 2004b).

Some of the highest HIV rates are found in Karnataka's northern districts. In one of these, Bagalkot, the India-Canada Collaborative HIV/AIDS Project (ICCHAP) has carried out population-level surveys and more focused studies of sex workers and their clients, providing one of the few detailed pictures of HIV/ AIDS epidemics outside India's large urban centers. Across the district, prevalence is estimated at 2.9 percent; in the rural areas it is half again as high as in the urban areas (3.6 percent vs. 2.4 percent). Among agricultural workers, HIV infection (6.2 percent) was more than twice the district mean. Prevalence among adult men was a third higher than that among women (3.3 percent vs. 2.5 percent). However, among those 15–19 years of age, prevalence was more than five times greater among women than men (3.2 percent vs. 0.6 percent), likely reflecting marked inequalities of power and a substantial level of cross-generational sexual relations. Knowledge of HIV/AIDS, its causes, and prevention measures is generally poor, especially in rural areas. Only 6 percent of rural women claim to have ever seen a condom (KSAPS et al. 2004; Blanchard, Reza-Paul, and Ramesh 2004).

Poverty, indebtedness, abandonment, and widowhood were the most common reasons women cited for entering commercial sex work. Many women in northern Karnataka enter through the *devadasi* or temple dancer tradition. They are typically younger and have more clients than other sex workers, are more likely to be illiterate, rural-based, and less able to influence the conditions under which sex is exchanged. Sex work is conducted in a variety of locations in urban and rural areas: at home, in lodges or brothels, at roadsides, or in other public places. In the urban areas of Bagalkot district, female sex workers were estimated to represent 1.1 percent of the 89,000 women aged 15–49, and their clients 20.4 percent of the 93,000 men (Foss et al. 2004; KSAPS et al. 2004; Blanchard et al. 2005).

The scenario modeling that follows considers the links between food and livelihood insecurity and two situations of risk: seasonal migration and commercial sex work. Others, which may be of epidemiologic significance but for which there is limited research to draw on in this context and are not modeled, include transactional sex of an occasional, possibly seasonal nature, early marriage, and the sexual vulnerability of women left behind when men migrate. I return to these issues in the Discussion.

Methods

In the context of HIV/AIDS, epidemiologic models have frequently been used to assess an intervention's contribution to prevention in a specific locale, both among the individuals targeted and among those to whom they would have otherwise transmitted the infection (i.e., secondary prevention) (Grassly et al. 2001). Such models have also been used to estimate the effectiveness of a suite of individual prevention measures in halting the spread of HIV/AIDS at national, regional, and global levels (Stover et al. 2002). The AIDS Strategic Intervention Simulation Tool

(ASIST), a mathematical model and user interface (Ferguson et al. 2002), has been used in both applications. Here ASIST is used in a strategic sense to assess the contribution of a structural intervention, WSD, in different scenarios based on the context of northern Karnataka.

The model underlying ASIST is formulated as a set of ordinary differential equations. These describe a population of adults divided according to HIV status: either susceptible or in any of five stages of infection, from incubation to full-blown AIDS. The population is further stratified by sex, sexual activity class, and whether individuals are covered by control interventions. Heterosexual partnerships and mother-to-child transmission are the only infection routes considered by ASIST. The sexual activity classes, defined for the population being modeled, are characterized by the rate of partner change and the number of sex acts per partnership per year. Sexual mixing is represented by means of an "assortativity" factor, where 1 implies that people choose their partners at random among the activity classes and 0 that they choose them only from within the same activity class. When a partnership occurs across activity classes, the number of sex acts is determined by the highest-activity individual. Adolescents are recruited to the population as susceptible adults, and individuals die at a rate determined by life expectancy and HIV/AIDS status.

A viral and a bacterial sexually transmitted infection are modeled in parallel with HIV, and prior infection with either increases the likelihood of HIV transmission. Five control interventions can be modeled by ASIST. Skills-based education reduces the rate of partner change and thus infection risk for both HIV and the other STIs. Correct use of condoms likewise increases protection against all three infections, and treatment of the bacterial STI reduces HIV risk at the same time. On the other hand, antiretroviral therapy is specific to HIV, slowing progression from one infection stage to another and reducing viral shedding. ASIST can also be used to explore the impact of a hypothetical microbicide whose efficacy and rate of uptake can be varied. Ferguson et al. (2002) provide a more detailed description of the model.

The baseline scenario draws on the epidemiologic and demographic characteristics of Bagalkot district. It envisages the adult population of such a district divided into three interacting sexual activity classes: a high-activity class, which includes both rural and urban sex workers and their clients; and an urban and a rural class, both with lower levels of sexual activity. Sex workers are assumed to have 460 different partners per year, the mean in northern Karnataka (KSAPS et al. 2004), and their clients nine new partners per year, near the lower end of the range calculated by Foss, Vickerman, and Watts (2004). The rural men who join this activity class are migrants (though not all migrants are necessarily in this class). Men in the rural class are assumed to have one-third as many new partners as migrants, as Washington et al. (2004a) found in rural Rajasthan, that is, three new partners per year. Men in the low-activity urban class are assumed to have two new partners per year, in line with the lower prevalence in urban areas. Women in both urban and rural low-activity classes are assumed to have a new partner only once in 20 years, based on data from Bhattacharjee et al. (2004) that suggest that most of the relationships women in Bagalkot have outside of marriage occur before marriage. Sex workers and their clients are assumed to have two sex acts per partnership in a year, and men and women in the low-activity rural and urban classes 52 acts per year, in line with survey results in Bagalkot (Foss, Vickerman, and Watts 2004).

The urban population is assumed to consist of 186,000 adults 15–49 years of age, of whom 20,045 (19,000 men, 1,045 women) are in the high sexual activity class (Foss et al. 2004).[3] The rural adult population is assumed to be 455,400, based on the 29 percent/71 percent urban/rural distribution of Bagalkot's population (Census of India 2001). In the baseline scenario, 25 percent of the rural population are assumed to migrate, a relatively modest rate in comparison to the situations referred to in the previous section, and join the high-sexual-activity class. Women are assumed to be 5 percent of these high-activity migrants, as in the urban areas.

ASIST is designed to assess specific individually oriented interventions and imposes several limitations when adapted to assess structural ones such as WSD. Scenarios in which, for example, migration levels are altered can be simulated only as different runs of the model, assuming that the intervention had been in place at the beginning of the epidemic. In contrast, condom distribution and the other predefined interventions can be introduced at any point. ASIST also offers only limited capacity to model different patterns of interaction among the sexual activity classes by means of the assortativity factor described earlier. The baseline scenario uses 0.8 for this factor, reflecting a situation in which migrants return relatively frequently, such as seasonally, to their rural homes (Washington et al. 2004a), and urban high-activity men and women often maintain concurrent relationships with their spouses or partners.

Other model parameters are given in Table 14.1.

Results

Figure 14.1 illustrates the effect on HIV prevalence in the urban and rural population of WSD in place from the beginning of the epidemic, which consistently reduces migration by 40 percent, the top end of the range among Andhra Pradesh watersheds cited by Hanumantha Rao (2000). WSD targeted at the areas managed by 200,000 adults (44 percent of the rural population) reduces the peak prevalence

Table 14.1 Simulation parameters other than those described in the text

Demography:		Viral STDs:	
Fertility rate (per woman, per year)	0.1332	Transmission rate M→F/ F→M	0.07 / 0.01
Natural death rate (in the absence of AIDS)	0.0154 (equivalent to life expectancy 65 years)	Enhancement of viral STD transmission caused by HIV infection, by HIV stage I–IV	1 / 1 / 4 / 12
Child aging rate (1/age at sexual debut)	0.0666		
Simulation settings:		HIV:	
Steps per sample	1	Transmission rate M→F/ F→M	0.0005 / 0.00025
Tolerance	10^{-6}	Relative infectiousness by stage	3 / 1 / 2 / 4
Epidemiology:		Progression rates of each incubation stage	4 / 0.114 / 1 / 2
Year HIV epidemic started	1985 (First Indian AIDS case reported 1986)	Vertical transmission, by incubation stage	0.25 / 0.25 / 0.25 / 0.25
Bacterial STDs:		Cofactor enhancement of HIV infectiousness: Symptomatic bacterial STD/asymptomatic bacterial STD/viral STD	2 / 2 / 2
Transmission rate M→F/F→M	0.5 / 0.25		
Recovery rate (per year) symptomatic/ asymptomatic	12 / 12		
Proportion males symptomatic/ asymptomatic	0.9 / 0.1	Cofactor enhancement of HIV susceptibility: Symptomatic bacterial STD/asymptomatic bacterial STD/viral STD	4 / 4 / 3
Proportion females symptomatic/ asymptomatic	0.4 / 0.6		

Note: These are the ASIST default values unless otherwise noted (Ferguson et al. 2002).

by 6.3 percent; targeted at the areas managed by 400,000 adults (88 percent of the rural population), it reduces peak prevalence by 14 percent. However, prevention of infection is a better measure of impact, and these efforts are more effective in these terms, particularly in the early stages of the epidemic: over the first 15 years (1985–2000), the 200,000-person effort averts 12.8 percent of infections, the 400,000-person effort 27.3 percent.

A modest economy of scale is evident: the 200,000-person effort averts 6 percent more infections over the first 15 years than would be expected from a linear extrapolation of an effort targeting 10,000 people. The scale effect for the 400,000-person effort is 12.7 percent.

This scenario envisages a fairly free mixing of the urban and rural population, particularly of high-sexual-activity individuals, as might occur in an area with good roads and transport. A contrasting scenario is of a relatively isolated rural popula-

Figure 14.1 Effect of watershed development on the prevalence of HIV at two levels of effort in targeting the rural population

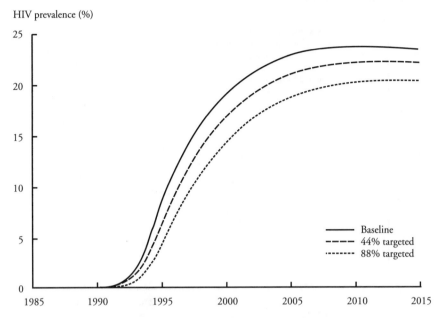

Note: The population consists of 455,000 rural and 186,000 urban adults linked by high-sexual-activity migrants. WSD is assumed to reduce migration by 40 percent.

tion that has its "own" group of high-activity men and women, as might occur around a rural industry or plantation. The number of infections averted by a given level of WSD effort is quite similar in this "isolated" and the "integrated" baseline scenario. However, in the integrated case, urban people share in the benefits: with 400,000 rural adults targeted by WSD, 14.4 percent of the infections prevented in the first 15 years are in the low-sexual-activity urban class. I return to this issue below.

The baseline scenario assumes that high-sexual-activity women constitute 5 percent of rural migrants and that WSD reduces migration to the same extent for both men and women. Figure 14.2 illustrates the sensitivity of results to changes in these assumptions, when the initial level of migration (25 percent of the rural population) and WSD's impact on migration overall (40 percent reduction) are held constant.

Over the first 15 years of the epidemic, WSD targeted to 88 percent of the population averts 31.4 percent fewer infections than in the baseline scenario when

Figure 14.2 Infections averted by watershed development

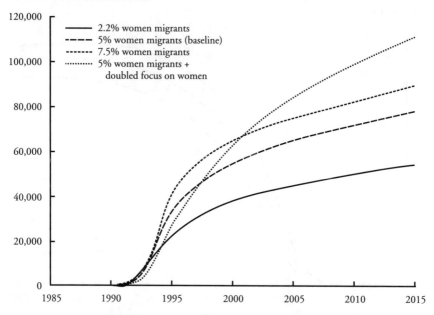

Cumulative HIV infections averted

Note: Infections averted by watershed development, assuming different proportions of high-sexual-activity women among migrants and different proportions of the benefits of the program accruing to women. WSD is targeted at 400,000 adults (88 percent of the rural population) and reduces migration by 40 percent.

women constitute 2.2 percent of migrants and 17.6 percent more than the baseline when they constitute 7.5 percent of migrants. This highlights the importance of understanding women's involvement in distress migration in particular situations. The difference between the 2.2 percent and 7.5 percent cases involves 2,100 women, just 0.7 percent of the adult female population, but the difference in infections averted over 15 years is 27,400.

The effect of targeting the benefits of WSD more to women, doubling the proportion of women among those who are able to remain in the low-risk rural class, is ambiguous. Fewer infections are averted in the earlier years, but many more after about 12 years. This appears to be because men, who are the majority of migrants in these scenarios, play a key role as "bridges" between the high-activity class where HIV prevalence is greatest and the initially low-prevalence rural areas.

The impacts of WSD on HIV prevention considered so far have been inadvertent and unintended side effects. How might WSD complement formal HIV/AIDS control programs? Here I consider some epidemiologic aspects, returning in the next section to institutional ones.

Under the conditions of the baseline scenario, a condom promotion program that is in place at the beginning of the epidemic and that results in sex workers using condoms with 50 percent of their clients, similar to levels found in Karnataka (KSAPS et al. 2004), is able to maintain prevalence at relatively low levels, at least for the first 20 or so years (Fig. 14.3). A delay of five years in implementing the program, however, allows HIV to reach higher prevalence sooner. The consequences of the delayed public health response are mitigated to an extent if the rural area has benefited from WSD.

This can be seen more clearly from the infections averted (Fig. 14.4). Over the first 20 years of the epidemic, the five-year delay in implementing condom promotion results in more than 100,300 extra infections. The cost of delay is almost

Figure 14.3 Effect on HIV prevalence of watershed development and condom promotion, delayed or not by five years after the beginning of the epidemic

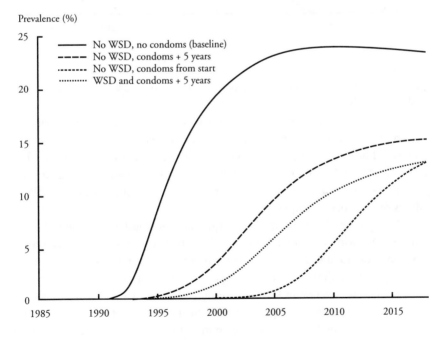

Figure 14.4 Infections averted by watershed development and condom promotion, delayed or not by five years after the beginning of the epidemic

Cumulative infections averted

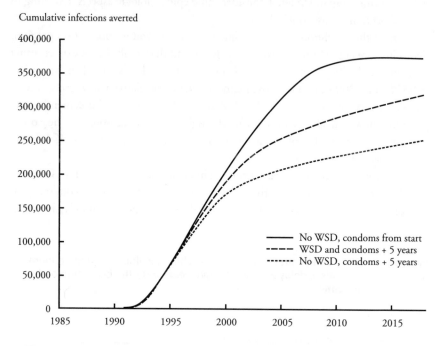

halved (54,600 extra infections) if the delay occurs in an area where WSD has been in place from the start.

There is a synergistic interaction between WSD and condom promotion: the proportion of infections averted when both are implemented together is greater than would be expected from their individual effects. In the above case, the effect amounts to 23,300 infections over 20 years. This appears to result from their complementary modes of action: condoms reduce the risk from unsafe sex; WSD reduces the number of people at risk.

Although the objective was not to reproduce the Bagalkot situation, the scenario of WSD with condom promotion delayed by five years provides a reasonable approximation to the district's current pattern of infection: overall prevalence below 5 percent in 2003 and around 50 percent among sex workers.

The cost effectiveness of WSD in averting infection, with or without condom promotion, is illustrated in Figure 14.5. As in the above scenario, condom promotion is delayed by five years after the start of the epidemic. The analysis draws on cost estimates from Maharashtra (John Kerr pers. comm.) of Rs.2,686/person where NGOs implement WSD and Rs.3,753/person where NGOs and government agencies jointly implement the program (US$62/person and US$87/person, respectively, in 1999). The costs illustrated for situations where WSD and condom distribution are both present are for the portion of infections averted by WSD.

In the absence of condom promotion, WSD implemented by NGOs or by NGOs and government jointly would avert infections at a cost of $1,000 per infection after 13 and 23 years, respectively. In the presence of condom promotion, it would take 21 and 36 years for the NGO or NGO and government programs to reach the $1,000 per infection level. For comparison, condom distribution among high-risk women in Kenya averted HIV infections at a cost of $1,060 per infection (Creese et al. 2002). And Stover et al. (2002) estimate the cost-effectiveness of the expanded global prevention program, which draws only on individually focused interventions, at $1,000 per infection averted, and likely more, in the 2001–10 period.

Figure 14.5 Cost-effectiveness of watershed development in the presence or absence of condom promotion delayed by five years after the start of the epidemic

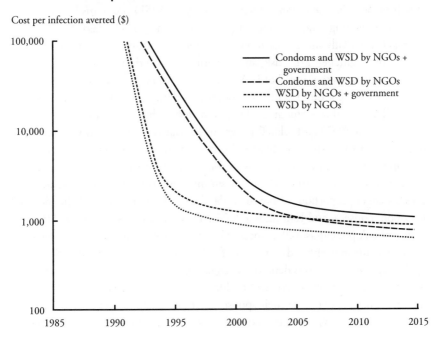

Discussion

These results suggest that some watershed development programs may currently be making a significant but entirely inadvertent contribution to the prevention of HIV/AIDS, in some situations at a cost comparable to single-purpose preventive measures. They may also be helping to mitigate the effects of delay in implementing those measures. The scenarios explored in this chapter are based on what is, in the Indian context, a high-prevalence area and assumes a level of effectiveness in reducing migration at the top end of what is likely achieved in most large-scale WSD programs. It assumes as well that this impact is sustained for a considerable period. There is little evidence available concerning the longevity of WSD efforts, save for pioneering "success stories" such as Sukhomajri and the *Pani Panchayats* in Maharashtra, which continue to operate successfully after more than 25 years (Kerr 2002). The scenario developed here therefore approaches a "best case."

As pointed out earlier, WSD has often failed to achieve broad-based participation in decisionmaking and equitable sharing of the fruits of environmental improvement. Water harvesting and soil conservation have benefited the landed and especially those with fields in the lower reaches of the watershed. Sustained increases in employment after the construction phase and improvements in the resources, often from common land, on which women, landless, *adivasis,* and other groups depend have been meager or nil in many areas. More of the landless say they have been harmed than helped in some large WSD programs by the restrictions on harvesting fodder and forest products (Shah 2001a,b; Kerr 2002). Where distress has actually increased among those most at risk of being pushed into situations of heightened HIV risk, and disparities of wealth have grown, WSD may be contributing to the spread of HIV. This is the "worst case" scenario.

Work on the ground is urgently needed to clarify these predictions. It should be possible to add assessment of changes in risky behavior to current or planned evaluations of WSD and related programs at relatively little cost. Greater clarity is needed on the impact of distress. Discussion in India usually revolves around migration and its hazards, whereas in southern and eastern Africa the emphasis is on transactional or "survival" sex, often involving more limited movement and possibly larger proportions of the rural population (Loevinsohn and Gillespie 2003; Bryceson, Fonseca, and Kadzandira 2004). To what extent is that more diffuse situation of risk present as well in specific Indian situations, and how is it affected by improvements in livelihood as a result of WSD and other efforts? Similarly, distress is often an important consideration when families contract early marriages for their daughters. Young women married to older men are at heightened risk of contracting HIV and STIs because their spouses are more likely to be infected than men their own age. Socially isolated and with limited autonomy and access to information, they have little ability to negotiate when and under what conditions sex occurs (Bruce and Clark 2004). Is there evidence that this situation of risk too has been reduced where livelihoods have become more secure? Clearer understanding of the HIV risks faced by different kinds of migrants, for example, those who move either more or less voluntarily, is also needed. Finally, more flexible model frameworks are required that can be used to assess the consequences of various patterns of migration and of interaction between and within rural and urban populations.

Beyond the unintended effects considered so far and the epidemiologic synergies suggested in the last section, how can WSD support HIV/AIDS control efforts in a more active sense? I believe the most important opportunities lie in the institutions that WSD has fostered at different levels. There is growing recognition of the importance of participatory groups, based on an affinity of interests, at the smallest scale that give voice to the concerns of those often not heard—women, landless, *adivasis*—in associations or councils at the watershed and wider scales (Fernandez 2003). These affinity-based groups can also provide health workers a means to reach people whose knowledge of HIV/AIDS and how to avoid it is often slight, though they may be among the most at risk. These groups provide their members a valuable forum for discussion.

The prospect of another form of synergy, between AIDS education and natural resource management, opens when people better understand the risks they face and when they see that there are means close to hand, such as WSD, that can help them avoid them. In much of eastern and southern Africa the opposite has been the case: many people with good knowledge of the health hazard are, for economic and other reasons, unable to act on it (Ngwira, Bota, and Loevinsohn 2002; Campbell 2003). Knowledge of the risks and of the means to avoid them is crucial but not sufficient when, as in a watershed, access to resources depends on the decisions of others.

How does responding to HIV/AIDS support or undermine achievement of the objectives that WSD programs are currently pursuing? Increasingly, equity is seen as *the* critical issue by government agencies as well as NGOs (Hanumantha Rao 2000; Kerr 2002). Failure to ensure equitable sharing of benefits threatens the participation that underpins the local adaptation of WSD, its productivity and sustainability (Fernandez 2003). There would seem therefore to be a shared interest in equity. Yet equity remains the hardest of objectives to achieve, particularly in large-scale programs. HIV/AIDS may help shift the balance. The scenarios explored in this chapter suggest that failure to achieve equitable sharing of benefits now has further consequences, infection risks, that are shared by all within the watershed and beyond, in the larger epidemiologic basin defined by people's movement and relationships. The challenge for those working with decisionmakers within and beyond the watershed will be to make these links clear and present in situations where many still do not have personal experience of AIDS. Handled clumsily, the attempt could backfire, particularly where AIDS-stigma is widespread and may attach to groups already marginalized.

In India, something of a tradition has evolved of learning from the experience of small-scale, pioneering efforts and intensive NGO-led projects in areas such as WSD and Joint Forest Management. The process has certainly not always been smooth or as rapid as some may have wished, but—through mechanisms including advocacy by the NGOs and their civil society partners; policy reviews; training of government and NGO cadres, sometimes together; and seconding of experienced NGO staff to government departments and programs jointly implemented by government and NGOs—there has been a general ratcheting up of practice and the emergence of more supportive policy. This experience and these mechanisms may well prove critical to the development of WSD and related programs as bio-structural interventions that consciously seek the synergies between human health and sustained, equitable management of natural resources.

Acknowledgments

I am grateful to Willo Pequegnat at the National Institute of Mental Health, Bethesda, Maryland, for making the ASIST model available, to Charlotte Watts, Anna Foss, and Peter Vickerman at the London School of Hygiene and Tropical Medicine for unpublished epidemiologic data from Karnataka, to John Kerr at Michigan State University for data on the cost of implementing WSD, and to him and Wenny Ho, Amsterdam Institute for Social Research, for helpful discussion.

Notes

This chapter was originally presented at the International Conference on HIV/AIDS and Food and Nutrition Security, Durban, South Africa, April 14–16, 2005.

   1. Some NGOs, such as Social Centre in Maharashtra, aim not at stopping migration but at reducing its pernicious aspects and enabling the poor to benefit from its income-diversifying potential.

   2. Across all four of the southern states, HIV infection at STD clinics was 7–27 percent greater among rural than urban attendees (PFI/PRB 2003).

   3. The small adjustments from the breakdown cited earlier are necessitated by ASIST, which assumes a 50/50 sex ratio.

References

Abbot, J., P. J. Lerotholi, M. Mahao, and M. Lenka. 2005. *From condoms to cabbages: Rethinking agricultural interventions to mitigate the impacts of HIV/AIDS in Lesotho.* Paper presented at the

Conference on HIV/AIDS, Food and Nutrition Security, April 14–16, 2005, Durban, South Africa.

Bhattacharjee, P., U. Rani, S. Moses, and J. Blanchard. 2004. *A population-based approach to HIV prevention in vulnerable rural communities of Karnataka, India.* Paper presented at the XVth International AIDS Conference, Bangkok, August 2004, Abstract number: ThPeE8208. http://www.ias.se/ejias/.

Blanchard, J., S. Reza-Paul, and B. M. Ramesh. 2004. *Should geographical intervention replace targeted intervention: A community prevalence study from Bagalkot district of Karnataka, India.* Paper presented at the XVth International AIDS Conference, Bangkok, August 2004, Abstract C12180. http://www.ias.se/ejias/.

Blanchard, J. F., J. O'Neil, B. M. Ramesh, P. Bhattacharjee, T. Orchard, and S. Moses. 2005. Understanding the social and cultural contexts of female sex workers in Karnataka. India: Implications for prevention of HIV infection. *Journal of Infectious Diseases* 191 (Suppl. 1): S139–S146.

Bruce, J., and S. Clark. 2004. *The implications of early marriage for HIV/AIDS policy.* New York: Population Council.

Bryceson, D. F., J. Fonseca, and J. Kadzandira. 2004. *Social pathways from the HIV/AIDS deadlock of disease, denial and desperation in rural Malawi.* CARE International in Malawi.

Campbell, C. 2003. Letting them die: Why HIV/AIDS prevention programmes fail. London: James Currey.

Creese, A., K. Floyd, A. Alban, and L. Guinness. 2002. Cost-effectiveness of HIV/AIDS interventions in Africa: A systematic review of the evidence. *Lancet* 359: 1635–1642.

Decosas, J., F. Kane, J. Anarfi, K. Sodii, and H. U. Wagner. 1995. Migration and AIDS. *Lancet* 346: 826–828.

Ferguson, N., G. P. Garnett, S. Riley, M. Fishbein, W. Pequegnat, and E. Sover. 2002. *NIMH/ASIST: AIDS strategic intervention simulation tool.* Bethesda, Md.: National Institute of Mental Health. www.nimh.nih.gov.

Fernandez, A. 1994. *The interventions of a voluntary agency in the emergence and growth of people's institutions for the sustained and equitable management of micro-watersheds.* Bangalore, India: MYRADA.

———. 2003. *People's institutions managing natural resources in the context of a watershed strategy.* Bangalore, India: MYRADA.

Foss, A., P. Vickerman, B. M. Ramesh, S. Moses, J. Blanchard, and C. Watts. 2004. *The potential impact of microbicides in Bagalkot District, Karnataka, India: Model projections and implications for product promotion.* London: International Family Health. www.ifh.org.uk.

Foss, A., P. Vickerman, and C. Watts. 2004. *The potential impact of microbicides in Bagalkot District, Karnataka, India: Model inputs, calculations and assumptions.* Technical document for Family Health International [unpublished paper available from the authors].

Grassly, N. C., G. P. Garnett, B. Schwartlander, S. Gregson, and R. M. Anderson. 2001. The effectiveness of HIV prevention and the epidemiological context. *Bulletin of WHO* 79 (12): 1121–1132.

Hanumantha Rao, C. H. 2000. Watershed development in India: Recent experience and emerging issues. *Economic and Political Weekly* 35 (45): 3943–3947.

Joy, K. J., and S. Paranjape, with A. K. Kirankumar, R. Lele, and R. Adagale. 2004. *Watershed development review: Issues and prospects.* Bangalore: Centre for Interdisciplinary Studies in Environment and Development.

KSAPS (Karnataka State AIDS Protection Society), ICCHAP (India-Canada Collaborative HIV/AIDS Project), Population Foundation of India, and Population Reference Bureau. 2004. *HIV/AIDS in Karnataka: Situation and response.* Bangalore, India: KSAPS.

Kerr, J. 2002. *Watershed development projects in India: An evaluation.* Research Report 127. Washington, D.C.: International Food Policy Research Institute.

Loevinsohn, M. E., and S. Gillespie. 2003. *HIV/AIDS, food security and rural livelihoods: Understanding and responding.* RENEWAL Working Paper no. 2/IFPRI Discussion Paper no. 157. http://www.ifpri.org/divs/fcnd/dp/papers/fcndp157.pdf.

Loevinsohn, M. E., G. Meijerink, and B. Salasya. 2001. Developing integrated pest management with Kenyan farmers: Evaluation of a pilot project. In: *Assessing the impact of participatory research and gender analysis,* eds. N. Lilja, J. A. Ashby, and L. J. Sperling. Cali: CIAT, pp. 231–247. http://www.prgaprogram.org/modules/DownloadsPlus/uploads/PRGA_Publications/quito.pdf.

Mosse, D., S. Gupta, M. Mehta, V. Shah, J. Rees, and the KRIBP Project Team. 2002. Brokered livelihoods: Debt, labour, migration and development in tribal western India. *Journal of Development Studies* 38 (5): 59–88.

NAC (National AIDS Commission). 2003. HIV sentinel surveillance report 2003. Lilongwe, Malawi: NAC and Ministry of Health and Population.

Ngwira, N., S. Bota, and M. E. Loevinsohn. 2002. *HIV/AIDS, agriculture and food security in Malawi: Background to action.* RENEWAL Working Paper 1. Washington, D.C.: IFPRI. http://www.ifpri.org/renewal/plans.htm.

Parker, R. G., D. Easton, and C. H. Klein. 2000. Structural barriers and facilitators in HIV prevention: A review of international research. *AIDS* 14 (suppl 1): s22–s32.

PFI (Population Foundation of India) and PRB (Population Reference Bureau). 2003. HIV/AIDS in India: The hard-hit states. Fact sheets for Tamil Nadu, Karnataka, Andhra Pradesh, and Maharashtra. Delhi. www.prb.org.

Rafique, A., and B. Rogaly. 2003. *Internal seasonal migration, livelihoods and vulnerability in India: A case study.* Paper presented at the Regional Conference on Pro-Poor Policy Choices in Asia, Dhaka, Bangladesh, June 22–24, 2003. www.livelihoods.org.

Shah, A. 2001a. *Who benefits from participatory watershed development? Lessons from Gujarat, India.* Gatekeeper Series no. 97, London: International Institute for Environment and Development.

———. 2001b. Water scarcity induced migration: How far can watershed projects help? *Economic and Political Weekly* 36 (35): 3405–3410.

Singh, K. 1994. *Managing common pool resources: principles and case studies.* Delhi: Oxford University Press.

Srivastava, R., S. K. Sasikumar, and V. V. Giri. 2003. *An overview of migration in India, its impact and key issues.* Paper presented at the Regional Conference on Migration, Development and Pro-Poor Policy Choices in Asia, June 22–24, 2003, Dhaka, Bangladesh. www.livelihoods.org.

Stover, J., N. Walker, G. P. Garnett, J. A. Salomon, K. A. Stanecki, P. D. Ghys, N. C. Grassly, R. M. Anderson, and B. Schwartlander. 2002. Can we reverse the HIV/AIDS pandemic with an expanded response? *Lancet* 360: 73–77.

Sumartojo, E., L. Doll, D. Holtgrave, H. Gayle, and M. Merson. 2000. Enriching the mix: Incorporating structural factors into HIV prevention. *AIDS* 14 (Suppl. 1): s1–s2.

Turton, C. 2000. *Enhancing livelihoods through participatory watershed development in India.* Working Paper 131, London: Overseas Development Institute.

UNAIDS. 2004. *Report on the global AIDS epidemic 2004.* Geneva: Joint United Nations Programme on HIV/AIDS. www.unaids.org/bangkok2004/report.html.

Washington, R. G., D. Singh, A. Adrien, J. F. Blanchard, S. Moses, and R. Rajdoctor. 2004a. *An evidence-based approach to understanding and addressing rural-to-urban migration in India.* Paper presented at the XVth International AIDS Conference, Bangkok, August 2004, Abstract TuPeD5238. http://www.ias.se/ejias/.

Washington, R. G., J. F. Blanchard, S. Moses, V. Gurnani, D. Bidari, S. M. Jangay, and B. M. Ramesh. 2004b. *The rapidly emerging epidemic of HIV in Karnataka.* Paper presented at the XVth International AIDS Conference, Bangkok, August 2004, Abstract C11783. http://www.ias.se/ejias/.

Chapter 15

Mainstreaming HIV and AIDS into Livelihoods and Food Security Programs: The Experience of CARE Malawi

Scott Drimie and Dan Mullins

Introduction

It is now well recognized that household food insecurity in Southern Africa can be properly understood and addressed only if HIV/AIDS is factored into the analysis. Analysis of linkages between food security and HIV/AIDS show that the relationships work in both directions and are systemic, affecting all aspects of livelihoods (Haddad and Gillespie 2001). Effective analysis and action to influence the causes and outcomes of HIV/AIDS requires a contextual understanding of livelihoods (SADC FANR Vulnerability Assessment Committee 2003).

This raises significant challenges for organizations designing or modifying food security and livelihoods interventions in a context of HIV and AIDS. HIV/AIDS mainstreaming into livelihoods can support prevention of new infections as well as improve resilience to the impacts of AIDS. Recognizing this reality and the importance of HIV/AIDS mainstreaming, organizations such as CARE Malawi have been researching the situation for several years and developing programs that seek to address the epidemic through new ways of doing core business.

The key question posed by this chapter is how a mainstreamed food security or livelihoods program is different from other nonmainstreamed programs. This chapter reviews the experience and lessons learned in CARE Malawi, which have evolved over the past five years. Some of the lessons involve framing expectations, having clear foundations, using appropriate approaches and tools, and working and learning in partnership with others.

The Intertwined Relationship between Livelihoods (and Food Security) and HIV/AIDS

CARE's overall approach is based on livelihoods analysis; food security is addressed as a subset of livelihoods. Livelihoods security can be defined as adequate and sustainable access to income and resources to meet basic needs and realize basic rights. It includes adequate access to food, potable water, health facilities, educational opportunities, housing, and time for community participation and social integration. Secure livelihoods are based on ownership of or access to resources that are used in productive activities to offset risks, ease shocks, and meet contingencies (Chambers and Conway 1991).

More narrowly, people enjoy food security when they have access to sufficient, nutritious food for an active and healthy life. Achieving this involves availability (ensuring that a wide variety of food is available in local markets and fields), access (people are able to produce or purchase sufficient quantities of foods that are nutritionally adequate and culturally acceptable at all times), and utilization (food is stored, prepared, distributed, and eaten in ways that are nutritionally adequate for all members of the household, including men and women, girls and boys.)

At a household level, there is a two-way relationship between livelihoods and HIV/AIDS. Insecure livelihoods exacerbate the risk and vulnerability environment for HIV/AIDS. At the same time, illness and death associated with AIDS undermine livelihoods options (Box 15.1).

Vulnerable people are forced to make decisions, often involving trade-offs among basic needs. For example, a family with insecure livelihoods but with a fair amount of food on hand may have to sell stocks of food in order to raise cash for school fees or medical care, even though they know they will have to buy back food later at a higher cost. In this environment, insecure livelihoods exacerbate the risks and vulnerabilities of HIV and AIDS. Lack of options can push some people into activities or situations that put them and others at high risk of HIV, such as sex work. Lack of food, money, and health care are key factors in rapid progression from HIV infection to onset of AIDS. People with insufficient resources find it harder to properly take medications, including antiretrovirals. Finally, those with weak livelihoods are more vulnerable to social and economic impacts of illness and death in their families and communities.

Baylies notes that HIV/AIDS can, on one hand, be treated in its own right as a shock to household food security, but on the other, it has such distinct effects that it is a shock like none other (Baylies 2001). Among others, AIDS tends to strike people in their most productive years, leading to loss of assets and reduced options for livelihoods activities in the household.

Box 15.1 The Intertwined Relationship between Food (In)security and HIV/AIDS

Insecure livelihoods exacerbate the risk and vulnerability environment for HIV/AIDS through:

- increased risk of HIV infections

- faster progression from HIV infection to onset of AIDS

- difficult environments for proper treatment of HIV

- increased socioeconomic impacts of AIDS

Illness and death associated with AIDS in turn undermine livelihoods options by:

- weakening or destroying human capacity (human skills, knowledge, experience, and labor)

- depleting control and access to other key assets: financial, social, natural, and physical

- constraining options for productive activities, reducing participation in community activities, and increasing time needed for reproductive and caring activities

---

An understanding of the negative two-way relationship between livelihoods and HIV/AIDS opens up opportunities. Policymakers, government officials, and development practitioners can pursue livelihoods objectives in ways that also address major aspects of HIV and AIDS.

There are various definitions of AIDS mainstreaming. Rather than debate these, this chapter addresses some of the main concepts needed to make livelihoods and food security programs relevant to the realities of HIV and AIDS. The challenge for analysts, policymakers, donors, and implementers is to understand how the rural socioeconomy is being affected; how development interventions have intended and unintended impacts on the course of the epidemic; how those at risk and affected are being supported, undermined, or ignored; and, consequently, how development policy and programming should be modified to better achieve their objectives. Because of the long-wave nature of the AIDS epidemic, the full impact of the disease will not manifest until the next several decades (Barnett and Whiteside 2002). For this reason, efforts to address the social and economic causes and consequences of HIV and AIDS must be flexible and based on an approach of continued learning and improvement.

The Experience of CARE Malawi

CARE Malawi runs a broad portfolio with strong emphasis on improving livelihoods security, with programs in such areas as agricultural development, microsavings, and social protection. These are complemented by work on the health and education sectors as well as on decentralization. Over the past 5 years, the team has gone through a process to help the staff, local partners, and communities to better understand the relationships between HIV/AIDS and agriculture and livelihoods and to develop systematic approaches to mainstreaming HIV/AIDS in all its work.

There has never been interest in shifting CARE's focus from agriculture or livelihoods to HIV programs such as condom distribution or health care. However, the focus and understanding of "mainstreaming" developed over time. From the start, CARE tried to identify its comparative advantage and where it could add the greatest value. There are many other organizations, mostly local, that are better placed and better equipped to carry out the "traditional" responses to HIV/AIDS: home-based care, condom distribution, behavior change communications, and so on. In the first initiatives, the emphasis was primarily on learning how HIV/AIDS undermines the ability of affected households to engage in and benefit from agriculture. This has widened beyond looking at the impacts of AIDS to include a stronger focus on how various responses can reduce risk of transmission, prolong healthy living, and mitigate impacts. This involves a range of nonagricultural issues, such as food distributions, safety nets, and infrastructure programs. CARE Malawi now pays close attention to both the risk and vulnerabilities associated with illness and mortality and seeks to support the resilience of those at risk of being affected.

The process has involved a large number of diverse efforts over several years: field research (Shah et al. 2002; Frankenberger et al. 2003; Bryceson, Fonseca, and Kadzandira 2004; Pinder 2004), participation by staff and managers in several workshops and conferences, significant investment in CARE's internal HIV/AIDS workplace policy for its own staff (which guides education and access to services and improves staff skills and confidence to work effectively in an HIV/AIDS context), membership in food distribution consortia with other agencies, creation of a "mainstreaming working group" comprising a mix of senior managers, program and support staff, midterm modifications of existing programs, development of livelihoods programs that explicitly recognize HIV/AIDS as major features of the risk and vulnerability environment, development of training and resource materials on HIV/AIDS and livelihoods, for use with community-based organizations, and a review of lessons learned in the process of mainstreaming HIV/AIDS into livelihoods work.

This effort is still ongoing, with continually evolving ideas and initiatives. It is clear that there is no simple leap from "nonmainstreamed" to "mainstreamed" work. However, the review of CARE Malawi's process recently helped staff to reflect on their progress and to identify some key lessons, which are outlined below (Drimie and Mullins 2005).

CARE Malawi has defined mainstreaming HIV/AIDS as carrying out the organization's core business in ways that better address the causes and consequences of HIV/AIDS as well as addressing the epidemic through all elements of the organization, including within the workplace and throughout all programming. The latter involves strategic planning, all stages of the program cycle from situation analysis and project design to implementation, monitoring, and evaluation (Care Malawi HIV/AIDS Thematic Team 2004). It involves development of partnerships, program work in communities, and policy analysis and advocacy. CARE Malawi emphasizes that "if a development programme does not recognize the fact [that HIV/AIDS affects all aspects of society], then it will be 'mopping with the tap running' or treating the symptoms of a problem without addressing the cause" (Care Malawi HIV/AIDS Thematic Team 2004).

Using HIV/AIDS Objectives to Guide Mainstreaming in Food Security Work

If HIV mainstreaming is to succeed, those involved in food security programs, including staff, community members, and other organizational partners, must understand basic facts about the disease. For people without public health backgrounds, the HIV/AIDS epidemic can seem a vast, faceless problem about which they simply do not know what to do. One of the simplest and most practical approaches used by CARE entails learning about four main objectives of work on HIV and AIDS: prevention, positive living, treatment support, and mitigation of social and economic impacts. The staff, partners, and community members then review each of these in turn to consider how their work in food security and economic livelihoods could potentially help achieve each of these objectives:

- *Prevention:* increasing options for safe secure sources of food and nutrition security and reducing risk of new infections

- *Positive Living:* enabling longer, healthier life for those with HIV through improved access to nutritious food and to reliable income

- *Treatment Support:* facilitating access and adherence to proper treatment through improved access to nutritious food and to reliable income

- *Impact Mitigation:* improving resilience of community and family members to social and economic impacts of illness and death through improved access to nutritious food and to reliable income

In August 2004, CARE Malawi program staff reviewed their work and identified examples of how programs have been modified to make them more relevant to the causes and consequences of HIV and AIDS. Some of these involve partnerships with both local and international agencies.

CARE staff reviewed their main programs and noted how each might contribute to one or more objectives related to HIV and AIDS:

- Reducing risk of HIV infection
  - Supporting and mitigating the impact of HIV/AIDS for livelihoods enhancement (SMIHLE): Skills training for adolescent girls to increase options for safe, secure incomes
  - Consortium for southern African food security emergency (C-SAFE): food aid targeting at-risk women and girls, to help avoid survival sex
  - Partnership in capacity-building in education (PACE): advocacy for zero tolerance of abuse of female students

- Improving positive living with HIV
  - Central regional livelihood security project (CRLSP): village savings and loans that include affected and nonaffected households, to increase access to financial assets
  - CRLSP: supporting production and preparation of nutritious field crops and vegetables

- Improving access and adherence to treatment
  - C-SAFE: food aid targeting at-risk women and girls, to help avoid survival sex

- C-SAFE: targeted food aid to encourage people to complete full course of TB treatment
  - National AIDS Commission umbrella program for small grants (NAC-UP): using HBC to link families to agricultural and health care interventions

- Mitigating social and economic impacts
  - C-SAFE: food aid targeting at-risk women and girls
  - NAC small grants: writing wills and disseminating information on inheritance law, to strengthen access and control over resources for widows and orphans
  - Hope for African children initiative (HACI): providing skills training for youths such as carpentry, bricklaying

These examples represent new ways of intentionally using livelihoods work to address risk, morbidity, and mortality. The review by CARE brings together several interventions that are under way in different geographic areas; a similar process could be used to identify how various government and nongovernmental initiatives are jointly addressing HIV and AIDS in a single community or district.

CARE Malawi: Lessons Learned about Mainstreaming HIV/AIDS

How is a "mainstreamed" program any different from a program that does not mainstream? This simple question is crucial if we are to go beyond simply using the jargon at conferences and workshops and in program documents and publicity pieces.

However, there is no one simple answer: there seem to be some general approaches, but as with any program, the details depend on the sector and the situation. Indeed, some of the points below have been identified and discussed by a number of organizations: CARE's experience further confirms some and helps build the basis of practical experience. Many of these lessons simply underscore good principles of development programming, which are made even more crucial in areas that have heavy burdens of HIV and AIDS:

- Framing expectations

- Clear foundations: in the workplace and in the program

- Helpful approaches and tools

- Working and learning with others

The following sections discuss each of these in turn.

Framing Expectations: Mainstreaming Is a Process of Learning, Synthesizing, and Acting; Not a Single Event

Those embarking on "mainstreaming" need to be clear from the start: this is a long-term process, not a single event that can be planned, conducted, completed, and left behind. The Malawi experience provides one example of a process that is long term, involving education, skills development, and new ways of thinking and working, so that staff and partners automatically seek to understand and address risks and vulnerabilities associated with HIV and AIDS. The process in CARE Malawi has involved a number of diverse events and initiatives, and ongoing efforts to ensure that all involved actually learn from these opportunities.

However, having a number of initiatives is only part of the process: if the lessons learned are not properly synthesized and used to modify existing work and guide new work, the collection of initiatives no more ensures "mainstreaming" than a collection of raw foodstuffs ensures good, nutritious meals or than one good meal ensures food security. Those embarking on a journey of mainstreaming should be prepared to invest some time, energy, and thought in the process.

Clear Foundations: In the Workplace and in the Program

CARE's experience strongly supports that of several others: organizations need to address HIV/AIDS in the workplace as well as in programs. Both are necessary, neither one is sufficient on its own, and in fact, they can and should be mutually supporting.

From Personal to Professional: The Workplace as Foundation for Program Work

At the start of its mainstreaming efforts, CARE Malawi found that staff did engage in initial efforts to learn about HIV and AIDS in communities, but their actual knowledge of HIV and AIDS, and at times some of the attitudes demonstrated, were not always conducive. Further, given the high adult prevalence in Malawi, it was clear that CARE's staff were themselves at risk, that some of the 130 staff probably were already living with HIV (even if they did not know it themselves), that others were ill, and that many were dealing with HIV and AIDS personally in their families and communities outside of work.

Besides impacts on staff themselves, illness and death in the workforce undermine the organization. Common impacts of HIV and AIDS include greater absenteeism, reduced productivity, increased financial costs, higher staff turnover, lower morale, and falling levels of experience and quality (Mullins 2002).

One cannot expect managers, staff, or partners in communities or other agencies to critically analyze and address issues that they do not understand or issues with which they are personally uncomfortable. Staff who are informed and comfortable, who know how to address HIV and AIDS in their own lives, will be much better placed to address these issues in their work. Such a process of internal reflection on HIV/AIDS deepens understanding and knowledge as well as the implications of HIV/AIDS for individuals and members of society.

However, this does not mean that an organization must have complete "success" in HIV workplace interventions before starting to mainstream HIV/AIDS into its core programs. HIV workplace issues and HIV mainstreaming in programs (sometimes referred to as internal and external mainstreaming) can be mutually reinforcing. The overall emphasis is to help staff gain confidence and ability in all aspects, from the personal to the professional.

CARE set up a team to review risk and impacts of illness and death, both as they affect staff and their families and as they affect the overall organization. The team, comprised of a mixture of managers, program staff, and support staff at various levels, went on to draft a policy. This laid out the approach, including such interventions as staff education, reviewing other staff health policies, negotiating with an external specialist to provide subsidized medical care, reforming the performance management system, assessing budgets and financial planning, and undertaking human resources workforce planning.[1]

This process seems to have helped: staff now routinely talk about HIV and AIDS, the overall level of correct knowledge has improved (from guards and drivers to support staff to program managers). CARE's staff as a whole seem more personally and professionally able to engage with the issues than was the case five years ago.

Build on Comparative Advantage: Focus on the Core Business

The organization should start by focusing on its core business. It may later turn to other fields but should in no case overlook the possible comparative advantages and opportunities of its existing experience. In the case of CARE Malawi, the focus has been largely on livelihoods work. The new element of mainstreaming HIV and AIDS means that these livelihoods objectives should be achieved in ways that also help achieve key objectives of work on HIV and AIDS: prevention, positive living, treatment support, and impact mitigation.

This is very different from the approach of continuing to run livelihoods programs in much the way they were done before HIV came on the scene and merely adding on a new, poorly integrated element such as HIV awareness raising or condom distribution. The focus on core business helps people understand their comparative advantage. It also helps guard against the tendency to drop one's existing work completely in order to take on new work, such as shifting from food security programs to home-based care. The focus on comparative advantage might encourage people to design food security programs that complement and support home-based care.

Helpful Approaches and Tools

Once managers and staff are clear that they are embarking on a long process that will involve attention to HIV in the workplace as well as in programs, they can benefit from simple frameworks, approaches, and tools. CARE Malawi found several that were helpful. The livelihoods approach helps to understand livelihoods risk, vulnerabilities, and opportunities holistically; by building an explicit HIV/AIDS lens into the process, users pay particular attention to the links between health and livelihoods.

Adopt a Livelihoods Approach: Focus on Risk, Vulnerability, and Resilience

CARE uses a livelihoods approach to guide analysis of risk and vulnerabilities and to help identify opportunities and options. This approach helps one to understand livelihoods risk, vulnerabilities, and options in systematic, holistic ways. It guides users to start with the household as the initial unit of analysis but then encourages them to analyze livelihoods at various levels: similarities and differences within households (for example, how do gender and age influence control or access over resources, and roles and responsibilities), between households in a community (for example, diverse assets, competition, and collaboration), and external influences (such as policies, economic systems, social and cultural factors, and climate).

This analytic approach helps identify aspects of livelihoods that increase risk of and vulnerability to illness and death and guides users to understand how various factors influence livelihoods and resilience. By pushing analysis beyond the individual and household level, it helps understanding of broader systemic influences ranging from gender inequity in control over assets such as land to policies that marginalize the most vulnerable, such as agricultural extension policies that focus on serving those who have the ability to demand support from extension agents. No single organization or department can respond to all the issues identified, so the livelihoods approach calls for prioritization and partnerships. I-LIFE,[2] for example, proactively strengthens linkages among organizations that have relevant, complementary skills.

Communities consistently identified the most vulnerable as those with severe health problems (including HIV/AIDS), households caring for chronically ill persons, households hosting orphans, child-headed households, elderly-headed households, and female widowed households. However, this tendency to target types of people rather than actually looking at vulnerability is problematic. Not all female-headed households are vulnerable; some families headed by the elderly are actually fairly secure. Although discussions may begin with a focus on types of people, the livelihoods approach can guide analysis to go further, to a better understanding of who is actually at risk or vulnerable, why, and how to improve their options and resilience.

Start with HIV/AIDS Lens, Move to "Health and Development" Lens

To focus the use of livelihoods analysis, CARE Malawi started to use an "HIV/AIDS lens" (Fig. 15.1). This is not a separate tool but rather refers to explicit efforts by staff and managers to make sure that they consider HIV and AIDS while doing their work. The HIV/AIDS lens helps move from understanding to responding (Loevinsohn and Gillespie 2003), guiding use of livelihoods analysis by encouraging continual analysis of key questions: (1) how does the risk of HIV and impacts of morbidity and mortality affect this situation, and (2) how do livelihoods, and our interventions, affect risk of HIV transmission, progression to AIDS, and impacts of HIV and AIDS?

Some argue that such a lens is not actually needed if people use the livelihoods approach fully and properly. Livelihoods analysis always should include attention to human capacity, to control and access over resources, to options for livelihoods

Figure 15.1 HIV/AIDS lens

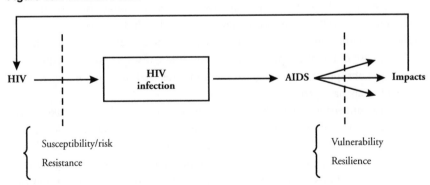

Source: Gillespie and Kadiyala (2005).

activities, and to external influences; implications of and for health should in principle always be part of the analysis. However, in practice, we have seen that many users of the livelihoods approach overlook the role of health as a key feature of the risk and vulnerability environment.

CARE Malawi's workplace policy underpins this "lens" by helping make discussion of HIV/AIDS a normal, daily occurrence. Managers and staff now routinely discuss HIV and AIDS, refer to risk of infection and impacts of ill health, and have conducted livelihood assessments with explicit focus on understanding the bidirectional relationship between HIV/AIDS and food security for both I-LIFE and SMIHLE.

There is an important caveat: Experience has shown that an overly direct focus on HIV and AIDS may actually get in the way. Initial efforts tried to target "people with AIDS"; this is highly problematic for many reasons. Most people with HIV do not know their serostatus. Among those who do know their status, their family and caregivers are seldom publicly open about it. Finally, there is no obvious reason why support should be given to people with or affected by HIV and AIDS, yet not to those with other chronic or critical health problems.

Some community members are uncomfortable talking about AIDS but are keen to discuss other very real health issues, ranging from sexually transmitted infections to malaria. This also reflects the fact that AIDS, though a major problem, is one of many health issues confronted by people in Malawi. The HIV/AIDS lens provided an important initial way of making programs more relevant. However, over time, this should be broadened into a better understanding of how livelihoods and health influence one another more broadly, with HIV/AIDS as one crucial aspect.

Address Stages of HIV/AIDS Timeline
The vulnerability of individuals, households, communities, and institutions varies with the stages of HIV/AIDS: from the risk of infection, progression from infection to onset of AIDS, and impacts on those affected including survivors. The risks and vulnerabilities vary over time: from the perspective of an individual or family (at each phase different people are affected in different ways and may require different types of support) and at a given point in time, a community or even a single household may have people in different phases.

A basic understanding of this reality is important. It can help one take a challenge that seems overwhelming and make it manageable by breaking it down in to bite-sized chunks. Rather than having to respond to the totality of the pandemic, staff and communities can start by analyzing how livelihoods increase or decrease risk of new infections among specific people and develop appropriate responses. They can move on to analyze in turn various situations: how to support positive living by people with HIV, how to facilitate access to and proper use of ART, and how to mitigate social and economic impacts (Greenaway and Mullins 2005).

In February 2005, CARE Malawi ran a workshop for members of 10 community-based organizations and faith-based organizations that undertake a range of activities, such as awareness-raising, home-based care, agricultural production, and support for income generation. After discussing the HIV timeline, they used stickers to indicate where their current activities were focused. They realized that the bulk of their activities involved awareness-raising for prevention and efforts to mitigate impacts, with far fewer activities in the areas of positive living and supporting access to treatment; these were identified as gaps that needed to be addressed.

Table 15.1 uses the timeline and notes just a few possible livelihoods interventions that could be undertaken by different organizations, including community groups, to address specific people at various stages of the timeline.

Working and Learning with Others

The causes and consequences of the epidemic are so diverse that no single organization can have much impact by itself. CARE Malawi has engaged in a variety of efforts to work and learn with others to help build a broad front of civil society, government, and private sector responses to HIV and AIDS.

Partnerships to Provide a Range of Complementary Services

CARE Malawi programs support local partners in project activities and through strengthening community institutions. This includes facilitating improved knowledge on the relationship between HIV/AIDS and food security, strengthening CBOs to manage food security activities that mitigate the impact of the epidemic, and enhancing linkages among different sectors to facilitate responsive service delivery with HIV/AIDS as a core concern. The CORE Initiative small grants program, run in tandem with the NAC small grants, is developing resource materials on HIV and livelihoods for use by CBOs and village development committees.

The timeline presented below can be a valuable tool to help diverse organizations (government, NGOs, CBOs, private sector, faith-based organizations) in a single community to assess who is best placed to address which aspects. This can lead to a range of complementary services provided by various organizations with complementary skills.

In addition to merely cooperating with others, some CARE programs explicitly seek to strengthen linkages among organizations. For example, SMIHLE facilitates communication and joint planning among local churches, orphan care and home-based care groups, village AIDS committees (VACs), funeral committees

Table 15.1 Examples of program interventions at various states

Intervention	Before HIV infection	Asymptomatic	Symptomatic	Death	Survivors
Targeting	Teenage girls at risk	Women with HIV	PWHAs, caregivers	Widow/er, orphans	Survivors
Objectives	Prevent new infections	Positive living	Care and support, impact mitigation	Mitigation: protect assets	Prevention and mitigation
Interventions	Safe livelihood, skills development	Nutrition, income	Nutrition, income food aid	Legal aid: inheritance	Safe livelihood, skills development
Methodology	Girls' youth groups	Build in all livelihoods work	Targeted support	Target vulnerable households	Targeted support
Potential partners	VCT, IEC, school	Support groups, treatment literacy	Clinics, HBC, child care	HBC, paralegals	Child care, paralegals

and local health clinics, and agricultural development initiatives. The CORE Initiative provides small grants and capacity-building support to CBOs and faith-based organizations and intentionally brings together a mix of those working on health and on livelihoods in order to stimulate sharing, learning, and complementary approaches.

Lessons about the successes and difficulties encountered with efforts to mitigate the impact of HIV/AIDS will be shared and lessons used to review and improve advocacy efforts of the Civil Society Agricultural Network (CISANET), which represents a broad network of civil society agencies and advocates for a rights-based approach to communities.

Identify Strategic Entry Points
This entails identifying and agreeing on the key issues to address and strategic entry points for operationalizing programs. For example, agricultural extension workers should play to their comparative advantage through addressing causes and consequences of HIV in agriculture, rather than acting as HIV educators. In Uganda each key service sector (health, education, agriculture, labor) outlined its own approach and requirements for a scaled-up community mobilization plan because the impact of HIV is felt most keenly at the community and household level (Butcher 2003). Because most responses have occurred at this level, a coherent community mobilization strategy enabled different sectors to respond to the epidemic while playing to their comparative advantages.

CARE Malawi has also used community mobilization as its major entry point for most programs. For example, in the CLRSP organizational capacities and partnerships were developed and strengthened with community-based organizations at the group village head level and with government agricultural field staff partners. Similarly, SMIHLE intends to prioritize participatory techniques to mobilize communities, particularly in identifying "vulnerable" people or groups, establishing and supporting local management structures of CBOs and for participatory monitoring and evaluation with beneficiaries and government structures.

CARE Malawi's relationship with the National AIDS Commission through the "Umbrella Programme" (NACUP), which is a grant-making and capacity-building intervention at the district and community level, is another key strategic entry point for eventually mainstreaming HIV into all programs. NAC intends to strengthen the capacity of local governments, in particular district AIDS coordination committees (DACCs) and city AIDS coordinating committees (CACCs) to take on a greater role in supporting community-based action. The main role of the contracted umbrella organizations is to support these committees in aspects of planning and managing the various initiatives by communities in responding to the epidemic.

CARE Malawi has been contracted as the umbrella organization for the Lilongwe district and city.

Research, Reflection, and Integrating Lessons Learned
Programming should explicitly document, learn from, and build on lessons about the relationship between livelihoods and HIV/AIDS and on evidence of success or failure. This requires an active reflection process as programs are developed, a comprehensive monitoring and evaluation framework, and specific efforts to document, learn, and share.

For example, CARE Malawi's most coherent mainstreamed program is called Supporting and Mitigating the Impact of HIV/AIDS for Livelihood Enhancement (SMIHLE). SMIHLE builds and consolidates previous livelihoods programs such as the Central Region Livelihoods Security Programme (CRLSP). The lessons from this project should be shared with and used by other CARE projects and exchanged with other agencies that might take different approaches.

In the words of one member of its staff, SMIHLE is "our mainstreamed programme, which is a process we have learnt as programmes have unfolded . . . until now mainstreaming has not been formalised."[3]

Another example is called Improving Livelihoods through Increasing Food Security (I-LIFE). This is based on the collective experience of a consortium working in the sectors of agriculture, marketing, health and nutrition, HIV/AIDS, and decentralization. I-LIFE explicitly builds on lessons learned to improve the quality of programming, which implies a learning and reflection process as experiences are channeled into proposal design and ultimately implementation. This process is partly intended to build confidence among staff as they reflect on their own successes in dealing with the issues arising around HIV/AIDS.

The SMIHLE proposal drew heavily on research from a number of sources including previous livelihood and HIV/AIDS assessments carried out by CARE Malawi.[4] Similarly, a core pillar of the I-LIFE proposal was that it was built on a better understanding of the relationship between HIV/AIDS and food security to adequately address the long-term needs of vulnerable rural households. Ongoing research was identified as a core component of the sustainability of the program. The I-LIFE Technical Working Groups are intended to collaborate across technical sectors in order to initiate research that would improve program quality. For example, the HIV/AIDS and Agriculture Technical Working Groups intend to conduct action research on crop production and socioanthropological relationships, seeking to design cooperative crop production models that enable HIV/AIDS-affected households to maintain and potentially increase their incomes while improving their nutritional status. With greater understanding of the links between HIV/

AIDS and agriculture, the I-LIFE Consortium should be well placed to assess how agricultural knowledge is shared among populations affected by HIV/AIDS and how to strengthen efforts for cooperative agricultural production.

Monitoring and Evaluation

Appropriate monitoring and evaluation systems should be employed to ensure that beneficiaries, implementers, policymakers, donors, and other stakeholders have the information on whether interventions are working or not. However, the development of appropriate indicators to accurately gauge impact has been difficult in practice. Indeed, recent literature on this issue indicates the difficulty of unscrambling the effects of AIDS on rural communities and food security from economic, climatic, environmental, and governance developments. The apparent impact on food production, access, and use occurs in concert with a series of other factors, including erratic weather patterns, widespread poverty, poor governance, ill-advised economic policies, failed markets, and the compounding force of HIV/AIDS (Drimie 2004). Suggestions to develop appropriate monitoring and evaluation (M&E) systems include:

- use a livelihoods approach to understand particular risks and vulnerabilities in the local socioeconomic environment, the level of HIV/AIDS prevalence, and to guide and assess locally relevant interventions

- integrate health, demographic, and agricultural production indicators into an M&E framework

- develop a core impact assessment methodology, similar to environmental impact assessments (EIAs), which will provide information that can be used to compare the impacts of projects between projects and different localities and countries

CARE Malawi is mainstreaming HIV/AIDS into food security, health, and education programs, identifying core indicators of success in each sector and ensuring active participation of people who are affected or at risk in the monitoring of progress. Questions include: are the new interventions more accessible and more directly relevant, and are they actually benefiting more now than before the programs were "mainstreamed"? Participatory monitoring entails ensuring people are involved not just in feeding in information and data to managers but actually discussing the issues at local level and changing the program as needed.

Challenges and Opportunities

A number of challenges and opportunities have been identified by CARE Malawi staff, including uneven understanding within the team and insufficient evidence of success in reducing risk of infection and vulnerability to impacts of morbidity and mortality. Given multiple types of risk and vulnerability, broad lack of awareness of HIV status, and stigma, proxy indicators are commonly used (O'Donnell 2004).[5] There are issues of attribution as well as problems of assessing success in, for example, infections averted. More work on how to monitor success as well as evidence of actual success is needed.

Scaling up is another challenge. Moving beyond pilot projects and mainstreaming must be standard operating procedure in all programs, in all sectors, all the time. This entails ensuring that all analysis and program design automatically addresses the issues of risk of HIV infection and impacts of AIDS. To enable this to happen, donors must be on board to support and facilitate this process. No one organization can do everything; partnerships are essential. Capacity often needs significant strengthening in a range of areas ranging from technical skills in food security and livelihoods to basic understanding of HIV and AIDS, participatory approaches, organizational management, and so on. Building a successful mainstreamed program in a handful of organizations in a limited number of communities can provide valuable lessons and may improve the lives of hundreds or even thousands of people, but this is a minor step in the face of the larger pandemic. CARE Malawi is increasingly working with community organizations in a range of sectors and facilitating learning and sharing among them. Some of them are starting with experience in HIV and AIDS and learning about food security, others are starting from a food security perspective and learning about HIV and AIDS, but all are learning about how to better respond to the epidemic using their core strengths. CARE, other NGOs, donors, and government must work together to modify work in entire sectors.[6]

Government–Civil Society Partnerships

Government and civil society bring potentially complementary skills and resources to the picture. However, they need to establish a common agenda and practical working relationships. Overstretched staff on both sides, bureaucratic delays, changes in national priorities or ignorance of government priorities, and resource allocation decisions are but a few of the issues that must be tackled.

Building a More Systematic Approach

CARE and others in Malawi have gathered experiences over several years, based on a number of interlinked activities: research, staff training, participation in workshops and conferences, development of an internal HIV/AIDS workplace policy, creation of a "mainstreaming working group," and a review of lessons learned in the process of mainstreaming HIV/AIDS into livelihoods work. These have enabled modifications of existing programs and development of new programs that explicitly recognize HIV/AIDS as major features of the risk and vulnerability environment. CARE Malawi now has the opportunity to distill these into a more systematic approach to mainstreaming in all future programs. This should include staff development processes to help deepen relevant skills and information, allowing for normal staff turnover. All strategic plans and all processes of program design, implementation, and monitoring should consider tools such as livelihoods analysis and the HIV/AIDS lens.

Summary

Mainstreaming HIV/AIDS is good development practice. The tendency by some to frame it as "different" or "difficult" actually makes it less likely that governments, NGOs, CBOs, and faith-based organizations will actually take steps to understand and address the risk and vulnerability associated with HIV and AIDS. Mainstreaming requires a "back to basics" approach and better application of social science: participatory approaches, understanding of differentiation within communities, an explicit focus on vulnerability and opportunities, and attention to the influences of factors far beyond the household. The use of such approaches as livelihoods analysis, with an HIV/AIDS lens, can help us to rethink livelihood targeting and design of interventions (Abbot 2004). The initial focus on HIV/AIDS should gradually broaden to a more inclusive understanding of the two-way relationships between health and development.

In effect, mainstreaming HIV/AIDS requires programmers to return to some of the main principles and tools of development work. They need to work smartly, strategically, and systematically in thinking about HIV and AIDS as major influences on risk and vulnerability in order to effectively use development approaches in the midst of the epidemic.

Notes

1. As identified by Mullins (2002), there is a great range of information and guidance on addressing HIV/AIDS in the workplace. For example see the International Labor Organization: "An ILO code of practice on HIV/AIDS and the world of work," Geneva, June 2001.

2. Improving livelihoods through increasing food security (I-LIFE) is being implemented by a consortium of seven NGOs covering eight districts in Malawi.

3. Interview, CARE Malawi offices, August 20, 2004.

4. From early reports back from Shah et al. (2002), Bryceson, Fonseca, and Kadzandira (2004), and Pinder (2004).

5. For a debate and discussion on the use of proxy indicators, see Mdladla et al. (2003), SADC FANR Vulnerability Assessment Committee (2003), and Marsland (2004).

6. The experience gained under the CRLSP and other programs have not only influenced CARE's future programming but also Malawi's Poverty Reduction Strategy Paper (PRSP) and the Malawian government's Food Security and Nutrition Policy. CARE's livelihoods and HIV/AIDS program is intended to continue to influence, support, learn from, and monitor these government programs (SMIHLE Proposal, 2004, p. 3).

References

Abbot, J. 2004. *Rural livelihood interventions for households affected by HIV/AIDS.* Prepared by CARE-Lesotho, South Africa, for DFID Zimbabwe, February.

Barnett, T., and A. Whiteside. 2002. *AIDS in the twenty-first century: Disease and globalisation.* New York: Palgrave/Macmillan.

Baylies, C. 2001. *The impact of AIDS on rural households in Africa: A shock like any other.* Institute of Social Studies, United Kingdom.

Bryceson, D., J. Fonseca, and J. Kadzandira. 2004. *Social pathways from the HIV/AIDS deadlock of disease, denial and desperation in rural Malawi.* Lilongwe: CARE International and RENEWAL (Regional Network on HIV/AIDS, Livelihoods, and Food Security). www.ifpri.org/renewal/studies.htm.

Butcher, K. 2003. *Lessons learned from mainstreaming HIV into the poverty eradication action plan in Uganda.* DFID Uganda, October, p. 9.

Care Malawi HIV/AIDS Thematic Team. 2004. *CARE Malawi HIV/AIDS mainstreaming strategy.* Unpublished report. Lilongwe: CARE Malawi.

Chambers, R., and G. Conway. 1991. *Sustainable rural livelihoods: Practical concepts for the 21st century.* IDS Discussion Paper no. 296. Brighton, U.K.: University of Sussex Institute of Development Studies.

Drimie, S. 2004. *The underlying causes of the food crisis in the southern African region: Malawi, Mozambique, Zambia, and Zimbabwe.* Pretoria: Oxfam-GB Southern Africa Regional Office.

Drimie, S., and D. Mullins. 2005. *Mainstreaming HIV and AIDS into livelihoods and food security programmes: An analysis of CARE Malawi programmes,* February.

Frankenberger, T., K. Luther, K. Fox, and J. Mazzeo. 2003. Livelihood erosion through time: Macro and micro factors that influenced livelihood trends in Malawi over the last 30 years. Tango International for CARE Southern and Western Africa Regional Management Unit (SWARMU), March.

Gillespie, S. R., and S. Kadiyala. 2005. *HIV/AIDS and food and nutrition security: From evidence to action.* Food Policy Review 7. Washington, D.C.: IFPRI.

Greenaway, K., and D. Mullins. 2005. *The HIV/AIDS timeline as a program tool: Experiences from CARE and C-SAFE.* Paper for IFPRI Conference "HIV/AIDS, Food and Nutrition Security," Durban, South Africa, April.

Haddad, L., and S. R. Gillespie. 2001. Effective food and nutrition policy responses to HIV/AIDS: What we know and what we need to know. *Journal of International Development* 13 (4): 487–511.

Loevinsohn, M., and S. Gillespie. 2003. *HIV/AIDS, food security and rural livelihoods: Understanding and responding.* Food Consumption and Nutrition Division Discussion Paper no. 157. Washington, D.C.: International Food Policy Research Institute.

Marsland, N. 2004. *Development of food security and vulnerability information systems in southern Africa: The experience of Save the Children UK.* Unpublished paper, Save the Children UK.

Mdladla, P., N. Marsland, J. Van Zyl, and S. Drimie. 2003. *Assessment methodologies: Integration of HIV/AIDS related indicators: Examples from the field.* United Nations Regional Inter-Agency Coordination and Support Office, Technical Consultation on Vulnerability in the Light of an HIV/AIDS Pandemic, September 9–11, 2003, Johannesburg, South Africa.

Mullins, D. 2002. *What can it look like to mainstream HIV and AIDS?* Oxford: Oxfam UK.

O'Donnell, M. 2004. *Food security, livelihoods & HIV/AIDS: A guide to the linkages, measurement & programming implications.* London: Save the Children UK.

Pinder, C. 2004. *Economic pathways for Malawi's rural households.* CARE Malawi, May.

SADC FANR Vulnerability Assessment Committee. 2003. *Towards identifying impacts of HIV/AIDS on food security in southern Africa and implications for response: Findings from Malawi, Zambia and Zimbabwe.* Harare, Zimbabwe.

Shah, M., N. Osborne, T. Mbilizi, and G. Vilili. 2002. *Impact of HIV/AIDS on agricultural productivity and rural livelihoods in the central region of Malawi.* CARE International in Malawi.

Chapter 16

Measuring the Impact of Targeted Food Assistance on HIV/AIDS-Related Beneficiary Groups: Monitoring and Evaluation Indicators

Kari Egge and Susan Strasser

Background, Objectives, and Methodology

In October 2005, the Consortium for the Southern Africa Food Security Emergency (C-SAFE) transitioned to its final year of a regional "developmental relief" program. Yet, members continued to collaborate on this specific learning activity given their common objectives of improving monitoring and evaluation (M&E) for HIV/AIDS-related beneficiary groups. C-SAFE's strategic objectives included (1) improving and maintaining nutritional status, (2) protecting productive assets, and (3) improving community resilience to food security shocks.

As part of its targeted food aid (TFA)[1] program, C-SAFE provides food assistance to four HIV/AIDS-related beneficiary groups. The chronically ill (CI) is used by all three members as a proxy for HIV/AIDS,[2] and several of C-SAFE's members link TFA to medically oriented interventions such as Prevention of Mother to Child Transmission (PMTCT), Tuberculosis-Directly Observed Therapy, and Antiretroviral Therapy (ART).[3] Throughout implementation, the issue of how to measure impact of food aid on individuals receiving ART or tuberculosis (TB) drugs, mothers and infants enrolled in PMTCT programs, and the chronically ill has been discussed and debated. Although C-SAFE regularly monitors household food security using various tools, and in some programs measures nutritional status of children under 5; measuring the impact of food on these four HIV/AIDS-related groups remains a challenge.

For individuals receiving ART or TB drugs, and those in PMTCT programs, C-SAFE members monitor whether food was received but generally do not gather additional information. Many clients are being weighed regularly by health-service providers, and a range of other indicators are being used to monitor progress, though C-SAFE staff have not generally taken advantage of this information or systematically applied other (livelihoods or nutrition) indicators to measure whether there is demonstrable change as a result of food aid. The most common measure of "success" has been program uptake and treatment adherence. Monitoring of the chronically ill is similar, with limited or no data gathered to demonstrate the impact of food aid.

As C-SAFE members and others expand their involvement in such programming, it is important to build an evidence-based understanding of the attribution of food aid to the quality of life and physical status of these beneficiaries, not only to better justify the provision of such assistance but also to improve the design and implementation of targeted food assistance programs to beneficiaries.

To assist consortium members, a study was commissioned by C-SAFE Learning Spaces[4] in November 2004. A review of the literature was completed in December 2004, and field research in Malawi, Zambia, and Zimbabwe in February 2005. The researchers summarized current knowledge and practices and offered advice about appropriate, practical methods for monitoring the impact of targeted food assistance on HIV/AIDS related beneficiary groups.

Objectives

The aim of this research was to investigate current practices for measuring the impact of TFA on four HIV/AIDS-related beneficiary groups: (1) the chronically ill (CI); (2) women and infants engaged in PMTCT programs; (3) individuals on ART; and (4) individuals on TB treatment. This was done through a review of the literature followed by interviews and observational visits to HIV/AIDS-related food aid programs in Malawi, Zimbabwe, and Zambia. Recommendations for measuring the impact of TFA are provided based on the literature review and fieldwork.

Methodology

The literature review included a search of academic and relief and development agency databases. When saturation of the literature was achieved, papers were scrutinized for information on nutritional status and the impact of TFA in the context of HIV and AIDS. Because the literature is limited, a wider review was done, including disease progression, nutrition, treatment impact, and psychosocial issues. Because of the lack of available papers in peer-reviewed journals, the "gray" literature was also reviewed.

Information was also gathered through key informant interviews, group discussions, observational visits, and collection of current monitoring and evaluation tools. In each study country, a local representative identified appropriate field sites and stakeholders. For each intervention type, analysis focused on objectives, strengths and weaknesses of current practices, gaps, and recommendations for integrating impact measurements into future activities. A total of 66 individuals from 29 different agencies were interviewed across the three countries.

For further details on persons and organizations interviewed, recommended indicators, and tools for consideration, please refer to the full paper with annexes at www.c-safe.org.

Results

Review of the Literature

This work highlights the paucity of studies addressing TFA to people living with HIV/AIDS (PLWHAs) and almost complete lack of documentation on measuring impact of food aid on PLWHA. Practical tools to assess TFA's impact on households and nutritional outcomes for PLWHA are not widely available.

The literature review began with AEGIS.COM news briefs from June 2002. Common themes included food relief (supplements) as long-term care or recovery, the concept of a "new variant famine," chronic illnesses' negative impact on household food security, the unmet needs of orphans and vulnerable children (OVC), multiple targets and entry points, denial and stigma, and gender inequity (women as caregivers, girls leaving school to care, etc.).

Although many organizations advocate for incorporating food aid into HIV/AIDS programming, there is a serious lack of empirical evidence on how best to evaluate the impact of programs on participants who are HIV positive or living with AIDS (IFAD 2001; FAO 2003; USAID PVO Steering Committee 2003; Canahuati 2004; FANTA 2004a,b). Despite the lack of experience in how to evaluate the impact of TFA on HIV/AIDS participants, this review has identified a number of starting points and potential indicators to pilot for use in measuring impact changes from TFA programs. Findings geared to individual and household levels are outlined below.

Assessing Individual Impacts

Nutritional status. Anthropometric measures are important assessments and one of the few quantitative measurements that are practical for field measurement. The literature provides guidance on how to use anthropometric indicators to measure program impact. Miller (2003) suggests that nutritional status can be assessed through vigilant weight monitoring and that disease progression can be monitored through serial measurements of mid–upper arm circumference (MUAC), triceps skin folds, and other anthropometry (FANTA 2000). These recommendations are supported by the Highly Active Antiretroviral Therapy (HAART) and HARVEST program in Kenya, which monitors weight in an effort to link food security with ART outcomes (FANTA 2004a).

In the few research studies measuring the impact of food aid on PLWHA, body mass index (BMI),[5] MUAC, and weight measurements were the most common indicators, though head circumference, weight for height, bioelectrical impedance analysis (BIA), body circumferences, and skin-fold measurements were also used to measure nutritional impacts of TFA programs (Swanson 1998; Maina et al. 2005; Ochieng Owingo 2005; Torreblanca and Kim 2005). Organizations are experimenting with handgrip strength as an easily administered proxy for nutritional status using mechanical handgrip dynamometers. Used primarily with elderly populations, handgrip has been positively correlated to BMI, MUAC, and arm muscle area (Chilima and Ismail 2001).

HIV/AIDS brings problems in interpretation of anthropometric measurements that compromise their value as indicators of TFA impact. Even in ideal conditions where HIV-positive children receive over the recommended daily allowance (RDA) of calories and protein, inferior growth may be seen, and HIV-positive adults with no enteric pathogens have shown diminished skin-fold thickness and lower weight than HIV-negative adults despite equal food intake (Miller 2003). Nutritional status and growth may be impaired because of malabsorption and a metabolism that can exceed one's ability (or appetite) to consume, so although the food aid may be enhancing the food security of the family and even helping the PLWHA nutritionally, the BMI or MUAC measurements would not reflect this. Therefore, it is difficult to interpret anthropometric measurement trajectories because the impact of TFA may be reduced weight loss versus weight gain as is normally anticipated.

Anthropometric indicators also show change subsequent to other subclinical health measures, so by the time there are measurable changes, other important health changes have already occurred, and the impact of food aid may not be detectable. In relation to MUAC, lipodystrophy may make that measurement unreliable for PLWHA who are on certain forms of ART.

The literature therefore shows that anthropometric measurements are useful components but alone would not provide the level of understanding needed to assess a TFA program's impact and could be misleading. What are required are program indicators that are sensitive to a variety of HIV/AIDS effects (FAO/WHO 2003).

Strength and stamina. The return of strength and ability to be productive are possible indicators of TFA impact (WFP 2004). Yet, it would be important to control for the availability and use of medical treatment. A handgrip dynamometer could be used to measure changes in strength as a result of TFA programs, though little has been published to test this instrument with PLWHA.

Diarrhea prevalence. Diarrhea prevalence in young children (under 24 months of age) is another possible proxy measure of health and improved food security (Swindale 2004). Another study supports a significant association between malnutrition and diarrhea incidence (Measurement Excellence and Training Resource Information Center 2005).

Treatment uptake and efficacy. For individuals on TB treatment or ART, a commonly mentioned impact of TFA programs was an increase in treatment uptake and a decrease in default rates.

Treatment completion (tuberculosis) and treatment adherence. For PLWHA on TB treatment or ART, a commonly mentioned impact of TFA programs was an increase in treatment acceptability and ease of adherence with drug regimens. One study has shown that among a small sample of treatment interrupters, lack of money for food is seen as a barrier to treatment adherence (Rowe et al. 2005). Despite this, further studies are needed to better understand and document the impact of food security on TB treatment completion and adherence to HAART.

Quality of life. Current literature abounds with studies on quality of life (QOL) among PLWHA. Interviews with health workers and TFA field staff support exploring the use of QOL tools. QOL is a multifaceted concept that considers the impact of impairments, function, perceptions, and social opportunities (Robinson 2004). Numerous studies have been done using QOL measures with HIV-positive persons (Jacobson, Wu, Feinberg, and Outcomes Committee 2003; Mast et al. 2004; Preau et al. 2004), and a number of tools exist (Ferrans and Powers 1992; Wu et al. 1997; Webster, Cella, and Yost 2003; RAND Health 2004). However, there is nothing published that looks directly at the impact of food assistance on QOL for PLWHA. One unpublished pilot study has been done in South Africa on QOL and food, and another has looked at ART-related nutritional problems and QOL (Fields-Gardner and Keithley 2001). QOL measures offer a richer assessment of the impact of TFA, including physical, social, and psychological components. These benefits will need to be weighed against time needed to complete QOL assessments and translation and training requirements.

Other scales [Karnofsky and Disease Stage Scale, the WHO/Zubrod or Eastern Cooperative Oncology Group (ECOG) Scale] that were originally developed to measure physical functioning levels for patients with cancer (Karnofsky and Burchenal 1949; Oken et al. 1982; Lanksy et al. 1987) are now used to assess health and physical ability of PLWHA. These scales focus on physical functioning. There is a scale used in medical oncology for children that is based more on observation, called the Lansky scale, but it does not appear in research conducted in the developing world context related to HIV/AIDS (Oken et al. 1982). The World Health Organization (WHO) recommends Karnofsky as a tool to monitor clinical status for patients on antiretroviral (ARV) treatment (WHO 2002). Finally, strength and stamina issues are often incorporated into QOL indices.

Assessing Household Impact
It is acknowledged that food aid impacts all household members as the individual and household are intrinsically linked. Therefore, food aid programs usually measure household-level impact. However, a demonstrated impact at the household level does not necessarily imply that there is also impact for the targeted individual.

The link between HIV/AIDS and household food insecurity has been documented.[6] Therefore, although there are no tested examples presented in the literature, the level of household food insecurity is a potential indicator to use to measure the impact of food aid on PLWHA. In addition to using individual level measurements (e.g., BMI) of all household members to measure household impact, a composite measure of household food insecurity level has been used to measure impact of food aid. Known household responses that could be used include sale of assets (productive and nonproductive), dietary changes, hiring in and out of household labor, and withdrawal of children from school (FANTA 2000). Swindale has identified multiple household indicators to measure food insecurity, such as dietary diversity, asset retention, as well as anthropometry, demographics, and diarrhea prevalence in young children (Swindale 2004).

Another distinction that could be made involves categorizing households based on the type of impact of AIDS, such as chronic illness, death, or support of orphans. This could be broken down into impacts on human, financial, social, physical, and natural capital (O'Donnell 2004). Indicators already included in many data collection tools measuring food security include number of meals eaten per day, quantity or number of foods eaten in the past 24 hours, dietary diversity indices, consumption of luxury items, amount of land planted, and expenditure on food. Examples of indices, which may be useful, are the Experiential Household Food Insecurity Scale (EHFIS), Household Dietary Diversity, Household Asset Index (Canahuati 2004), and Coping Strategy Index (Maxwell et al. 2003).

An issue to consider when assessing impact is the bidirectional nature of chronic illness and food security. Chronic ill health may serve as a cause of food insecurity as well as a consequence of food insecurity (WFP 2003). HIV disease is related to food security at the individual, household, and community levels. For example, during times of food insecurity individuals may skip meals, which potentially could exacerbate chronic illness. In turn, subsequent infection and illness reduce an individual's ability to improve his or her household food security.

Results of Field Research

Current Practices and Impressions of Impact Measurement

As in the literature review, the primary finding from the field was that indicators to measure the direct impact of food aid on PLWHA are not prevalent. Although C-SAFE partners have a great deal of experience monitoring receipt of food aid and food security status of targeted households, most do not have systems to measure the impact of food aid on PLWHA.

Although anthropometric, clinical, and performance measures are collected at the clinic level, they do not inform food programming, and often information is collected only on a qualitative or anecdotal basis. C-SAFE partners are collecting fairly extensive information on household coping strategies, assets, use of food aid, and vulnerability levels. However, this information generally is not analyzed in a manner that is able to tease out the direct impact of food aid on particular subgroups of beneficiaries. In general, C-SAFE programs are not analyzing individual health outcomes, survival, QOL, or nutritional status but focus on the household level. Anecdotal information exists in relation to the impact of food aid on the individual and household, but neither agencies nor health facilities have systems of sufficient rigor or regularity to support reported observations. This is not necessarily a result of the lack of capacity or interest, as staff stated they wanted to learn more about the impact of food aid on CI beneficiaries, but C-SAFE was neither mandated nor funded to collect this level of data, so M&E frameworks were not designed to do so.

Although no quantitative data exist to demonstrate the impact of food aid on PLWHA in C-SAFE programs, almost all beneficiaries and stakeholders gave anecdotal evidence of positive impacts of food aid: weight, improved health, and food consumption. After receiving food, beneficiaries experienced improved body weight, strength, ability to work, and overall well-being. For example, a Malawian woman with Kaposi's sarcoma reported:

It was good to receive [the food aid]. I ate three meals a day compared to once a day before. [Before], I was dependent on visitors to bring food. I could not have employed someone to do the gardening. [With food aid], I had money to spare for other things, to buy fish, eggs, vegetables, and relishes. I was able to plant beans and maize.

Another couple on ART explained:

Before food aid I had many challenges. I was sick, had stomach aches, heart palpitations, headaches, and pneumonia. I started on ARVs and then got C-SAFE food. With drugs and food my physical problems decreased, I had less diarrhea, I gained a lot of energy and could move around and get involved. I had enough strength to mold bricks and construct a house. I could increase the gardening. [Since the food has been stopped,] I have an increased problem taking the medications, and my weight has decreased.

Before food support the wife's reported weight was around 40 kilograms; with the ART and food support, she went to 61 kilograms. She is still on ART, but with no food support, she now weighs 47 kilograms.

Clinicians reiterated impact of food aid on health, treatment adherence, and nutritional status. In Zimbabwe, a hospital matron commented on HIV-positive support members (none of whom are on ART) who received TFA with corn soy blend:

I could see improvement in their general disposition and less complaints about their conditions. I also noticed people gaining weight. Now, at TB days each month, weight has dropped, and there are less people attending [since food aid stopped in October].

Although BMI was consistently proposed as an impact measure, interviewees raised concerns regarding capacity and equipment to accurately collect BMI. The quality of weight scales and height measurement were questioned. Indicators tracking health status, program uptake, drug efficacy, and strength or stamina were also commonly mentioned alongside household food security measures. When queried about QOL issues such as mental health and ability to conduct daily activities, interviewees felt that these were things that food aid does impact but that are not normally tracked. None mentioned handgrip strength, BIA, head circumference, or skin-fold measurements.

The work involved in collecting additional impact information would not be extensive because much is already being collected or partially collected. Clinics routinely collect weight, symptoms, visit frequency, treatment regimes, clinical outcomes, and information that could be adapted to performance indicators such as the Karnofsky and ECOG. Yet, it did not appear that this information is retrieved or used by TFA programs. Although cooperation between medical services and NGOs exist (such as clinics providing beneficiary lists to NGOs), linkages between monitoring and evaluation systems and data sharing are few. Both value integrating their information and expertise, but little partnership currently exists.

Field Practices and Proposed Indicators by Program
Targeted food assistance to tuberculosis programs.   Interviewees proposed the following indicators: mortality, adherence and default rates, weight, BMI, morbidity, stamina, and length of hospital stay. Unlike the other groups, research has been conducted on the impact of food aid on TB programs. According to the head of the Malawi TB program, food aid is a priority in treatment and reducing mortality. Although more than half of TB patients on admission were found malnourished, with food support there was a dramatic reduction in early mortality (Zachariah et al. 2002). Using food as an incentive for adherence was also mentioned, and WFP (Zimbabwe) is looking at adherence to TB treatment as an effect of food aid.

Most interviewees expected food aid to increase weight gain, reduce symptoms, and enhance productive capacity. Others mentioned that although TB patients may complete the treatment, many of them remain malnourished; thus, without food assistance they are too weak to farm or actively return to daily activities. Another potential indicator mentioned was decreased hospital stay. The TB program at Chikankata Hospital (Zambia) found that malnutrition on admission significantly increases the length of stay for TB patients, and staff anticipates that food support would contribute to recovery.

Targeted food assistance to ART programs.   Interviewees mentioned the following indicators to measure the impact of food aid on ART recipients: mortality/prolonged survival, drug adherence and efficacy, weight/BMI, morbidity/symptoms (e.g., diarrhea), productivity, quality of life (QOL).

The relationship between nutritional status (usually measured through BMI) and survival was also mentioned. Research in Malawi showed that a BMI less than 16 was predictive of high mortality (50 percent of patients died within 6 months of going on ART) when coexisting with anemia, poor functionality, and CD4 below 50.[7] It was implied that nutritional status could be enhanced through food aid; thus, when it is coupled with ART a positive synergy could result.

Using food aid as an incentive for adherence was frequently mentioned. Field staff reported communities asking "how are we to take these drugs if we have nothing in our stomachs?" implying that without food, they could not take the prescribed drugs because the drugs would not work or they would get sick. When the issue was proposed to medical professionals and beneficiaries, though, their opinion was that generally people are so grateful to be on ARVs and feel the benefits are so substantial that adherence is already high. The head of HIV/AIDS (Malawi–Ministry of Health) said that from crude adherence monitoring (measuring the number of pills left in bottles brought back each month by patients), default rates in government-sponsored ART programs is less than 5 percent.

Several interviewees predicted an enhanced efficacy of ARV drugs with the availability of food. Again, most clinical practitioners did not support this suggestion but were also unaware of research to refute it. Some doctors explained that the ARVs were deliberately chosen because they do not need to be taken with food and should not be affected by the food security status of the patient. Several practitioners mentioned that even for severely malnourished patients, the recommendation is not to wait for weight gain but to concurrently treat malnutrition while giving ART because experience has shown that the drugs are still effective even when the patient is malnourished.

Weight gain measured through BMI was commonly suggested as something that should be measured to show the impact of food aid on ART program participants and would not be burdensome. Because ART drugs are dosed by weight, patients are weighed regularly and recorded on master cards. National guidance in Malawi calls for BMI to be measured on ART patients to enable referral to feeding programs (for BMI less than 16, patients are referred to therapeutic feeding; for BMI 16–18.5, to a supplemental feeding program, though these referral options may not reliably exist).

Symptoms, productive capacity levels, and QOL scales were posed as additional indicators to demonstrate the impact of food support. Interviewees felt that many PLWHA live in such food-insecure situations that although ART is a key intervention, nutritional support is also needed to fully benefit from improved CD4+ counts. ART protocols consistently identify "good nutrition" as an integral part of a comprehensive care package. In order to provide self-care, resume productive activities, and reduce reliance on caregivers, improved nutrition is required. Symptoms, especially diarrhea, were predicted by interviewees to decline with the addition of food aid to the ART regime. Finally, when probed, most interviewees felt that QOL indicators that included daily activities, mental outlook, and productive capacity would also be well received and informative.

Targeted Food Assistance to the Chronically Ill

Potential indicators for measuring the impact of food aid on the chronically ill were: weight change/BMI, symptoms (e.g., diarrhea), productivity, quality of life, household assets, coping strategies, attendance/school performance, and need for caregivers.

Weight change was the primary indicator that stakeholders proposed for measuring impact in this group. Chronically ill beneficiaries reported impacts such as; "giving strength" and "(I have) gained weight, my skin is healthier, (I have) strength to walk." Issues related to collecting weight and BMI data were similar to those mentioned previously. If patients are well enough to get to a health center, weight will be recorded on the patient retained clinic card, but for homebound patients, there may be access, equipment, and data collection constraints.

Symptom reduction, particularly diarrhea, was also cited as something field workers felt would result from food aid. Not everyone agreed, however, as some medical practitioners felt the reduction in symptoms was more likely the result of treatment than food.

As mentioned under other programs, QOL was mentioned as important indicators of impact. It was predicted that with food aid, PLWHA would be able to get out of bed, take care of themselves, and get involved in household and farming activity. Individuals mentioned that the ability to buy sugar, soap, and other basic household goods also enhanced daily life and improved the mental health of recipients. The assurance of continued food assistance also reportedly reduced targeted beneficiaries' worry and stress within the household.

In addition to individual impacts, household impacts were identified; with food aid, caregivers were not needed as much and were able to return to work, reducing the sale of assets and increasing household production/income. Food security and coping strategy indicators were also recommended, as were increased attendance and performance at school due to improved ability of the household to pay for school fees, better nutrition, and decreased need for children at home.

Catholic Relief Services (CRS)-Zambia is currently investigating the impact of nutritional supplementation on the QOL and anthropometric status of HIV+ home-based care (HBC) program clients over a six-month period. Dependent variables include BMI, QOL scores, MUAC, and dietary diversity.

Targeted Food Aid to PMTCT Clients
With regard specifically to PMTCT programs, participants proposed the following indicators: weight change/BMI, symptoms (e.g., diarrhea), productive capacity levels, quality of life, coping strategies, program uptake (increased testing, disclosure, attendance at counseling sessions), maternal weight change, BMI and MUAC, birth outcomes and infant weight, level of mixed feeding, exclusive breastfeeding, weaning (timing and success), length of exclusive breastfeeding, and duration of the weaning period.

M&E systems have already been developed for PMTCT programs regionally. However, most of these systems focus on program uptake and outcomes (women receiving voluntary counseling and testing, mother–infant dyads receiving Nevi-rapine, and number of children testing positive at 18 months) and do not focus on the impact of food assistance. Respondents felt the need to substantially improve monitoring of nondrug prevention measures and to include nutritional and behavioral indicators in the current PMTCT M&E plans.

It was widely agreed that food aid attached to PMTCT programs would increase program participation. If food aid were linked to HIV status, disclosure would also be inadvertently increased, though this raises ethical issues on the use of food.

As with all food aid interventions, it was predicted that PMTCT participants would gain weight and improve their nutritional status. Because there are links between maternal nutritional status and birth outcomes, numbers of LBW children born to HIV-positive mothers, weight gain during pregnancy, BMI during lactation, and infant growth were all mentioned as potential indicators to measure impacts.

Infant feeding practices such as the level of mixed feeding, exclusive breast-feeding, and accelerated weaning behavior are a great concern to many involved in PMTCT. Insufficient energy for the mother to exclusively breastfeed, lack of house-hold food security, and low availability of proper weaning foods were examples of inhibitors to exclusive breastfeeding and accelerated weaning, thus increasing the risk of vertical transmission. Indicators of food aid impact on PMTCT could therefore include incidence of mixed feeding and duration of the weaning period (e.g., duration of mixed feeding) for HIV positive mothers. Indicators proposed would reflect the type of PMTCT food assistance and counseling provided. Currently, there are no indicators which measure exclusive breastfeeding or quality of weaning practices.

Other impacts previously mentioned such as QOL, productive capacity, and coping strategies were also brought up by PMTCT stakeholders as indicators that could be used to examine food aid impacts on PMTCT participants.

Issues That Could Affect Measurement

A number of general concerns were raised that could affect data collection and measurement of impact: time, equipment, training, experience, and existence of indicators and assessment tools; the tools to measure expected impact either do not exist or have not been fully tested. For example, the need to be realistic about the long-term and potentially cyclical needs of CI households was discussed. For this reason, NGOs are trying to develop assessment tools that can identify when to inter-vene with food support and when to "pull back." The concept of identifying a "trigger point" for both safe graduation and increased vulnerability are needed. Finally, the availability of staff that can design and complete studies of the complexity that will be necessary to show causal attribution of food aid to individual and household impact are a concern.

Discussion

Proposed Indicators

This research highlighted the dearth of evidence, in print and in the field, that measures the impact of food aid on PLWHA. Current M&E systems are not designed to evaluate this impact. Despite the lack of evidence, numerous testimonials from HIV-positive beneficiaries and program staff gave examples of impacts on the chronically ill. Nobody expressed doubt about the importance of food aid as a key component of comprehensive HIV/AIDS services. From a literature review,[8] discussions with technical staff, and experience from traditional food aid evaluations, a framework of suggested indicators to measure the impact of food aid on individuals and households living with HIV/AIDS are proposed.

According to the review of the literature and field research, anticipated improvements from food aid at the household and individual levels are increased daily food consumption, money available for other needs, and household food security. These improvements generate a cascade of changes that are believed to result in increased weight, energy, treatment adherence, school attendance, immunity, medical treatment, QOL, productive capacity, and ultimately survival. In addition, there is an anticipated increase in programmatic uptake (Fig. 16.1).

Because many indicators are difficult to collect (and to interpret), this chapter considers a short list of indicators. Yet C-SAFE does not purport that they are the most appropriate in all cases. They are simply those thought to be the most feasible and relevant given C-SAFE's operating environment and capacity. The indicators highlighted in Figure 16.1 are: anthropometrics (BMI, MUAC, weight for age, and percentage weight change), treatment adherence and default rates (TB, ART), infant feeding protocols, coping strategies, mental health, productivity, ability to perform daily living activities, need for caregivers, and program uptake.

A decision as to which of the indicators to use will depend on the relationship with food aid, biological plausibility, and their perceived feasibility for partners.

Some medically oriented impacts such as viral load were not included because they would require extensive clinical examinations not deemed to be realistic. Obviously, if these data are available, they could be used. Other medically oriented impacts suggested, such as diarrhea incidence and drug efficacy, were not included.

With indicators that are high up the flow chart (Fig. 16.1), it will be difficult to separate out the impact of food aid from other factors influencing that variable.

Figure 16.1 Potential impact of food aid on persons living with HIV and AIDS

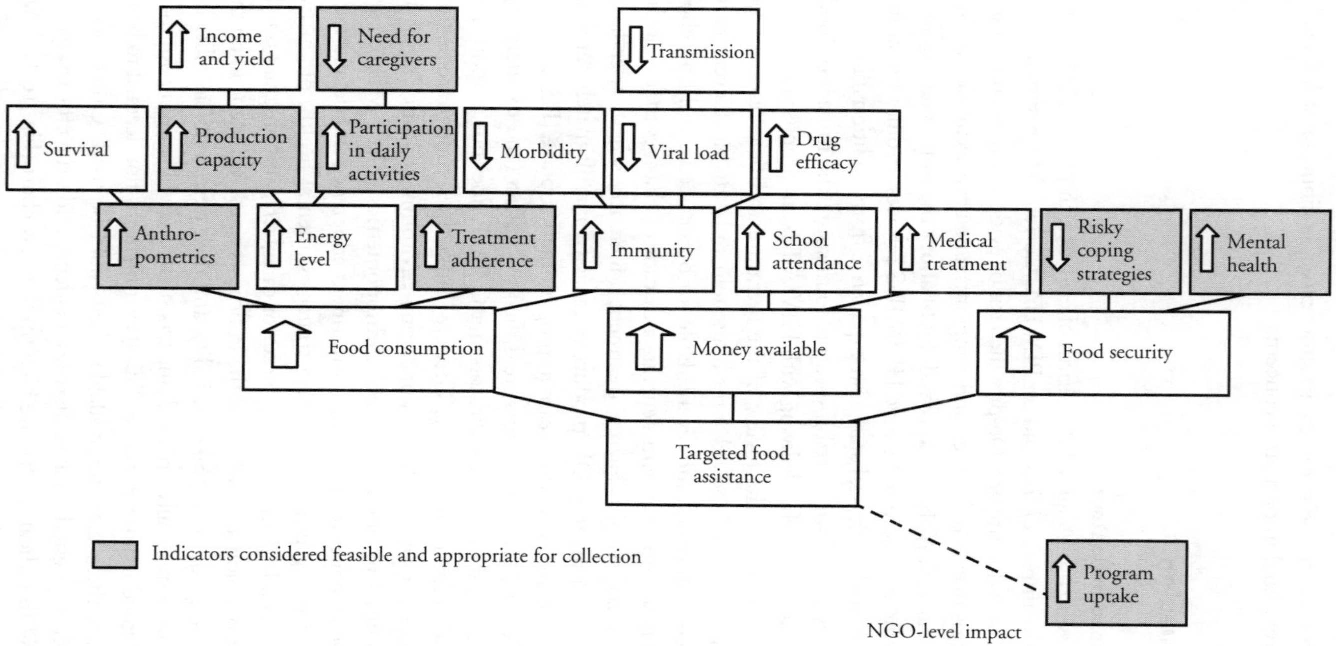

Survival → Anthropometrics

Income and yield → Production capacity

Need for caregivers → Participation in daily activities

Energy level

Treatment adherence

Anthropometrics

Transmission → Drug efficacy

Morbidity → Viral load

Immunity

School attendance

Medical treatment

Risky coping strategies

Mental health

Food consumption

Money available

Food security

Targeted food assistance

Program uptake

NGO-level impact

☐ Indicators considered feasible and appropriate for collection

■ (shaded box legend)

So the farther away the potential impact is listed away from food aid, the less likely an indicator measuring those impacts would be recommended. The impact of increased money available to the household (because less money is being spent on food) is more difficult to attribute directly to food assistance, as there are many other reasons why a household has more money available to it besides food aid. School attendance, for example, was not recommended for collection because of the difficulty in collecting quality data and the number of other factors that could influence attendance.

It is not feasible to use all indicators. Implementers will have to examine program objectives and capacities to determine what indicators to use. Indicators are recommended by program type (Table 16.1). Lesser-known and more experimental indicators (handgrip strength, BIA, and head circumference) were not included.

Challenges to Evaluating Impact

Establishing a framework to measure the impact of food aid on PLWHA is not simple. Constraints include data collection capacity, complexity of study design and analysis, financial resources, and limited understanding of the interplay between HIV and micro- and macronutrients. Also intrahousehold distribution, sales, and food sharing will all be uncontrollable variables.

Proving causal attribution of an impact to food aid is difficult because of HIV disease complexity and numerous factors influencing beneficiaries' experiences.

Table 16.1 Indicators for consideration to measure impact of TFA by program type

| Indicators for consideration in measuring impact | Program type | | | | |
| | | | | PMTCT | |
	TB	ART	CI	Mother	Child
1. Anthropometrics					
BMI	X	X	X	X	
Percentage of weight change		X	X	X	
MUAC				X	
Weight for age					X
Weight for height					X
2. Treatment adherence	X	X		X	
3. Risky coping strategies		X	X	X	
4–6. Quality of life					
Mental health	X	X	X	X	
Activities of daily living	X	X	X	X	
Productive capacity	X	X	X	X	
7. Need for caregivers		X	X		
8. Program uptake	X			X	

Morbidity, mortality, length of hospital stay, and community ability to care are influenced by many factors, and only an extensive and rigorous evaluation design could sort out whether an impact was related to food aid versus rainfall, government policy, quality of local medical facilities, and similar issues.

Potential confounders must be identified and collected in baseline and monitoring tools, particularly if a cross-sectional survey design is used rather than a baseline-evaluation model. Research is needed to better understand independent variables relevant to collect to show causal attribution of food aid. One confounding variable is continued wasting even for beneficiaries on ART (Miller 2003). Other variables include ART side impacts such as nausea, vomiting, metabolic complications of treatment (derangement of lipid and glucose metabolism) (Shevitz and Knox 2001) and prolonged recovery times (Sandige et al. 2004).

Key control variables include, but are not limited to, demographic information (e.g., gender, age, ethnicity, location, household size), program inputs (e.g., quantity of food and commodities received and for what duration), treatment received (e.g., ARVs, breastfeeding counseling, cotrimoxazole), stage of disease and CD4 count at onset and completion of research period, and signs and symptoms experienced by PLWHA during research period. If these variables are not controlled for, it will not be possible to determine what impact came from food aid and what came from other sources.

Recommendations

Neither the literature review nor the field research found significant evidence of TFA impacts being measured among PLWHA. The following recommendations therefore do not reflect validated research but, rather, ideas from TFA technical staff:

- Pilot the indicators noted in the Discussion section of this chapter at select sites of C-SAFE, Improving-Livelihoods through Increasing Food Security (I-LIFE), and similar NGO food aid programs targeting PLWHA to measure program impact.

- Indicators measuring program inputs, activities, and outcomes are also needed as monitoring tools and to help interpret impact indicators but are not discussed in this chapter.

- Include suggested indicators into future C-SAFE and I-LIFE surveys and eventually integrate these indicators into future project M&E systems.

- In established end-use monitoring, postdistribution monitoring, and community and household surveillance collection tools, link data already collected such as coping strategies, school participation, and program uptake to participation in food aid programs.

- Establish M&E partnerships between health centers and with district-level, central governmental, and food aid programs serving similar populations and determine mutual areas of interest in order to share information.

- Share lessons learned among C-SAFE partners, the wider UN/NGO network, and health service providers.

The literature review identified two research priorities for evaluating the impact of food aid on PLWHA: (1) mixed (qualitative and quantitative) studies of optimal dietary advice with the outcomes such as quality of life, morbidity, disease progression, and survival time (CRCHS, WHO, AED-SARA Project 2003), and (2) quantitative studies of optimal nutrition support and outcomes such as body composition, morbidity (especially diarrhea), CD4 counts, viral load, disease progression, survival time, and MTCT (rate) (CRCHS, WHO, AED-SARA Project).

Notes

1. The term targeted food assistance (TFA) is used by the C-SAFE members to include individual or household rations, dry or wet distribution methods, and "supplemental" and "complementary" feeding. TFA is distinct from general food distributions (GFD) and food for assets (FFA). It refers to targeted feeding to specific vulnerable groups such as the chronically ill (a proxy for HIV/AIDS).

2. To date, C-SAFE has used chronic illness as a proxy for AIDS as defined by an individual experiencing persistent and recurring illness lasting three months or more, which has reduced that person's level of productive capacity.

3. A summary of C-SAFE's better practices in TFA, which cites examples of these types of programs, was published by the C-SAFE Learning Center in 2005. The document also provides guidance for linking food aid with medical interventions. *Targeted Food Assistance in the Context of HIV/AIDS* is available at www.c-safe.org.

4. Learning Spaces was housed by the Regional Program Unit of C-SAFE through September 2005. This initiative provided a vehicle for learning among consortium members and other stakeholders on key themes such as HIV/AIDS and food security, food aid targeting, and lessons learned from working in a consortium format.

5. Body mass index is calculated as kilograms of mass divided by height (in meters) squared.

6. Documents include *Targeted Food Assistance in the Context of HIV/AIDS, Food Aid and Chronic Illness: Insights from the Community and Household Surveillance Surveys,* and others.

7. Personal communication with Dr. Mina Hosseinipour, UNC Project, Tidziwe Clinic, Lilongwe Central Hospital, Lilongwe, Malawi.

8. A limitation of this work was the lack of published research available at the time of this study. A review of the gray literature was therefore used, and thus, the exploratory nature of this work and the recommendations that emanate from it are acknowledged.

References

Canahuati, J. 2004. *Basic principles for food assisted programs in the context of HIV/AIDS.* Presented at Entebbe, Uganda, November 2–5, 2004. www.fantaproject.org/publications/hiv_foodaid2004. shtml.

Chilima, D. M., and S. J. Ismail. 2001. Nutrition and handgrip strength of older adults in rural Malawi. *Public Health Nutrition* 4 (1): 11–17.

CRCHS, WHO, AED-SARA Project. 2003. Providing nutritional care and support for people living with HIV/AIDS: guidelines for policy makers and programme managers in the African region. Arusha, Tanzania: CRCHS.

FANTA. 2000. *Potential uses of food aid to support HIV/AIDS mitigation activities in Sub-Saharan Africa.* Washington, D.C.: FANTA.

———. 2004a. *AMPATH: Academic model for the prevention and treatment of HIV/AIDS.* Washington, D.C.: FANTA. Retrieved December 20, 2004, from www.fantaproject.org/events/ampath04. shtml.

———. 2004b. *HIV/AIDS and food aid: Assessment for regional programs and resource integration.* Washington, D.C.: FANTA.

FAO. 2003. *Incorporating HIV/AIDS considerations into food security and livelihood projects.* Rome: FAO.

FAO/WHO. 2003. *Living well with HIV/AIDS.* Rome: FAO.

Ferrans, C., and M. Powers, 1992. Psychometric assessment of the quality of life index. *Research in Nursing and Health* 15: 29–38.

Fields-Gardner, C., and J. K. Keithley. 2001. Management of ARV related nutritional problems: Challenges and future directions. *Journal of the Association of Nurses in AIDS Care* 12: 79–84.

IFAD. 2001. Strategy paper on HIV/AIDS for East and Southern Africa. Rome: IFAD.

Jacobson, D. L., A. W. Wu, J. Feinberg, and Outcomes Committee of the Adult Clinical Trials Group. 2003. Health-related quality of life predicts survival, cytomegalovirus disease, and study retention in clinical trial participants with advanced HIV disease. *Journal of Clinical Epidemiology* 56: 874–879.

Karnofsky, D. A., and J. H. Burchenal. 1949. The clinical evaluation of chemotherapeutic agents in cancer. In: *Evaluation of chemotherapeutic agents,* ed. C. M. MacLeod, p. 196. New York: Columbia University Press.

Lansky, S. B., M. A. List, L. L. Lansky, C. Ritter-Sterr, and D. R. Miller. 1987. The measurement of performance in childhood cancer patients. *Cancer* 60: 1651–1656.

Maina, G., C. Field-Gardner, E. Murphy, S. Kugonsa-Isingoma, and J. Kulabako. 2005. *Nutritional impact of the Title II feeding program targeting people living with and affected by HIV/AIDS in Uganda.* Working paper prepared for the International Conference on HIV/AIDS and Food and Nutrition Security, April 14–16, Durban, South Africa.

Mast, T. C., G. Kigozi, F. Wabwire-Mangen, R. Black, N. Sewankambo, D. Serwadda, R. Gray, M. Wawer, and A. W. Wu. 2004. Measuring quality of life among HIV-infected women using a culturally adapted questionnaire in Rakai district, Uganda. *AIDS Care* 16: 81–94.

Maxwell, D., B. Watkins, R. Wheeler, and G. Collins. 2003. The coping strategies index: a tool for rapidly measuring food security and the impact of food aid programs in emergencies. Nairobi, Kenya: CARE and World Food Programme.

Measurement Excellence and Training Resource Information Center. 2005. *Critical review of health related quality of life-HIV (HRQOL-HIV).* http://www.measurementexperts.org//instrument/instrument_reviews.asp?detail=14, November 20.

Miller, T. L. 2003. Nutritional aspects of HIV-infected children receiving highly active antiretroviral therapy. *AIDS* 17: S130–S140.

Ochieng Owino, V. 2005. Modification of complementary foods in Zambia. *Field Exchange* 25: 12.

O'Donnell, M. 2004. Food security, livelihoods, and HIV/AIDS: a guide to the linkages, measurement and programming implications. London: Save the Children UK.

Oken, M. M., R. H. Creech, D. C. Tormey, J. Horton, T. E. Davis, E. T. McFadden, and P. P. Carbone. 1982. Toxicity and response criteria of the Eastern Cooperative Oncology Group. *American Journal of Clinical Oncology* 5: 649–655.

Preau, M., C. Leport, D. Salmon-Ceron, P. Carrieri, H. Portier, G. Chene, B. Spire, P. Choutet, F. Raffi, M. Morin, and the APROCO Study Group. 2004. Health-related quality of life and patient–provider relationships in HIV-infected patients during the first three years after starting PI-containing antiretroviral treatment. *AIDS Care* 16: 649–661.

RAND Health. 2004. *HIV-PARSE baseline questionnaire.* Retrieved December 27, 2004, from www.rand.org/health/surveys/MR342/MR342.html.

Robinson, F. P. 2004. Measurement of quality of life in HIV disease. *Journal of the Association of Nurses in AIDS Care* 15: 14S–19S.

Rowe, K. A., B. Makhubele, J. R. Hargreaves, J. D. Porter, H. P. Hausler, and P. M. Pronyk. 2005. Adherence to TB preventive therapy for HIV-positive patients in rural South Africa:

Implications for antiretroviral delivery in resource-poor settings? Department of Internal Medicine, Mayo Clinic, U.S.A. *International Journal of Tuberculosis and Lung Disease* 9 (3): 263–269.

Sandige, H., M. J. Ndekha, A. Briend, P. Ashorn, and M. J. Manary. 2004. Locally produced and imported ready-to-use food in the home-based treatment of malnourished Malawian children. *Journal of Pediatric Gastroenterology and Nutrition* 39 (2): 141–146.

Shevitz, A. H., and T. A. Knox. 2001. Nutrition in the era of highly active antiretroviral therapy, *Clinical Infectious Diseases* 32: 1769–1775.

Swanson, B. 1998. Bioelectrical impedance analysis (BIA) in HIV infection: Principles and clinical applications, *Journal of the Association of Nurses in AIDS Care.* 9 (1): 49.

Swindale, A. 2004. *Assessing the potential for food aid interventions in high HIV prevalence contexts.* Presented at Entebbe, Uganda, November 2–5, 2004. Retrieved from www.fantaproject.org/downloads/pdfs/hfa04_3p.pdf.

Torreblanca, A., and E. Kim. 2005. WFP recipients' weight gain at reach out clinic. *Field Exchange* 25: 6.

USAID-PVO Steering Committee on Multisectoral Approaches to HIV/AIDS. 2003. *Multisectoral responses to HIV/AIDS: A compendium of promising practices from Africa.* Washington, D.C.: USAID.

Webster, K, D. Cella, and K. Yost. 2003. The functional assessment of chronic illness therapy (FACIT) measurement system: Properties, applications and interpretation. *Health and Quality of Life Outcomes* 1: 79.

WFP. 2003. *Programming in the era of AIDS: WFP's response to HIV/AIDS.* Rome: WFP.

———. 2004. *WFP and food-based safety nets: concepts, experiences and future programming opportunities.* (WFP/EB.3/2004/4-A). Rome: WFP.

WHO. 2002. *The use of antiretroviral therapy: a simplified approach for resource-constrained countries.* WHO Project: ICP HIV 001. New Delhi: World Health Organization, Regional Office for South-East Asia.

Wu, A. W., D. A. Revicki, D. Jacobson, and F. E. Malitz. 1997. Evidence for reliability, validity and usefulness of the Medical Outcomes Study HIV health survey (MOS-HIV). *Quality of Life Research* 6: 481–493.

Zachariah, R., M. P. Spielmann, A. D. Harries, and F. M. Salaniponi. 2002. Moderate to severe malnutrition in patients with tuberculosis is a risk factor associated with early death. *Transactions of the Royal Society of Tropical Medicine and Hygiene* 96 (3): 291–294.

Chapter 17

Junior Farmer Field and Life Schools: Experience from Mozambique

Carol Djeddah, Rogério Mavanga, and Laurence Hendrickx

Background

In the last 20 years HIV/AIDS has progressed from seemingly isolated small epidemics to a more generalized epidemic. In countries hard hit by the epidemic, HIV/AIDS continues to contribute to the problems faced by youth. A serious consequence of the AIDS epidemic is the growing number of AIDS orphans. In 2003 there were a total of 43 million orphans in Sub-Saharan Africa, of whom 12.3 million were orphaned by AIDS. It is estimated that in the region, by 2010, orphans from all causes will total 50 million, of whom 18.4 million will have lost one or both parents to AIDS (UNAIDS/UNICEF/USAID 2004). Recent data suggest that in some highly HIV/AIDS-impacted countries the prevalence of orphans is higher in rural than urban areas (UNICEF 2003).

Mozambique has a high HIV prevalence, with the majority of new infections occurring among those under 29 years old. The 2004 *Report on the Global AIDS Epidemic* (UNAIDS 2004) shows an adult (15–49 years old) HIV prevalence rate of 12.2 percent out of a total population of around 18.8 million people (MISAU/INE 2004). The 2005 update is estimating that national adult HIV prevalence is rising to over 16 percent, with HIV spreading fastest in provinces that contain the country's main roads linked with Malawi, South Africa, and Zimbabwe. Among pregnant women in Caia (Sofala Province), HIV prevalence rose almost threefold from 7 percent in 2001 to 19 percent in 2004. Overall, the highest HIV prevalence levels are found in Mozambique's central (Sofala, Manica) and southern (Gaza, Maputo) provinces, where national (weighted) prevalence was over 18 percent and

20 percent, respectively, in 2004 (UNAIDS/WHO 2005). Life expectancy in 2004 was as low as 38.1 years, compared to 46.4 without HIV/AIDS. In Mozambique, in 2003, the total number of children orphaned by all causes (including AIDS) was estimated to be 1.5 million from an under-18 population of 9.8 million.

In addition to experiencing trauma, orphans and children who are made vulnerable by HIV/AIDS (OVCs) are more likely to be at risk of malnutrition, disease, abuse, stigmatization, and sexual exploitation. In a situation of chronic illnesses and deaths from AIDS, agricultural education and knowledge are not passed to the younger generation, leaving children with few agricultural and life skills with which to survive. From a farm-household perspective, food security is diminished: both the quantity and quality of food diminish, and orphans often go hungry or are malnourished (Du Guerny 1998). Furthermore, orphaned children are growing up without the necessary knowledge for their future livelihoods.

Manica Province

The central province of Manica covers an area of 61.661 square kilometers; it has nine districts and 34 administrative posts and an estimated population of 1.1 million. It has boundaries with Tete, Gaza and Inhambane, and Sofala provinces in the north, south, and east, respectively, and with Zimbabwe in the east. The province is crossed by two important corridors (Beira and Tete), connecting Mozambique to countries such as Zambia, Zimbabwe, and Malawi, which have HIV prevalence rates that are even higher than Mozambique. A third corridor (Mossurize) crosses the south of the province and is an important transport route for workers working in South African mines and on Zimbabwean tea, sugar cane, and tobacco plantations. It is one of the provinces that suffered most during the 16-year civil war. In addition, two traditional death rites that aid the spread of HIV, ritual sex and widow inheritance, are most commonly practiced in Manica and Tete. The combination of these factors explains why the province has one of the country's highest HIV prevalence rates.

Junior Farmer Field and Life Schools: A New Approach to Meet OVCs' Needs

All these factors led the province of Manica to be chosen as a pilot province of the Junior Farmer Field and Life School program (JFFLS), as a joint initiative by the government of Mozambique and two UN agencies: the Food and Agriculture Organization of the United Nations (FAO) and the World Food Programme (WFP). The project arose as an attempt to respond to the growing needs of orphans and vulnerable children. This is done by introducing a medium- and long-term strategy to empower orphans and vulnerable children in order to improve their livelihoods and long-term food security, agriculture knowledge, life skills, and self-esteem.

JFFLS are designed specifically to empower orphans and other vulnerable children aged between 12 and 18 years living in communities highly impacted by HIV/AIDS. A JFFLS seeks to improve the livelihoods of vulnerable boys and girls and provide them with future opportunities while minimizing the risk of adopting negative coping behaviors. The knowledge and skills acquired by the young girls and boys are also helping them to develop positive values regarding gender equality and human rights. Life skills represent an important part of the curriculum in order to demonstrate ways in which the crop cycle is similar to the human life cycle (JFFLS 2005b). This approach is an adaptation of the following successful methodologies developed by FAO and WFP to teach agricultural knowledge and skills to farmers in difficult circumstances.

The Farmer Field School Approach

The concept of the Farmer Field School (FFS) is based on experiences of the Integrated Pest Management Programme in Asia, which pioneered the concept in the early 1980s (Gallagher 2003).[1] The underlying principle behind the field school is that farmers can become experts in their own field.

Farmer Field Schools provide an exceptional "school without walls" for farmer learning, discussion, and experimentation on agricultural strategies for improving their food and livelihood security. Field schools are based on sound community-based adult-education practices and are an effective way of transferring knowledge (both local and external) through learning by doing using the Agro-Ecosystem Analysis (AESA).

They are organized by community-based groups of 25–30 farmers under the facilitation of an extension worker. The "classroom" is actually a plot of land where farmers carry out studies without personal risk, allowing them to make management decisions that they might not otherwise attempt in trials on their own fields. Besides offering technical skills, the Farmer Field Schools empower farmers and provide an excellent vehicle for organizing or strengthening groups, thus providing a basis for sustainability of group activities.

The Farmer Life School Approach

Farmer Life Schools (FLS) are based on the learning cycle of the Farmer Field School. In the Farmer Life Schools, originally developed by FAO and the United Nations Development Programme (UNDP) in Cambodia, farmers examine the problems that threaten their livelihoods, weigh available options, and make decisions about what action they should take. The issues addressed range from poverty, loss of land, pesticide use, family planning, alcoholism, domestic violence, and the attendance of children at school, to specific health problems such as dengue, malaria, and HIV/AIDS. The schools strengthen communities by helping farmers learn to analyze how their behavior exposes them to HIV/AIDS. They learn to farm more wisely and use the plants and herbs around them for both food and medicinal purposes, which may have been forgotten with the introduction of modern seeds and chemicals.

The core process is the linking of ecology, group organization, and student-centered learning applied through the Human Ecosystem Analysis (HESA), in which groups of farmers investigate various threats to their lives such as HIV/AIDS by understanding their strengths and vulnerabilities instead of depending on outsiders to come up with solutions to local problems (see Cambodian rice farmers et al. 2004).[2] The Farmer Life Schools seek to build on the risk assessment knowledge that farmers already have through a holistic approach. The ultimate goal is to enable them to become effective decisionmakers in their own lives, the lives of their families, and in their community network.

The Junior Farmer Field and Life School Approach

By adapting these methodologies to children, the concept of Junior Farmer Field and Life Schools (JFFLS) emerged as a combined approach with a potential to reach orphans and youth and as a practical learning mechanism for transferring knowledge and skills and enhancing self-esteem among OVCs who would otherwise have been marginalized and have fallen out of the normal social safety nets. It has been developed and tested in Mozambique, Zimbabwe, Kenya, Swaziland, and Namibia since November 2003 (JFFLS 2005b).

The JFFLS approach is based on an experiential learning process that encourages the group to observe, draw conclusions, and make informed decisions consistent with good agricultural and life practices. Using this approach enables OVCs to understand how knowledge and life skills can change their attitude toward their lives while understanding how to grow crops. As children analyze crop growth–related problems as a part of agroecosystem analysis, they analyze problems faced during their childhood.

In JFFLS, children undergoing training analyze livelihood and social problems and discuss the results with their peers. In situations where children have very limited access to information and facilities, organizing and facilitating children to play, think, discuss, and to capitalize on local resources to solve their problems represent a suitable strategy for developing empowerment and enhanced self-esteem. This part of the educational process is done through drama, theater, and other cultural methodologies.

Crucial to the learning process is the ability of facilitators to recognize and encourage innovation, inquiry, and initiative and to facilitate interaction among children. The process of experiential and self-discovery learning is driven by the learners themselves, and their knowledge is built around their own experiences. In the learning process, choices made through experimentation must satisfy three important conditions for change: they must be understood; they must work in field conditions; and they must be accepted by the young farmers.

Adaptation of the Model to Mozambique

The approach, inspired by the FFS and FLS methodologies, which were both successfully introduced in Asia, needed to be adapted to the reality of Mozambique, with its own sociocultural and economic characteristics.

In November 2003, the project was introduced as a pilot exercise in one urban and three rural faith-based organizations' (FBO) "open centers" near Chimoio, the provincial capital of Manica, as a partnership among FAO, WFP, and the provincial directorates of the Ministries of Agriculture, Education, and Women and Coordination of Social Action. The direct beneficiaries were around 100 children attending the open centers.

The following criteria were used for the partnership with the faith-based organization: located in area with high HIV prevalence (with a large number of orphans in the area), local organization working with or hosting orphans and vulnerable children, access to land to establish the "demonstration site," and a good relationship with the local community. Children were selected on the following basis: being maternal or paternal orphans regardless of the cause of death of the parent, aged between 12 and 18 years, local resident, with an equal number of boys and girls.

Food: WFP Partnership

While the JFFLS program provides orphans and vulnerable children with crucial farming and life skills, WFP supplies nutritious daily meals. Food plays a crucial role in the success of the JFFLS program by acting as a powerful incentive for orphans and vulnerable children to attend and have enough energy to participate. In Mozambique, 24 JFFLS are linked with primary schools where a school feeding program is part of the WFP and FAO partnership (WFP/UNESCO/WHO 1999). WFP has also contributed nonfood items to help with the construction of warehouses and kitchens at project sites as well as some agricultural tools on an ad hoc basis. The construction of warehouses and later feeding of the JFFLS pupils was achieved through the cooperation of school teachers, community members, and JFFLS trainers. Teachers and trainers were trained in food management during the JFFLS training. Although the warehouse management was mainly the responsibility of the school, community members ensured availability of firewood and water and were responsible for preparing the food. Adding the JFFLS to the school feeding program enabled a good control of the activity via the Ministry of Education and ensured co-ownership of the activity between the government and community.

In Mozambique, WFP provides meals to the school children and JFFLS children, consisting of 150 grams of cereals, 50 grams of pulses, 10 milliliters of vitamin A–enriched vegetable oil, and 3 grams of iodized salt. Not only does each child receive two nutritious meals a day, but their relatives and foster families do not need to provide for them on those days, easing the burden on overstretched household resources.

Children Fields: The Living Classroom

Each JFFLS site is a living classroom and should be a well-organized model, with high visibility. The fields show technical, educational, and environmental feasibility and show measurable, concrete results while increasing community understanding of the advantages and impacts on long-term food security and protection of children. The fields should be structured to stimulate and sustain national interest and facilitate the flow of funds (public and private) and resources in order to scale up the JFFLS to national level.

The site selection criteria are developed through an open and participatory process in which FAO, together with the community and local institutions, participated by proposing sites for consideration. The learning field should be safe for the children, 3 kilometers maximum from the children's households and schools, near major roads (for ease of community access and for demonstration), near sources of water or have access to irrigation, in areas most impacted by HIV/AIDS, and, finally, requiring no cost for the community.

The field structure (see Fig. 17.1) not only introduces children to food security and nutrition but goes beyond this by introducing them to the complexity of agricultural production as well as managing different time frames and objectives. The field contains staples (millet and maize) to fill the stomach, the nutritional garden (beans, carrots, sunflower, greens, tomatoes, and onions) for healthy growth, long-term crops such as cassava, pineapple, and sweet potatoes to introduce planning for the future, a small traditional space for indigenous and medicinal plants to include health care, and trees as a potential for agroforestry in contributing to resource-based livelihoods.

Training follows the seasonal cycle according to the agroecological zones. Children learn about field preparation, sowing and transplanting, weeding, irrigation,

Figure 17.1 The field structure

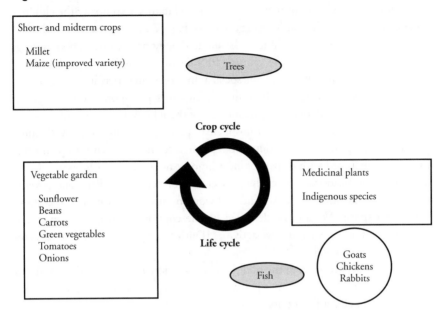

pest control, utilization and conservation of available resources, utilization and processing of food crops, harvesting, storage techniques, and marketing/entrepreneur skills. The curriculum has a practical agricultural bias covering both traditional and modern agricultural practices. The standard model of the school, with its emphasis on learner-centered and experiential learning, is adopted for a wide range of crops and medicinal plants. Activities include the introduction of livestock or fishery taking into consideration the diverse ecological and socioeconomic settings.

Besides agriculture, the curriculum also has a significant psychosocial component on life skills (self-awareness, assertiveness, HIV/AIDS prevention) as well as a sociological component focusing on gender equality and human rights.

In JFFLS, life skills are developed through creativity, using the local cultures (art, theater, dance, masks, etc.), thus facilitating the process of empowerment, self-knowledge, resilience, definition of identity and the capacity to define, and experiment risks and resources in a safe environment.

Participatory educational theater establishes bridges with the community and explores sensitive issues such as health and psychosocial problems, children's rights, gender roles in agriculture, and HIV/AIDS. It provides meaningful communication and enables the children to build trust, explore risks, solve problems, and develop more gender-equal attitudes.

The Interdisciplinary Team of Facilitators

An interdisciplinary team of men and women facilitators accompany the children in the field during the 1-year learning cycle (see Fig. 17.2). Each team is composed of one school teacher, who will take the methodology back to the school setting; one agriculturalist (a local extensionist, FFS facilitator, or JFFLS graduate) for improving agricultural skills; and one social animator as an expert in drama, dance, or other creative activities. Each team of facilitators is responsible for approximately 30 children, half of them girls and half of them boys. JFFLS learning groups are small in order to promote an atmosphere of participation and trust. As the program is scaled up, these core groups are replicated to meet demand. Implementation teams are linked with or part of local support networks (CBOs, local NGOs, faith-based organizations, the health and social sectors, etc.), guardians, and government services including social welfare and women, health, education and culture, youth, and sports. Volunteers identified by the community help to prepare the fields and perform labor-intensive activities. During the year, they also act as caregivers and prepare meals.

In a clear departure from the traditional instructional methods, JFFLS trainees attend school two or three times per week, guided by the interdisciplinary team. Sessions last for about five hours.

Appraisal, Lessons Learned, and Current Status

In 2004, the pilot exercise of four JFFLS in four open centers was expanded to 24 more schools, linked to the formal education system, thus covering nine districts in Manica Province as well as four districts in the neighboring province of Sofala.

In March 2005, after one year of activities, a joint assessment exercise (FAO/WFP) was conducted with the purpose of consolidating the achievements and lessons learned in the JFFLS in Mozambique and, more specifically, assessing the strengths, weaknesses, and opportunities of the JFFLS and its contribution to long-term, sustainable food security.

Two main typologies characterize the 28 pilot JFFLS: four schools associated with faith-based organizations, which started in late 2003, 24 schools linked to formal education and the WFP school-feeding program that commenced in late 2004. Within the 24 JFFLS there is a subcategory of 12 schools that are within commuting distance of a local FFS. Taking into account the distances across project locations and the need for adequate sampling within each typology group, field visits were arranged to 13 JFFLS sites representing a combination of these typologies.

The mission used semistructured interview techniques throughout its work in the field to gather information for the assessment. Interviews were also conducted individually with special stakeholders (e.g., village chiefs, facilitators, youth facilita-

Figure 17.2 The team

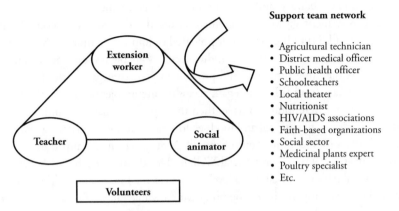

Support team network

- Agricultural technician
- District medical officer
- Public health officer
- Schoolteachers
- Local theater
- Nutritionist
- HIV/AIDS associations
- Faith-based organizations
- Social sector
- Medicinal plants expert
- Poultry specialist
- Etc.

tors, female OVCs), depending on information gained from the semistructured interviews with different groups.

The assessment team visited Mozambique in March 2005 and was composed of an FFS specialist, an HIV/AIDS and livelihoods diversification expert, and a social anthropologist accompanied by staff from FAO, WFP, and the Ministries of Education and Agriculture.[3] As a result of the assessment mission, the principal strengths and weaknesses of the JFFLS have been identified and are presented below.[4]

Strengths
The first strength identified was the empowerment process achieved through JFFLS (2005a).

> The inherent loss of survival knowledge can only be replaced, in part, by special efforts extended through experiential learning techniques to try and recreate the lost knowledge base and to develop the skills required by OVC in the areas of agriculture and life systems to become responsible, self-reliant citizens possessing a range of livelihood options.

To this end, discovery-learning and problem-solving approaches are emphasized in the JFFLS learning process as a "best practice" to reach orphans and youth; and as a practical learning mechanism for transferring knowledge, skills, and self-esteem among OVCs who would otherwise have been stigmatized and marginalized by their families or communities. In addition, through the participatory process of examining the problems that threaten their livelihoods and related agricultural production systems, and identifying local solutions to respond to those problems, the youths discover good agricultural practices in the areas of crop production, land husbandry, and natural resource management.

The assessment showed that graduates from the JFFLS, having gone through the FFS and FLS training, are better prepared to join the "senior" FFS. By bringing their experience from the JFFLS, they can be valuable resource persons in FFS training. At the same time, the FFS provide an "exit strategy" to the JFFLS program. Graduates from JFFLS can gain access to microprojects through the FFS.

The JFFLS were found to strengthen the capacity of national and local institutions to address nutritional and food security needs of OVCs. This was exhibited through the strong commitment of the different government ministries (Agriculture, Education, Women and Social Welfare, Health, and Youth and Sports) and the National AIDS Council, at all levels, as well as the functional multipartner collaboration. The program is collaborating with a whole range of other initiatives in the province and has contributed to a major impact of the program in the lives of the OVCs and the surrounding communities. Technical expertise from government services (such as extension staff and teachers), as well as from other FAO projects (such as in the area of conservation agriculture, NewCastle Disease Control), is being used as inputs for the JFFLS. There is also a strong demonstrated sense of community ownership of the program. Volunteers from the communities have been offering support to the children in the form of labor services and general caretaking. The community is also involved from the start in the selection of schools and beneficiaries. Volunteers from the community, including community leaders, are benefiting from the different training areas given by the program.

The learning process and methodology, introduced by the JFFLS, offers possibilities for other stakeholders to be used in the medium and long term, mainly in programs targeted at OVC. In addition, the expansion of the program within the formal education system provides an opportunity to reach more children and scale up the program on a national level. Furthermore, the JFFLS curriculum is being integrated into the 20 percent part of the primary school curriculum that can be decided on by the local school authorities.

The assessment team found that the nutritional needs of OVCs were reinforced through the establishment and implementation of food support programs for JFFLS youth and school children. The experience so far has shown that through the partnership with WFP, in particular the school-feeding program, both school enrollment and attendance in the communities are boosted. The JFFLS program has also attracted the interest of other children to agricultural activities. It is estimated that in this way, the project has had an indirect impact on three children per child participating in the JFFLS program.

Weaknesses and Constraints
However, during the approximately 1.5 years of its operation, the JFFLS program in Mozambique had to face the following weaknesses and constraints:

Training and curriculum development has been weak.   The program was initiated without clear guidelines in terms of content and learning objectives of the curriculum. As a result of this, the training of trainers (TOT) was conducted without proper learning materials. There is a need to elaborate materials that are specifically adapted for the teaching of children. Also, the duration of the TOT has been too short (two weeks); it should equal the duration of the cropping season (four months) in order to improve the transfer of knowledge, both its technical and methodological part. In addition, there has been high loss of trained personnel through high turnover (transfers of government officers) and deaths of government staff (extensionists and teachers).

JFFLS uses a participatory learning process. This is, however, a relatively new concept in Mozambique, where teaching is generally a top-down exercise, both in the education and the agricultural extension system. Participatory teaching methods have previously been introduced in the agricultural extension services, but its application has been limited. Moving from top-down teaching to participatory teaching requires a change in the mindset of the agricultural extension officers, from being a "teacher" to being a "facilitator"; this is a process that cannot be achieved in the short term. Moreover, the life skills and cultural part of the program has been less developed and has insufficiently been integrated into the agricultural activities, mainly because of lack of proper orientation of the social animators.

The illiteracy rates in the communities where the JFFLS are based are very high; this has been a limiting factor for achieving a strong linkage between the program and the community, as it limited the inclusion of community leaders and other potential key persons in the training programs.

Project planning and logistics.   Because the program requires an agricultural plot to be established, land has to be made available to the JFFLS. It is difficult for OVCs to obtain formal land ownership and entitlement to the land. The support of the faith-based organization has been essential; the linkage of the JFFLS to the formal education system has also proven to be fruitful in this regard. The problem is more difficult to solve for the graduates of the JFFLS (who are often still minors and therefore have no legal rights) once they leave the program and wish to start their own independent agricultural activities; often they find it difficult to access land and other capital resources. This has been compounded by the lack of "exit strategies." Because the program had only a very short time span, during which priority had to be given mainly to implementation, the possible "exit strategies" for the program have not sufficiently been explored. JFFLS graduates are equipped with agricultural knowledge and the capacity to define their livelihood options but have had insufficient access to resources to put their ideas into practice.

As explained above, the school feeding component has proved to be an essential support to the program. Problems have, however, been encountered by WFP in order to provide the necessary logistics to deliver the food inputs. This problem is mainly critical at the onset of the school year, as lack of provision of food to the school children has a direct impact on school enrollment and attendance, particularly in food-insecure and vulnerable areas.

Human resources were scarce, and the same officers were used by different projects and their partners. In order to overcome the insufficient number of extensionists and to make optimal use of these scarce resources, there is a need to better allocate the available staff to existing projects. In addition, the available resources necessary to implement proper monitoring (such as transport facilities) have been insufficient and irregular. Moreover, no adequate monitoring and evaluation system was set up at the time of the assessment mission.

The local socioeconomic context has been a restraining factor on the integration of gender-related issues in the program. In particular, it has been difficult to achieve equal participation by boys and girls. Dropouts of girls have been experienced as a result of early marriages and of the withdrawal of girls from the program in order to contribute to household-related tasks. This constraint was also linked to the weakness in the selection criteria used for the JFFLS. The initial target group of the program was mainly orphans. However, in areas that have in general a high level of vulnerability, children who are not orphans are equally vulnerable. Therefore, the selection criteria used needed to be adapted.

Way Forward

On the basis of the lessons learned from the pilot phase, the assessment team mission recommended that the following points be addressed before further scaling up of the program.

Training and Curriculum Development

The curriculum needs to be better developed in all aspects of the program: agriculture, culture, HIV/AIDS, and gender. Comprehensive, practical training materials, adapted to the specific needs of the target group, need to be prepared, and a training of trainers needs to be conducted over a period of 4 months. Special attention needs to be given to:

- The integration of the curriculum, both its agricultural and life skills parts, into the regular school curriculum. This is important not only in order to reach a greater number of children but to avoid using conflicting teaching methods within the same institution. Teachers involved in the JFFLS should use the same curriculum and teaching methodology outside the JFFLS activities.

- Ensure that trainings are conducted using a participatory, rather than a top-down, approach.

- When identifying new communities and beneficiaries within the communities for establishment of new JFFLS, stakeholder commitment and involvement need to be ascertained from the earliest stages. The objectives of the program need to be clearly explained to the beneficiaries themselves, the communities, and other stakeholders; the criteria for selection need to be identified together with the community; the FFS and FLS approach needs to be understood fully by the facilitators.

Exit Strategies and Sustainability

It is clear that more attention needs to be given to the development of an exit strategy to ensure sustainability of the program. The following issues were seen as crucial for Mozambique:

- The JFFLS approach should be integrated into the regular government activities of its respective ministries (agriculture, education, HIV/AIDS support programs) instead of being seen or implemented as a separate UN activity.

- There should be continued assistance to and follow-up of the child graduates. This should include not only technical assistance but facilitation of access to resources such as land and capital. The capacity that these graduates have gained to act themselves as facilitators, for example FFS, in life skills and HIV/AIDS prevention programs, should be fully used. Opportunities for these graduates to enroll as students in the agricultural training centers or other vocational training centers or even to join the civil service as extension agents or teachers, should be explored.

- More attention has to be given to the linkage of agricultural production to agroindustry and the marketing of agricultural produce. Transformation of agricultural produce, such as the extraction of oil from sunflower seeds, increases its marketing value. A more active cooperation with institutions that promote agroindustry and marketing needs to be sought.

• Ophans' livelihood options need also to be included in national action plans for addressing the needs of OVC.

At the regional level, the experience of Mozambique will inform the development of a regional strategic plan (RSP) to mainstream the lessons learned as a broad, regionwide institutional response using the JFFLS approach as one mitigation strategy to counter the impact of HIV and AIDS.

Notes

1. More information on IPM, FFS, and FLS can be found at www.fao.org/sd/erp/ and www.fao.org/hivaids/.

2. The manual describes the 16-week course designed to help the agriculture sector, AIDS programs, and nongovernmental organizations facilitate farming communities to face their local concerns, build their resilience, and thus reduce their vulnerability to HIV/AIDS.

3. The assessment team was composed of Owen Hughes (mission leader and FFS advisor), Maja Clausen (HIV/AIDS and livelihood diversification expert, FAO-TCER), Paolo Israel (social anthropologist consultant), Atanasio Rocha Augusto (senior program assistant, WFP Beira), Valentina Prosperi (UN fellow for HIV/AIDS and food security, FAO Maputo), Pedro Macome Jr. (school feeding/production coordinator, Sofala Province), and David Chihururu (school feeding coordinator, Manica Province).

4. Most of the findings were extracted from the assessment mission Report (JFFLS 2005a).

References

Cambodian rice farmers, O. Chhaya, J. du Guerny, R. Geeves, M. Kato, and L. Hsu. 2004. *Farmers' life school manual.* New York, Rome, and Boston: United Nations Development Programme, Food and Agriculture Organization of the United Nations, and World Education.

Du Guerny, J. 1998. Rural children living in farm systems affected by HIV/AIDS: Some issues for the rights of the child on the basis of FAO studies in Africa. SD Dimensions. http://www.fao.org/WAICENT/FAOINFO/SUSTDEV/WPdirect/WPan0026.htm. Accessed May 2006.

Gallagher, K. 2003. Fundamental elements of a farmer field school. *LEISA (Low External Input and Sustainable Agriculture)* 19: 5–6. http://www.farmerfieldschool.net/document_en/05_06.pdf. Accessed May 2006.

JFFLS (Junior Farmer Field and Life Schools). 2005a. Assessment mission report. Food and Agriculture Organization of the United Nations, Rome. Unpublished photocopy.

————. 2005b. Empowering orphans and vulnerable children living in a world with HIV/AIDS. Concept paper. Food and Agriculture Organization of the United Nations and World Food Programme, Rome. Unpublished photocopy.

MISAU/INE (Ministry of Health and National Institute of Statistics). 2004. *Demographic survey on HIV/AIDS in Mozambique.* Maputo.

UNAIDS (Joint United Nations Programme on HIV/AIDS). 2004. *Report on the global AIDS epidemic.* Geneva.

UNAIDS/UNICEF/USAID (Joint United Nations Programme on HIV/AIDS, United Nations Children's Fund, and United States Agency for International Development). 2004. *Children on the brink 2004.* A joint report on new orphan estimates and framework for action. Washington, D.C.: USAID.

UNAIDS/WHO (Joint United Nations Programme on HIV/AIDS and World Health Organization). 2005. *AIDS epidemic update.* http://www.unaids.org/epi/2005/doc/EPIupdate2005_html_en/epi05_00_en.htm. Accessed May 2006.

UNICEF (United Nations Children's Fund). 2003. A review of population-based household surveys from 40 countries in Sub-Saharan Africa. Paper presented at the conference, "Empirical Evidence for the Demographic and Socioeconomic Impact of AIDS," Durban, South Africa, March 26–28.

WFP/UNESCO/WHO (World Food Programme, United Nations Educational, Scientific and Cultural Organization, and World Health Organization). 1999. *School feeding handbook.* Rome: WFP.

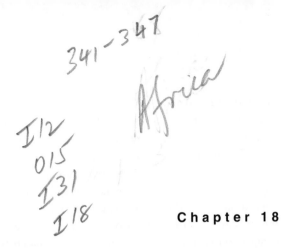

Chapter 18

HIV/AIDS, Nutrition, and Food Security: Looking to Future Challenges

Tony Barnett

The Challenge of ARV Rollout

Rollout of antiretroviral (ARV) therapy under the aegis of the WHO's "3 by 5" initiative, with funding from numerous donors via the Global Fund for TB, HIV/AIDS, and malaria, the U.S. PEPFAR and U.K. DFID, gives cause for hope for all those millions of people in Africa who are living with HIV/AIDS. Midway through 2005 nobody seriously believed that the target of 3 million people on treatment by year end would be achieved. However, it was a necessary goal at that stage. But for those concerned with meeting the challenge of HIV/AIDS impacts, increased antiretroviral therapy (ART) availability has to be seen for what it is: an opportunity to take a breath in the struggle against the impact of AIDS and think, and think hard, about what we do next.

The last 20 years have not shown any great success in confronting the impact of HIV/AIDS on nutrition and food security. Although this problem was identified as early as 1988 (Abel et al. 1988; Gillespie 1989) and explored through field research in 1989 (Barnett and Blaikie 1990), most if not all of the response has been to roll out policies that have been tried and tested in other, non-AIDS, situations, to try to apply existing "installed capacity," whether ideas, techniques, or institutions, rather than to recognize the specific nature of HIV/AIDS impact and respond to that. To use solutions to yesterday's problems to confront the new problems of today and tomorrow is to invite failure. This is even more the case in a world with ART. ART offers us a window of opportunity in which we must work hard to come up with new solutions appropriate to the new situation.

Viral Resistance

The danger that accompanies ART rollout is that potential transmission of viral resistance could quickly limit the effectiveness of antiretroviral treatment in Africa. There are two kinds of viral resistance, acquired and transmitted. Acquired viral resistance is seen where the viral population of an HIV individual's body adapts to the antiretroviral regimen he or she is receiving and is therefore able to increase its population, reflected in the individual's viral load despite treatment. In other words, the virus in that particular person evolves so as to be able to survive the medication being used to control it. Acquired resistance is bad news for the sick person, particularly as resistance to one medication often means that the virus is resistant to all medications in that class of drugs. In the absence of a second- or third-line treatment regimen, the individual prognosis is poor, and we should bear in mind that in most African countries, third-line treatments are not available.

The second type of resistance is transmitted resistance. This is bad news for the individual and is cause for concern at the population level. It means that already resistant forms of the virus may be transmitted between individuals, potentially creating an epidemic of drug-resistant HIV. Acquired resistance is already quite widespread in Europe and the United States, and around 20 percent of people treated for AIDS exhibit this form of resistance and have to have their treatment changed for this reason. Cases of transmitted resistance are rare, but they have made an appearance, most dramatically in New York in early 2005 (O'Rourke 2005; Smith 2005).

How the situation with regard to acquired resistance will play out is unclear. Thus, in a review of the situation, Wainberg concludes:

> Resistance to every HIV drug class is clearly emerging, and, alarmingly, transmission sometimes involves resistant strains that can cripple the effectiveness of combination chemotherapy. However, new agents, not cross-resistant with existing drugs, are being developed on a regular basis. This affords hope to patients who harbor viruses resistant to a variety of currently approved products. Whether the discovery of new agents keeps resistance at bay in the future is of obvious concern given the increasing reservoir of HIV patients worldwide that are being maintained on antiretroviral chemotherapy. (Wainberg 2004)

However, although this conclusion is sanguine and broadly optimistic, it strikes a note of caution. With regard to resource-poor settings, we cannot be so certain. First of all, we have to doubt whether the minimum level of compliance with treatment (95 percent)[1] can be met in many resource-constrained environments; second, we have to doubt whether the new pharmaceutical responses will be appropriate or available to people in resource-poor settings in time and at prices that will meet the rising curve of viral resistance.

The situation in regard to transmitted viral resistance at the population level is currently not at all well understood. Our understanding is largely dependent on modeling exercises (Blower et al. 2005). There is considerable uncertainty and debate as to the future development of transmitted viral resistance (Baggaley, Ferguson, and Garnett 2004). For the present it seems that we should err on the side of caution and assume that we will see viral resistance in resource-poor settings in the years ahead.

So, on both the acquired and transmitted viral resistance fronts, we should assume that ARTs provide a limited breathing space to think about how we proceed in our response to nutrition and food security issues in relation to the impact of AIDS. What should we do in the window that ARTs might provide if they were rolled out effectively, bearing in mind that this scenario is fairly unlikely in many countries where health infrastructure will just not meet the demands the ARV roll-out will place on it?

How Should We Respond to the Opportunity?

The problem is, we do not know what to do with the opportunities offered by that 5- to 10-year window. There is an urgent need for innovative solutions if we are not to waste them, but to develop these solutions we need to have a better understanding of the problem. Right now there is a real possibility that we will be responding to the wrong problem and the wrong story.

The impact of HIV/AIDS on nutrition and food security has tended to take a particular form; a particular story has been told. Early research (Barnett and Blaikie 1990) used field material from a number of sites in Uganda to suggest (1) the effects of AIDS on rural production in Uganda and possibly more broadly in Africa and (2) the methods that might be employed to explore the variability of the impact in production systems differentiated in terms of people, climate, soils, and temperature. Since then, many studies using mainly qualitative and participatory methods have confirmed a story of AIDS impact, which runs broadly as follows: AIDS causes rural labor shortages because of excess illness and death in the productive age group; this leads to a progressive decline of agricultural production and food availability as a result of reduction of cultivated land area and shrinkage of crop and livestock portfolios accompanied by decay of rural infrastructure and overall reduced rural production and productivity, and thus nutrition status of the population.

But we do not know whether and how far this story applies everywhere in Africa, let alone in other AIDS-affected rural communities globally. It is now of the greatest importance that we come to as clear an understanding as possible of the diversity of the AIDS impact on rural societies that depend predominantly on human labor. If we homogenize what is in reality a very diverse situation, we will come up with inappropriate solutions derived from a wrong analysis. For example, one frequently proposed solution has been to meet the labor shortage with a range of "labor-saving technologies" (LSTs). The problem here is that we do not have sufficient examples of successful LSTs that have been adopted in Africa in ordinary circumstances: there has been no African green revolution, let alone any examples of LST innovations appropriate to the new situation consequent on the impact of AIDS.

Because of this situation, there is a danger that attempts at impact mitigation could lead in the wrong direction if they are based on "simple stories," narratives of the epidemic and its impacts that have become accepted by policymakers, donors, opinion leaders, and the research community. The situation is that even so far into the epidemic, the third decade, we really do not have long-term evidence with the kind of detailed analysis necessary to understand the complexity and diversity of the impact of the epidemic on rural society in Africa. What we do have is a large and growing body of very uncertain "evidence" about what has been happening (this is reviewed in Gillespie and Kadiyala [2005]). Within that "evidence" it is hard to isolate the causal influence of HIV/AIDS from other underlying environmental and policy conditions. Indeed, the epidemic may be a tipping point factor, but in many circumstances, it may not be the sole reason for the effects that we are seeing. We are dealing with an extremely complex set of causal links, and these are likely to be different or nuanced from place to place.

What we know about HIV/AIDS impacts on rural societies, nutrition, and food security can be summed up as follows: seroprevalence figures provide a peek into the future, not an account of the present; there is an impact in most societies where seroprevalence levels have been high; it is without exception adverse and reaches beyond the individual into his or her household and community; but we do not know where it is worst and where it is less bad. Generalizations about the process in one place drawing on narratives derived from experience (often anecdotal) from elsewhere are probably unhelpful; policy responses based on general statements about "famine," "labor-saving technologies," "scaling up," and so on are likely to waste resources and fail to meet the needs of local communities. We must also be acutely aware that the development of the disease over eight to nine years in an individual, during which time their effectiveness is compromised, may not be long enough for adoption of innovation to take place. In communities severely affected by AIDS, the entire dynamic of innovation and adoption may be compromised.

The Challenge

So, in the limited window of opportunity that might be provided by ART rollout, were it widespread and effective, the challenge is to recognize the diversity of impact, to learn from local circumstances, and to aim to create large-scale responses that can cope with that impact.

This is difficult because governments, multilateral agencies, and bilateral agencies have great difficulty in dealing with diversity. Diversity has high overhead costs and requires constant learning capacity and institutional adaptation. Such an approach does not fit with the modus operandi of the major donors. It is very hard to have large programs that take into account the complexity of the situation. One size does not fit all, but it is hard for large organizations to take this into account. The situation does not ride well with the slow rate of innovation by large organizations.

The real challenges revolve around recognition of the following:

- The diversity of HIV/AIDS impact on food and nutrition security.

- The magnitude of the epidemic and its impact will span many decades in the most seriously affected countries.

- Long-term demographic changes alter the technical response possibilities: changed gender and age balances in a population will challenge existing and available intervention technologies, which are based on assumptions about the age and gender balance of "typical" communities.

- Community structure is likely to be weakened, and safety nets likely to break down.

- The contours of destitution may be redefined and include the very young and the very old, and among these women in particular. The numbers of destitute people in rural areas may increase. These will be people whose destitution reflects inability to access resources or decreased ability to use available resources as a result of weakened social, economic, and, in some cases, environmental infrastructure.

- In mature epidemics women are affected by HIV/AIDS more than men, and the gender balance is likely to alter. Thus, assumptions about the availability of women's labor and skills for household and farm work may not hold in the future.

- The crisis develops over a very long period and is a slow rather than abrupt crisis. It is thus not visible to the usual detection instruments. This means that there is a choice: (1) we can fail to act because the event is happening slowly (which is what has occurred so far), or (2) we can respond now so as to change the future.

Given the danger of viral resistance, we must act in relation to these realities now.

Note

1. This is generally held by clinicians to be the minimum level of compliance; see, for example, Ministry of Health, Malawi 2003; Garcia, Schooley, and Badaro 2003; Weiser et al. 2003.

References

Abel, N., T. Barnett, P. Blaikie, S. Cross, and S. Bell. 1988. The impact of AIDS on food production systems in east and central Africa over the next ten years: A programmatic paper, in *The global impact of AIDS*, eds. A. F. Fleming, M. Carballo, D. W. FitzSimons, M. R. Bailey, and J. Mann. New York: Allan R. Liss, and London: John Wiley.

Baggaley, R. F., N. M. Ferguson, and G. P. Garnett. 2004. *The epidemiological impact of antiretroviral use predicted by mathematical models: A review.* Unpublished paper, Imperial College, London.

Barnett, T., and P. M. Blaikie, with C. Obbo. 1990. *Community coping mechanisms in circumstances of exceptional demographic change: Final report to the Overseas Development Administration,* two volumes. London: Overseas Development Administration, and Norwich: Overseas Development Group, UEA.

Blower, S., E. Bodine, J. Kahn, and W. McFarland. 2005. The antiretroviral roll out and drug-resistant HIV in Africa: insights from empirical data and theoretical models. *AIDS* 19: 1–14.

Garcia, R., R. T. Schooley, and R. Badaro. 2003. An adherence trilogy is essential for long-term HAART success. *Brazilian Journal of Infectious Diseases* 7(5): 307–314.

Gillespie, S. 1989. Potential impact of AIDS on farming systems: A case study from Rwanda. *Land Use Policy* 6: 301–312.

Gillespie, S., and S. Kadiyala. 2005. *HIV/AIDS and food and nutrition security: From evidence to action.* Food Policy Review No. 7. Washington, D.C.: IFPRI.

Ministry of Health, Malawi. 2003. *Treatment of AIDS: Guidelines for the use of antiretroviral therapy in Malawi,* ed. 1. Malawi: National AIDS Commission.

O'Rourke, M. 2005. A single case of multidrug-resistant HIV and rapid disease progression. *AIDS Clinical Care.* http://aids-clinical-care.jwatch.org/cgi/content/full/2005/0301/1.

Smith, S. M. 2005. New York City HIV superbug: Fear or fear not? *Retrovirology* 2 (14). http://www.retrovirology.com/content/2/1/14.

Wainberg, M. A. 2004. The emergence of HIV resistance and new antiretrovirals: Are we winning? *Drug Resistance Updates* 7: 163–167.

Weiser, S., W. Wolfe, D. Bangsberg, I. Thior, P. Gilbert, J. Makhema, P. Kebaabetswe, D. Dickenson, K. Mompati, M. Essex, and R. Marlink. 2003. Barriers to antiretroviral adherence for patients living with HIV infection and AIDS in Botswana. *Journal of Acquired Immune Deficiency Syndromes* 34 (3): 281–288.

WHO Consultation on Nutrition and HIV/AIDS in Africa: Durban, South Africa, April 10–13, 2005

Participants' Statement

1. HIV/AIDS is affecting more people in eastern and southern Africa than the fragile health systems of the countries afflicted can treat, demoralizing more children than our educational systems can inspire, creating more orphans than communities can care for, wasting families, and threatening food systems. The HIV/AIDS epidemic is increasingly driven by and contributes to factors that also create malnutrition, in particular, poverty, emergencies, and inequalities.

2. In urgent response to this situation, we call for the integration of nutrition into the essential package of care, treatment, and support for people living with HIV/AIDS and for efforts to prevent infection.

3. We, the representatives of 20 countries in eastern and southern Africa and other participants, from organizations in the United Nations system, bilateral agencies, regional groups, nongovernmental organizations, academe, and other bodies, recognize that
   a. far-reaching steps need to be taken to reverse current trends in malnutrition, HIV infection, and food insecurity in most countries in the region, in order to achieve the Millennium Development Goals
   b. adequate nutrition cannot cure HIV infection but is essential to maintain a person's immune system, to sustain healthy levels of physical activity, and for optimal quality of life

c. adequate nutrition is also necessary to ensure optimal benefits from the use of antiretroviral treatment, which is essential to prolong the lives of HIV-infected people and prevent transmission of HIV from mother to child

d. there is a proliferation in the marketplace of unproven diets and dietary therapies, with exploitation of fears, raising of false hopes, and further impoverishment of those infected and affected by HIV and AIDS

e. exceptional measures are needed to ensure the health and well-being of all children affected and made vulnerable by HIV/AIDS, with young girls especially at risk

f. knowledge of HIV status is important to inform choices for reproductive health and child feeding.

Conclusions

After reviewing the scientific evidence and having discussed the programmatic experience on nutrition and HIV/AIDS, we come to the following conclusions.

Macronutrients

• HIV-infected adults and children have greater energy needs than uninfected adults and children. Energy needs increase by 10 percent in asymptomatic HIV-infected adults and children, and, in adults with more advanced disease, by 20 percent to 30 percent. For HIV-infected children experiencing weight loss, energy needs are increased by between 50 percent and 100 percent.

• There is no evidence to support a need for increased protein intake by people infected by HIV over and above that required in a balanced diet to satisfy energy needs (12 percent to 15 percent of total energy intake).

• Loss of appetite and poor dietary intake are important causes of weight loss associated with HIV infection. Effective ways of improving dietary intakes need to be developed and documented.

Micronutrients

Micronutrient deficiencies are frequently present in HIV-infected adults and children.

• Micronutrient intakes at daily recommended levels need to be assured in HIV-infected adults and children through consumption of diversified diets, fortified foods, and micronutrient supplements as needed.

- WHO's recommendations on vitamin A, zinc, iron, folate, and multiple micronutrient supplements remain the same.

- Micronutrient supplements are not an alternative to comprehensive HIV treatment including therapy with antiretroviral agents.

- More studies are needed to understand better the relationship between micronutrient supplementation and potential health benefits for people infected with HIV.

Pregnancy and Lactation
- Pregnancy and lactation do not hasten the progression of HIV infection to AIDS.

- Optimal nutrition of HIV-infected women during pregnancy and lactation increases weight gain and improves pregnancy and birth outcomes.

- HIV-infected pregnant women gain less weight and experience more frequent micronutrient deficiencies than uninfected pregnant women.

Growth
- HIV infection impairs the growth of children early in life. Growth faltering is often observed even before the onset of symptomatic HIV infection. Poor growth is associated with increased risk of mortality.

- Viral load, chronic diarrhea, and opportunistic infections impair growth in HIV-infected children. The growth and survival of HIV-infected children are improved by prophylactic use of cotrimoxazole, antiretroviral therapy, and early prevention and treatment of opportunistic infections.

- Improved dietary intake is essential to enable children to regain lost weight after opportunistic infection.

Infant and Young Child Feeding
- For HIV-uninfected mothers and mothers who do not know their HIV status, exclusive breastfeeding for six months is the ideal practice because of its benefits for improved growth, development, and reduced incidence of childhood infections. Safe and appropriate complementary feeding and continued breastfeeding for 24 months and beyond are recommended.

- The risk of transmission of HIV through breast milk is constant throughout the period of breastfeeding and is greatest among women newly infected or with advanced HIV disease.

- Exclusive breastfeeding is less associated with HIV transmission than mixed breastfeeding.

- WHO and UNICEF recommend that HIV-infected mothers should avoid breastfeeding when replacement feeding is acceptable, feasible, affordable, sustainable, and safe. These conditions, however, are not easily met for most mothers in the region.

- The safety of infant feeding can be improved with adequate support, but health systems and communities are not providing this support.

- Early cessation of breastfeeding is recommended for HIV-infected mothers and their infants. The age at which to stop breastfeeding depends on the individual circumstances of mothers and their infants. The consequences of early cessation on transmission, mortality, growth, and development need to be urgently studied. There is an immediate need to evaluate suitable ways of meeting nutritional needs of infants and young children who are no longer breastfed.

Interaction between Nutrition and Antiretroviral Treatment

- The lifesaving benefits of antiretroviral therapy are clearly recognized. To achieve the full benefits of such treatment, adequate dietary intake is essential.

- Dietary and nutritional assessment is an essential part of comprehensive HIV care both before and during antiretroviral treatment.

- Long-term use of antiretroviral agents can be associated with metabolic complications (e.g., cardiovascular disease, diabetes, and bone-related problems). Although the value of antiretroviral therapy far outweighs the risks, the metabolic complications need to be adequately managed. The challenge is how best to apply in Africa the extensive clinical experience in managing these types of metabolic disorders in HIV-infected adults and children.

- Interactions between nutritional status and antiretroviral treatment in chronically malnourished populations, severely malnourished children, and pregnant and lactating women need to be investigated.

- The effects of traditional remedies and dietary supplements on the safety and efficacy of antiretroviral agents need to be evaluated.

Recommendations for Action

Based on the foregoing scientific conclusions, we urge all concerned parties to make nutrition an integral part of their response to HIV/AIDS. We make the following recommendations for immediate implementation at all levels.

Strengthen Political Commitment and Improve the Positioning of Nutrition in National Policies and Programs

- Use existing, and develop new, advocacy tools to sensitize decisionmakers to the urgency of the problem, the consequences on development targets of neglecting the role of nutrition and not including it within the overall care and support package, and the opportunity to improve care.

- Advocate increased resource allocation and support for improved nutrition, in general, and tackling the nutritional needs of HIV-affected and infected populations.

- Prioritize the needs of children affected and made vulnerable by HIV/AIDS.

- Clarify and improve multisectoral collaboration and coordination among the agricultural, health, social services, education, and nutrition sectors.

Develop Practical Tools and Guidelines for Nutritional Assessment for Home, Community, Health Facility-Based, and Emergency Programs

- Validate simple tools to assess diet and use of supplements, including traditional and alternative therapies, nutritional status, and food security, so that nutrition support provided within HIV programs is appropriate to individual needs.

- Develop standard and specific guidelines for nutritional care of individuals and implementation of programs at health-facility and community levels.

- Review and update existing guidelines to include considerations of nutrition and HIV (e.g., guidelines on integrated management of adolescent and adult illness, antiretroviral treatment, and nutrition in emergencies).

Expand Existing Interventions for Improving Nutrition in the Context of HIV

• Accelerate the implementation of the global strategy for infant and young child feeding.

• Renew support for the Baby-friendly Hospital Initiative.

• Accelerate the fortification of staple foods with essential micronutrients.

• Implement WHO protocols for vitamin A, iron, folate, zinc, and multiple micronutrient supplementation and management of severe malnutrition.

• Accelerate training on, and use of guidelines and tools for, infant feeding counseling and maternal nutrition in programs to prevent mother-to-child transmission of HIV.

• Expand access to HIV counseling and testing so that individuals can make informed decisions and receive appropriate advice and support on nutrition, including in emergency settings.

Conduct Systematic Operational and Clinical Research to Support Evidence-Based Programming

• Develop and implement operational and clinical research to identify effective interventions and strategies for improving nutrition of HIV-infected and affected adults and children.

• Document and publish results and ensure access to lessons learned at all levels.

• Encourage scientific journals to give greater opportunity for publication of operational research and records of good practice.

Strengthen, Develop, and Protect Human Capacity and Skills

• Include funding for nutrition capacity development in plans for expanded treatment and care of people living with HIV and those affected by HIV/AIDS.

• Incorporate nutrition into training, including preservice training, of health, community, and home-based care workers, with development of specific skills such as nutritional assessment and counseling and program monitoring and evaluation. Such training should not favor particular commercial interests.

- Strengthen the capacity of government and civil society to develop and monitor regulatory systems to prevent commercial marketing of untested diets, remedies, and therapies for HIV-infected adults and children.

- Improve the conditions of service and coverage of health workers, especially dieticians and nutritionists, to deliver nutritional services.

- Identify and use local expertise to improve response to emergency conditions.

Incorporate Nutrition Indicators into HIV/AIDS Monitoring and Evaluation Plans

- Include appropriate indicators for measuring progress toward integrating nutrition into HIV programs and the impact of nutritional interventions in reporting the results of clinical and community-level surveillance and reporting of progress at national, regional, and international levels.

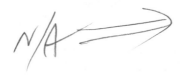

Contributors

Nigatu Alemayehu is a research and development officer with the Improving Productivity and Market Success (IPMS) Ethiopian Farmers Project at the International Livestock Research Institute, Addis Ababa.

Yirgalem Assegid is a research and development officer with the Improving Productivity and Market Success (IPMS) Ethiopian Farmers Project at the International Livestock Research Institute, Addis Ababa.

Linda A. Bailey is an assistant professor in the School of Public Affairs at Baruch College, City University of New York, U.S.A.

Tony Barnett is Economic and Social Research Council Professorial Research Fellow at the Development Studies Institute, London School of Economics.

Hans P. Binswanger is the chairman of Community and Enterprise Development Against Stigma, and a fellow at Tshwane University of Technology, Tshwane, South Africa.

Clare Bishop-Sambrook is an independent consultant based in Rome.

Virginia Bond is a research fellow at the London School of Hygiene and Tropical Medicine, and director of and senior social scientist with the ZAMBART Project, Zambia.

Deborah Fahy Bryceson is a research associate at the African Studies Centre, Oxford University.

Antony Chapoto is a research fellow with the Food Security Research Project, Lusaka, Zambia, and a professor in the Department of Agricultural Economics at Michigan State University, U.S.A.

Carol Djeddah is a consultant with the HIV/AIDS program of the Food and Agriculture Organization of the United Nations.

Cynthia Donovan is an assistant professor in the Department of Agricultural Economics at Michigan State University, U.S.A.

Andrew R. Dorward is reader in agricultural development economics at Imperial College, London.

Scott Drimie is an independent researcher based in Johannesburg, South Africa, and national coordinator of the Regional Network on HIV/AIDS, Rural Livelihoods, and Food Security (RENEWAL) South Africa.

Kari Egge is an independent consultant based in Minnesota, U.S.A.

Jodie Fonseca is an AIDS specialist with Save the Children, Washington, D.C. She was formerly HIV/AIDS advisor with CARE International, based in Lilongwe, Malawi.

David Galaty is a senior research analyst with Abt Associates Inc., Bethesda, Maryland, U.S.A.

Sarah Gavian is a senior research fellow in the Development Strategy and Governance Division of the International Food Policy Research Institute, Washington, D.C.

Berhanu Gebremedhin is a scientist with the Improving Productivity and Market Success (IPMS) Ethiopian Farmers Project at the International Livestock Research Institute, Addis Ababa.

Stuart Gillespie is a senior research fellow in the Food Consumption and Nutrition Division of the International Food Policy Research Institute, and director of the Regional Network on HIV/AIDS, Rural Livelihoods, and Food Security (RENEWAL). He is based in Geneva, Switzerland.

Guenter Hemrich is with the Food and Agriculture Organization of the United Nations, Rome.

Laurence Hendrickx was formerly emergency coordinator with the Food and Agriculture Organization of the United Nations, based in Maputo, Mozambique.

Thomas S. Jayne is professor, international development at Michigan State University, U.S.A.

Suneetha Kadiyala is a scientist in the Food Consumption and Nutrition Division, International Food Policy Research Institute, Washington, D.C.

Gilbert Kombe is principle associate and senior HIV/AIDS technical advisor at Abt Associates Inc., Bethesda, Maryland, U.S.A.

Michael E. Loevinsohn is the director of Applied Ecology Associates, Wageningen, the Netherlands.

Winford H. Masanjala is a senior lecturer in economics at the University of Malawi, Zomba, and is also affiliated with the Population Studies Center of the University of Pennsylvania, Philadelphia, U.S.A.

Rogério Mavanga is the Junior Farmer Field and Life Schools coordinator with the Food and Agriculture Organization of the United Nations, based in Chimoio, Mozambique.

Dan Mullins is the deputy regional director of the Southern and West Africa Regional Management Unit of CARE–USA, based in Johannesburg, South Africa.

Idrissa M. Mwale is an economist with the Ministry of Agriculture, Malawi.

Prabhu Pingali is the director of the Agricultural and Development Economics Division of the Food and Agriculture Organization of the United Nations, Rome.

Ken Polsky is the head of programs with Catholic Relief Services, Nigeria. He was formerly the regional technical advisor for livelihoods in southern Africa with Catholic Relief Services.

Shannon Senefeld is the HIV/AIDS monitoring and evaluation technical advisor at Catholic Relief Services.

Eileen Stillwaggon is associate professor of economics at Gettysburg College, Pennsylvania, U.S.A.

Susan Strasser is the regional technical advisor on HIV/AIDS for the Southern African Regional Office of Catholic Relief Services, based in Lusaka, Zambia.

Marcela Villarreal is the director of the Gender and Population Division with the Food and Agriculture Organization of the United Nations, Rome.

Gebremedhin Woldewahid is a research and development officer with the Improving Productivity and Market Success (IPMS) Ethiopian Farmers Project at the International Livestock Research Institute, Addis Ababa.

Index

Page numbers for entries occurring in figures are suffixed by an *f;* those for entries in boxes by a *b;* those for entries in notes by an *n,* with the number of the note following; and those for entries in tables by a *t.*